HIV and Endocrine Disorders

Editor

PAUL W. HRUZ

ENDOCRINOLOGY AND METABOLISM CLINICS OF NORTH AMERICA

www.endo.theclinics.com

Consulting Editor
DEREK LeROITH

September 2014 • Volume 43 • Number 3

ELSEVIER

1600 John F. Kennedy Boulevard • Suite 1800 • Philadelphia, Pennsylvania, 19103-2899

http://www.theclinics.com

ENDOCRINOLOGY AND METABOLISM CLINICS OF NORTH AMERICA Volume 43, Number 3
September 2014 ISSN 0889-8529, ISBN 13: 978-0-323-32321-5

Editor: Jessica McCool
Developmental Editor: Susan Showalter

Endocrinology and Metabolism Clinics of North America (ISSN 0889-8529) is published quarterly by Elsevier Inc., 360 Park Avenue South, New York, NY 10010-1710. Months of issue are March, June, September, and December. Periodicals postage paid at New York, NY and additional mailing offices. Subscription prices are USD 330.00 per year for US individuals, USD 581.00 per year for US institutions, USD 165.00 per year for US students and residents, USD 415.00 per year for Canadian individuals, USD 718.00 per year for Canadian institutions, USD 480.00 per year for international individuals, USD 718.00 per year for international institutions, and USD 245.00 per year for international and Canadian and foreign students/residents. To receive student/resident rate, orders must be accompanied by name of affiliated institution, date of term, and the signature of program/residency coordinator on institution letterhead. Orders will be billed at individual rate until proof of status is received. Foreign air speed delivery is included in all *Clinics* subscription prices. All prices are subject to change without notice. **POSTMASTER:** Send address changes to *Endocrinology and Metabolism Clinics of North America*, Elsevier Health Sciences Division, Subscription Customer Service, 3251 Riverport Lane, Maryland Heights, MO 63043. **Customer Service: Telephone: 1-800-654-2452** (U.S. and Canada); **1-314-447-8871** (outside U.S. and Canada). **Fax: 1-314-447-8029.** E-mail: **journalscustomerservice-usa@elsevier.com** (for print support); **journalsonlinesupport-usa@elsevier.com** (for online support).

Reprints. For copies of 100 or more, of articles in this publication, please contact the Commercial Rights Department, Elsevier Inc., 360 Park Avenue South, New York, NY 10010-1710; phone: +1-212-633-3874; fax: +1-212-633-3820; E-mail: reprints@elsevier.com.

Endocrinology and Metabolism Clinics of North America is covered in *MEDLINE/PubMed (Index Medicus)*, *EMBASE/Excerpta Medica, Current Contents/Clinical Medicine, Current Contents/Life Sciences, Science Citation Index, ISI/BIOMED, BIOSIS,* and *Chemical Abstracts.*

Contributors

CONSULTING EDITOR

DEREK LeROITH, MD, PhD
Director of Research, Division of Endocrinology, Metabolism, and Bone Diseases, Department of Medicine, Icahn School of Medicine at Mount Sinai, New York, New York

EDITOR

PAUL W. HRUZ, MD, PhD
Associate Professor of Pediatrics and Cellular Biology and Physiology; Director, Division of Pediatric Endocrinology and Diabetes, Washington University School of Medicine, St. Louis, Missouri

AUTHORS

THEA BREGMAN, MD
Physician, Department of Pediatrics, University of California Davis Medical Center, Sacramento, California

CAROLINE J. CHANTRY, MD
Professor, Department of Pediatrics, University of California Davis Medical Center, Sacramento, California

GEORGE P. CHROUSOS, MD
Professor, First Department of Pediatrics, "Agia Sofia" Children's Hospital, University of Athens, Athens, Greece

JULIET COMPSTON, MD, FRCP, FRCPath, FMedSci
Emeritus Professor, Department of Medicine, Addenbrookes Hospital, Cambridge Biomedical Campus, Cambridge, United Kingdom

SARA CROSS, MD
Division of Infectious Diseases, University of Tennessee Health Sciences Center, Memphis, Tennessee

JUDITH S. CURRIER, MD, MSc
Division of Infectious Diseases, Department of Medicine, David Geffen School of Medicine, University of California, Los Angeles, Los Angeles, California

ADRIAN DOBS, MD
Professor, Department of Endocrinology, Diabetes and Metabolism, Johns Hopkins University School of Medicine, Baltimore, Maryland

GEROME V. ESCOTA, MD
Division of Infectious Diseases, Washington University School of Medicine, St. Louis, Missouri

RUTH M. GREENBLATT, MD
Professor, Departments of Clinical Pharmacy, Medicine, Epidemiology and Biostatistics, University of California, San Francisco Schools of Pharmacy and Medicine, San Francisco, California

GIOVANNI GUARALDI, MD, PhD
Assistant Professor of Infectious Diseases, Infectious and Tropical Disease Unit, Department of Medical and Surgical Sciences of Mother, Child and Adult, Metabolic Clinic, University of Modena & Reggio Emilia, Modena, Italy

COLLEEN HADIGAN, MD, MPH
Laboratory of Immunoregulation, National Institute of Allergy and Infectious Diseases, National Institutes of Health, Bethesda, Maryland

STEEN B. HAUGAARD, MD, DMSc
Associated Professor; Consultant Physician, Department of Internal Medicine and the Clinical Research Centre, University of Copenhagen Amager Hvidovre Hospitals, Copenhagen S, Denmark

SARAH KATTAKUZHY, MD
Laboratory of Immunoregulation, Leidos Biomedical Research, Inc., Frederick National Laboratory for Cancer Research, Frederick, Maryland

THEODOROS KELESIDIS, MD, PhD
Division of Infectious Diseases, Department of Medicine, David Geffen School of Medicine, University of California, Los Angeles, Los Angeles, California

DONALD P. KOTLER, MD
Professor, Department of Medicine; Chief, Division of Gastroenterology and Hepatology, Mount Sinai St. Luke's, Mount Sinai Roosevelt Hospital, Icahn School of Medicine at Mount Sinai, Mount Sinai Health System, New York, New York

LINDSEY A. LOOMBA-ALBRECHT, MD
Assistant Professor, Section of Endocrinology, Department of Pediatrics, University of California Davis Medical Center, Sacramento, California

PAVAN K. MANKAL, MD, MA
Department of Medicine; Fellow, Division of Gastroenterology, Mount Sinai St. Luke's, Mount Sinai Roosevelt Hospital, Icahn School of Medicine at Mount Sinai, Mount Sinai Health System, New York, New York

WILLIAM G. POWDERLY, MD
Division of Infectious Diseases, Washington University School of Medicine, St. Louis, Missouri

VINCENZO ROCHIRA, MD, PhD
Assistant Professor of Endocrinology; Chair of Endocrinology and Metabolism, Unit of Endocrinology, Department of Biomedical, Metabolic and Neural Sciences, University of Modena and Reggio Emilia; Azienda USL of Modena, Modena, Italy

ANTHONY P. WEETMAN, MD, DSc
Department of Human Metabolism, University of Sheffield, Sheffield, United Kingdom

SWAYTHA YALAMANCHI, MD
Clinical and Research Fellow, Department of Endocrinology, Diabetes and Metabolism, Johns Hopkins University School of Medicine, Baltimore, Maryland

EVANGELIA D. ZAPANTI, MD, PhD
First Endocrine Department and Diabetes Center, Alexandra Hospital, Athens, Greece

Contents

Optimal nutrition is an important part of human immunodeficiency virus (HIV) care; to support the immune system, limit HIV-associated complications as well as maintain better quality of life and survival. The presentation and nature of malnutrition in patients with HIV has changed dramatically over the past 30 years from predominantly a wasting syndrome to lipodystrophy and, now, frailty. Nevertheless, we continue to see all 3 presentations in patient care today. The pathogenesis of poor nutrition in HIV-infected patients depends on caloric intake, intestinal nutrient absorption/translocation, and resting energy expenditure, which are features seen in all chronic diseases.

The pathogenesis of atherosclerosis in human immunodeficiency virus (HIV)-infected individuals is incompletely understood and appears to be multifactorial. Proatherogenic changes in blood and tissue lipids are associated with an increased risk of cardiovascular disease among HIV-infected subjects, and these changes may be both quantitative (dyslipidemia) and qualitative. In view of the pivotal role of dyslipidemia in the process of atherosclerosis, the increased incidence of dyslipidemia in HIV-infected individuals, and the emerging role of lipid abnormalities in systemic pathophysiologic processes such as immune activation, we review the contributions of dyslipidemia to cardiovascular risk in HIV infection.

As the modern era of combination antiretroviral therapy has increased life expectancy for individuals infected with the human immunodeficiency virus (HIV), type 2 diabetes mellitus and disorders of glucose metabolism have emerged as an important issue in the care of this population. Multiple mechanisms, both specific and nonspecific to HIV, underlie a significant prevalence. Although best-practice diagnostic testing remains unclear, the risks associated with diabetes in the setting of HIV are well characterized, ranging from organ-specific damage to socioeconomic decline.

As population-specific treatment data are limited, current guidelines serve as a basis for ongoing management.

Molecular mechanisms behind the defects in insulin production and secretion associated with antihuman immunodeficiency virus (anti-HIV) therapy and the development of HIV-associated lipodystrophy syndrome (HALS) are discussed in this article. Data suggesting insulin resistance on the beta cell and defects in first-phase insulin release of HALS patients are presented. Hepatic extraction of insulin, nonglucose insulin secretagogues and insulin-like growth factor release may exert influence on the demand of circulating insulin and on insulin secretion in HIV-infected patients. Finally, the paucity in understanding the incretin effects in HIV and HIV therapy in relation to insulin secretion is highlighted.

Androgen deficiency occurs frequently in men with human immunodeficiency virus (HIV) infection. Antiretroviral treatments had reduced the prevalence of male hypogonadism. The pathogenesis of testosterone (T) deficiency in HIV is multifactorial. Several mechanisms have been proposed; among them, drugs, fat redistribution, and a poor health status could explain the mechanism leading to gonadotropins inhibition and hypogonadotropic hypogonadism. The diagnosis of hypogonadism in HIV-infected men should be made based on clinical symptoms and a specific workup including T measurement. The interpretation of the results of biochemical testing is more difficult in men with HIV due to several confounding factors. T treatment should be offered to HIV-infected men with documented clinical hypogonadism and symptoms, especially if they are losing lean mass.

Most human immunodeficiency virus (HIV) infections among women occur early in reproductive life, which highlights the importance of understanding the impact of HIV on reproductive functions, and also the potential implications of reproductive function and aging on the course of HIV disease. Ovarian function is a crucial component of reproductive biology in women, but standard assessment methods are of limited applicability to women with chronic diseases such as HIV. Pregnancy can now be achieved without transmission of HIV to sexual partner or newborn, but complications of pregnancy may be more common in women infected with HIV than uninfected women.

The prevalence of vitamin D deficiency among HIV-infected persons is substantial and comparable to the general population. The factors associated with vitamin D deficiency are similar for both populations but additional factors (ie, use of certain antiretroviral agents) also contribute to vitamin D deficiency among HIV-infected persons. The adverse outcomes associated with vitamin D deficiency considerably overlap with non-AIDS defining illnesses (NADIs) that are increasingly becoming widespread in the aging HIV-infected population. However, there is scant evidence to support any causal inference. Further studies are warranted as efforts to identify and address modifiable risk factors contributing to NADIs continue.

Osteoporosis has emerged as an important co-morbidity of HIV infection and a modest increase in fracture risk has been documented. Bone loss from the spine and hip occurs after initiation of antiretroviral therapy but most data indicate that bone mineral density is stable in HIV-infected individuals established on long-term antiretroviral therapy. Assessment of fracture probability should be performed in individuals who have clinical risk factors for fracture. Adequate dietary calcium intake and vitamin D status should be ensured and in individuals with a high fracture probability, bisphosphonate therapy may be appropriate.

Thyroid abnormalities and nonthyroidal illness complicate human immunodeficiency virus (HIV) infection. Among the effects that result from HIV and other opportunistic infections, distinctive features of HIV infection include early lowering of reverse tri-iodothyromine (T3) levels, with normal free T3 levels. Later, some patients develop an isolated low free thyroxine level. After highly active antiretroviral therapy, the immune system reconstitutes in a way that leads to dysregulation of the autoimmune response and the appearance of Graves disease in 1% to 2% of patients. Opportunistic thyroid infections with unusual organisms are most commonly asymptomatic, but can lead to acute or subacute thyroiditis.

HIV infection induces hypothalamic-pituitary-adrenal (HPA) axis derangements. Partial glucocorticoid resistance has been observed in a subset of AIDS patients, possibly owing to HIV-induced altered cytokine secretion and action. Because glucocorticoids have immunomodulatory effects, the severity of the HPA axis disorder could play a central role in disease progression. The characteristic phenotype of AIDS patients (visceral obesity, lipodystrophy) may be owing to effects of HIV proteins on the HPA axis, including changes in glucocorticoid and insulin sensitivity of target tissues, as well as altered cytokine production and interaction with the HPA axis, genetic causes, comorbidities, and, possibly, use of antiretroviral agents.

Endocrine changes (including adrenal insufficiency, disorders of growth and puberty, thyroid dysfunction, metabolic abnormalities and osteopenia) accompany human immunodeficiency virus (HIV) infection in pediatric patients. The cause of these changes is multifactorial and includes direct viral effects of HIV, and effects of antiretroviral therapy. These effects may be of particular importance in childhood given the critical developmental processes that occur during this time period and the likelihood of prolonged exposure to the virus and medications.

ENDOCRINOLOGY AND METABOLISM CLINICS OF NORTH AMERICA

RELATED INTEREST

Infectious Disease Clinics of North America, Volume 28, Issue 3 (September 2014)
Updates in HIV and AIDS: Part I
Michael S. Saag and Henry Masur, *Editors*
Available at: http://www.id.theclinics.com/

VISIT THE CLINICS ONLINE!
Access your subscription at:
www.theclinics.com

Foreword

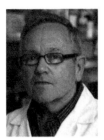

Derek LeRoith, MD, PhD
Consulting Editor

In this issue, Dr Hruz has compiled a number of articles related to the endocrinopathies associated with HIV-infected patients. Most endocrinologists are faced with these problems when called on to consult by colleagues who deal with these patients, given that antiviral therapy is so successful. As you read the individual articles, you will learn both the basic aspects of the endocrinopathies and the practical approaches to therapy.

In the opening article, we are exposed to an interesting phenomenon of a wasting syndrome, associated with sarcopenia leading to frailty. Before the advent of successful therapy, as described by Drs Mankal and Kotler, this was apparently a nutritional problem. Subsequently, with early HAART, there was associated lipodystrophy, and lately, with the chronicity of the disease, sarcopenia and frailty are quite evident. Each of these aspects is still evident today, and the effect on micronutrition and macronutrition, glucose metabolism need to be considered when health care providers what lifestyle interventions, such as diet and exercise are needed. Certain medications, such as rhGH for visceral obesity, are also occasionally indicated.

As discussed in the article by Drs Kelesidis and Currier, because HIV-infected individuals have prolonged survival, chronic medical conditions such as cardiovascular disease (CVD) have become of greater importance. They manifest many of the risk factors relating to this condition, namely, insulin resistance, hypertension, smoking, and hyperlipidemia. In addition, the HIV infection may induce an immune or inflammatory response that may be causative in the increased atherosclerosis. Thus, hypertriglyceridemia and low HDL are often found even in the absence of therapy. These alterations are also secondary to the successful antiretroviral therapy, adding to the risk of CVD. Fortunately, there are newer agents that have less of an effect on the lipid profiles. Nevertheless, health care providers need to be aware of these effects and monitor and treat accordingly.

With the advent of combination antiretroviral therapy, many millions of patients have survived the disease, and this has affected the long-term natural history. Indeed, as described by Drs Hadigan and Kattakuzhy, disorders of glucose metabolism and frank diabetes have become evident. In many studies, the incidence of diabetes in these patients may reach over 4% even in those without obesity. Initial therapies for HIV

Endocrinol Metab Clin N Am 43 (2014) xiii–xv
http://dx.doi.org/10.1016/j.ecl.2014.07.002
0889-8529/14/$ – see front matter © 2014 Elsevier Inc. All rights reserved.

endo.theclinics.com

included protease inhibitors that caused lipodystrophy and hyperlipidemia that may affect the incidence of diabetes. The viral infection itself may be a further etiologic factor, playing into the "inflammatory" process commonly seen in diabetes. Thus, early diagnosis and management of the diabetes are critical to avoiding complications in HIV-infected patients because these two chronic illnesses demonstrate significant interactions.

β-Cell insulin secretion is abnormal in HIV-infected individuals. Some studies have suggested that the overall insulin resistance these patients manifest is also seen in the β-cell where first-phase insulin secretion is particularly affected. As described by Dr Haugaard, patients with HIV-associated lipodystrophy syndrome are particularly prone to this effect, probably secondary to the generalized insulin resistance that occurs.

Hypogonadism, especially low testosterone, is quite common in HIV-infected men. As Drs Rochira and Guaraldi discuss, this is multifactorial. It may be secondary to infections of the testis, although probably more commonly secondary to poor health, excess fat, and drugs causing hypogonadotropic hypogonadism. When assessing the condition, one must consider that the higher SHBG in these patients may be elevated. On the other hand, replacement testosterone may be valuable especially to counteract the frailty and should be considered even on a trial basis before embarking on life-long therapy.

There are multiple aspects of HIV infection in women that may affect reproductive health. When high levels of viremia and low CD4 lymphocyte counts are evident, there is an associated reduction in fertility, although the exact cause is as yet unknown. Drs Yalamanchi, Dobs, and Greenblatt, in their article, further describe the possible mechanism whereby HIV infection may affect the hypothalamic-pituitary-ovarian axis, perhaps via immune responses. Nevertheless, with therapy today, women may be helped with fertility, and one can help partners and newborns to avoid the infection. Health care providers need to be cognizant of the fact that HIV-infected pregnant women show more complications in pregnancy.

Vitamin D deficiency is highly prevalent in HIV-infected individuals. In addition, as with the general population, this may be associated with many chronic disorders, such as diabetes, CVD, and osteoporosis. As discussed by Drs Escota, Cross, and Powderly, studies on replacement of vitamin D in the HIV-infected patient has not been convincing and, therefore, as with noninfected individuals, vitamin and calcium supplementation should follow general guidelines.

Dr Compston in her article discusses the relationship between HIV infection, treatment, and the risk of bone loss. Although there is a slight increase in bone loss following infection and certain medications, such as tenofovir, most of the bone loss is probably related to nutritional aspects, aging, and other medications, such as glucocorticoid therapy. Generally, recent data suggest that bone mineral density is generally quite stable in HIV-infected individuals not suffering from other disorders.

Dr Weetman describes the thyroid abnormalities that occur in HIV-infected patients. Extremely ill patients will of course develop euthyroid sick syndrome. However, in general, there some distinct characteristics of HIV infection: early, there is a lowering of reverse T3 levels, with normal free T3 levels; and later, some patients develop an isolated low free T4 level. As antiretrovirals allow for the reconstitution of the immune system, Graves may develop in up to 2% of cases. Finally, opportunistic infections have been shown to cause subacute thyroiditis.

A major effect of HIV infection is on the hypothalamic-pituitary-adrenal axis (HPA), described in the article by Drs Chroussos and Zapanti. Hypercorticolism and cortisol hypersensitivity may be caused by HIV involvement on the HPA, by either direct viral effects, inflammatory cytokines, or even cART. On the other hand, HIV and its therapy may uncover adrenal insufficiency. Overall, these effects may affect such comorbidities as lipodystrophy, insulin resistance, liver disease, and obesity. Thus, it behooves the clinician to be aware of these potential effects when managing these patients.

Of major concern is HIV infection in pediatric cases. This is a period of development that is crucial for later adult life. Drs Loomba-Albrecht, Bregman, and Chantry discuss how many of the developmental processes may be affected, such as growth, puberty, bone development, and adrenal disorders. Although the exact cause is not clear, both HIV itself and the medications may play a role in the causation. Appropriate therapy should be considered for each of the complications that develop, such as rhGH for growth, anabolic steroids for the treatment of hyperlipidemia and/or insulin resistance, and glucose lowering medications for metabolic changes. Ideally, these decisions should involve a multidisciplinary team.

Our sincere thanks to Dr Hruz and the authors for a very erudite and timely issue on a very important and growing topic that we all deal with in our practices.

Derek LeRoith, MD, PhD
Director of Research
Division of Endocrinology, Metabolism, and Bone Diseases
Department of Medicine
Icahn School of Medicine at Mount Sinai
One Gustave L. Levy Place
Box 1055, Altran 4-36
New York, NY 10029, USA

E-mail address:
derek.leroith@mssm.edu

Preface

HIV and Endocrine Disorders

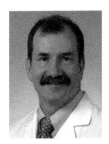

Paul W. Hruz, MD, PhD
Editor

With the development and clinical implementation of highly effective antiretroviral treatment regimens for HIV infection, this once fatal disease has now solidly transitioned to the status of a chronic illness. As such, HIV-infected patients are now living longer. Although this represents a crowning achievement of years of research and capital investment, affected individuals are experiencing many of the manifestations of aging at an alarming rate. This includes increased incidence of myocardial and metabolic diseases, such as diabetes, at younger ages than the HIV-uninfected population. As described in detail in this issue of *Endocrinology and Metabolism Clinics of North America*, interrelated adverse effects on multiple endocrine organs are now widely recognized. Causes are multifactorial and include environmental-related, disease-related, and treatment-related factors. Many of these disorders reflect an acceleration of the normal aging process. Although full mechanistic understanding of this complex disease phenotype has yet to be achieved, major strides forward have occurred within the past decade. This has included better understanding of the contributions of HIV infection itself, off-target drug effects, the role of chronic inflammatory changes, and influences of comorbid risk factors, such smoking and illicit drug use.

These advances have allowed targeted changes in therapeutic approaches, improved screening strategies, and the development of safer drugs. Nevertheless, there is still a need to study each of the observed metabolic changes and alterations of normal endocrine function in greater depth. Although great hope remains for the eventual development of safe and effective vaccines to prevent further virus transmission and the discovery of means to completely eradicate the virus from infected patients, those who are currently living with HIV will likely experience significant morbidity in the coming decades. For both the scientist and the clinician, it is anticipated that this collection of highly relevant and probing articles on endocrinopathies

Endocrinol Metab Clin N Am 43 (2014) xvii–xviii
http://dx.doi.org/10.1016/j.ecl.2014.07.001
0889-8529/14/$ – see front matter © 2014 Elsevier Inc. All rights reserved.

endo.theclinics.com

in HIV will provide a valuable reference for ongoing efforts to improve the lives of all patients affected by HIV infection.

Paul W. Hruz, MD, PhD
Division of Pediatric Endocrinology and Diabetes
Washington University School of Medicine
St Louis, MO 63110, USA

E-mail address:
hruz_p@kids.wustl.edu

From Wasting to Obesity, Changes in Nutritional Concerns in HIV/AIDS

Pavan K. Mankal, MD, MA[a,b], Donald P. Kotler, MD[a,c],*

KEYWORDS

- AIDS wasting syndrome • Malnutrition • Lipodystrophy • Frailty • HAART

KEY POINTS

- In the pre–highly active antiretroviral therapy (HAART) era, a wasting syndrome was the predominant nutritional alteration in human immunodeficiency virus/AIDS.
- The early HAART was complicated by the frequent development of a lipodystrophy syndrome related to medications, host factors, and disease characteristics.
- Frailty, associated with sarcopenia, is becoming a common nutritional and clinical problem in the current treatment era.

INTRODUCTION

An adage popular in the early part of the nineteenth century stated, *if you understand syphilis, you understand all of medicine*. In the latter part of nineteenth century the adage evolved to state, *if you understand tuberculosis you understand all of medicine*. In the current era, it can be said that *if you understand human immunodeficiency virus (HIV)/AIDS, you understand all of medicine*. These all are multifaceted diseases affecting multiple organ systems, and the implications span multiple levels within the health care system.

The history of HIV infection in the developed world can be divided into 2 eras, one preceding (1981–1996) and the other following (1996) the availability of highly active antiretroviral therapy (HAART). Much of the developing world remains in the pre-HAART

Disclosure: None.
[a] Department of Medicine, Mount Sinai St. Luke's, Mount Sinai Roosevelt Hospital, Icahn School of Medicine at Mount Sinai, Mount Sinai Health System, 1111 Amsterdam Avenue, New York, NY 10025, USA; [b] Division of Gastroenterology, Mount Sinai St. Luke's, Mount Sinai Roosevelt Hospital, Icahn School of Medicine at Mount Sinai, Mount Sinai Health System, 1111 Amsterdam Avenue, New York, NY 10025, USA; [c] Division of Gastroenterology and Hepatology, Mount Sinai St. Luke's, Mount Sinai Roosevelt Hospital, Icahn School of Medicine at Mount Sinai, Mount Sinai Health System, 1111 Amsterdam Avenue, New York, NY 10025, USA
* Corresponding author. Mount Sinai St. Luke's, Mount Sinai Roosevelt Hospital, 1111 Amsterdam Avenue, GI Division, S&R 12, New York, NY 10025.
E-mail address: dkotler@chpnet.org

Endocrinol Metab Clin N Am 43 (2014) 647–663
http://dx.doi.org/10.1016/j.ecl.2014.05.004   endo.theclinics.com

era, although the number of treated patients has increased progressively over the past 10 years. In contrast, untreated patients, either through the lack of diagnosis or unwillingness to adhere to treatment, continue to be seen in the developed world, including severely malnourished patients, similar to those seen in the pre-HAART era.

Nutritional consequences in HIV infection have been recognized since early in the epidemic. Protein-calorie malnutrition (wasting) with depletion of lean mass, fat, and micronutrients was the most common problem in the pre-HAART era and led to shortened survival and diminished quality of life.[1] The pathogenesis of wasting is multifactorial and related mainly to altered caloric intake, intestinal injury with nutrient malabsorption, and/or increased metabolic demands from the active infections.[2] Although the specific disease complications are limited to patients with AIDS or other immune deficiency states, the clinical-pathological correlations of malnutrition are the same as in nonimmune deficiency–mediated conditions. Also, as in non-AIDS patients, wasting exacerbates the immune deficits, promotes debility and dependency, and shortens the lifespan.[3] The success of HAART in reconstituting immune function and reducing morbidity ultimately allows HIV-infected individuals in North America to live as long as the general population.[4]

The widespread use of HAART has markedly improved clinical outcomes and decreased the prevalence of wasting. However, many treated patients develop a cluster of other nutritional alterations, including changes in body fat distribution, as well as dyslipidemia and insulin resistance, without wasting of muscle or other lean tissues.[5,6] The lipodystrophy syndrome, as it has come to be called, has attracted considerable clinical and experimental attention.[7,8] The causes are multifactorial, which led to a wide-ranging discussion about cause and effect and the relative roles of host, disease, and treatment in its pathogenesis.

The initial responders to the AIDS epidemic were in a unique situation in that they faced a brand new disease, with no evidence base for evaluation and management to help or hinder them. It soon became clear that the clinical manifestations represented disease complications and that the underlying disease and its causes had to be distinguished from the clinical complications of immune deficiency. For example, there was an initial reluctance by some surgeons to perform major surgery on patients with HIV/AIDS because of reports of poor clinical outcomes, whereas later observations showed that the poor results were related to protein calorie malnutrition and not to HIV/AIDS per se. The perceptions that progressive wasting is a universal phenomenon and that everyone with immune deficiency has intestinal dysfunction were subjected to clinical investigation and were shown not to be true.[9,10] In fact, the approach to nutrition in HIV/AIDS fits the classic clinical conundrum: How is what we are seeing the same as in other diseases, and how is it different?

Initially, there was little to go on other than the classic teachings of medicine. The situation fostered inductive reasoning as well as the performance of clinical trials to develop an evidence base. The response to HIV/AIDS was the first clinical condition in which nonmedical activists came to play an important role in the design and implementation of clinical trials, and they also played a crucial role in promoting acceptance and participation by HIV-infected people worldwide.

In this article, the authors describe the current knowledge on nutrition in the setting of HIV/AIDS, both in the presence and absence of antiretroviral therapy. The authors provide clinical descriptions and discuss pathogenic mechanisms, evaluation, and management of wasting and of lipodystrophy. The authors also briefly discuss the topic of nutritional assessment. The discussion of many topics, such as diabetes mellitus, cardiovascular disease, fat distribution, and so forth, is limited, as they are covered in greater detail elsewhere in this issue.

METHODS TO ASSESS NUTRITION

Although the high prevalence of weight loss and protein-calorie malnutrition was obvious from the earliest description of patients with AIDS, the only literature to guide the early clinicians was a subjective diagnosis of *slim disease* in a report from Africa. HIV/AIDS was one of the first diseases to be studied nutritionally using quantitative measures of body composition other than body weight.

Initial clinical studies, performed mainly on inpatients, demonstrated the weakness of using weight-based measures to estimate nutritional status.[1] Because of the wide ranges of premorbid body weights or body mass index (BMI) values as well as normal values, it may be difficult to detect wasting from a single measurement. The assessment of body weight provides no information about body composition: It cannot distinguish fat from muscle; it cannot distinguish lean mass from excess fluid, and it cannot detect micronutrient deficiencies at all. Body weight measurements were frequently difficult to interpret in patients with AIDS, especially hospitalized patients in whom wide swings in body weight resulted from diarrheal illnesses and from intravenous fluid administration. Quantitative measures of body composition had been developed more than 30 years before but had few clinical applications other than in examining the changes that occur during critical illness, aging, and obesity.

Wang and colleagues[11] organized body composition analysis by categorizing the measurements by level: atomic, molecular, cellular, tissue/organ, and whole body (**Table 1**). For example, the measurement of total body nitrogen by neutron activation analysis is part of the atomic level of measurement, whereas the measurement of total body water by isotope dilution is part of the molecular level of measurement and so forth. The 2 major rules of this organization are that the sum of all of the components within any level should equal the body weight and that one cannot use measurements from different levels in the same equation. However, one can derive predictive equations from one level to estimate the size of a compartment in another level (eg, total body protein = total body nitrogen $\times$ 6.25 or lean body mass = total body water/0.732).

Many techniques have been applied to the estimation of nutritional status in HIV/AIDS: (1) four-skinfold method, (2) hydrodensitometry, (3) neutron activation analysis, (4) bioelectrical impedance analysis (BIA), (5) dual-energy X–ray absorptiometry (DEXA), and (6) cross-sectional imaging (ie, computed tomography [CT]/magnetic resonance imaging [MRI]).[12–20] Because of their ease of use, BIA, DEXA, and CT/MRI have been used in clinical practice and research. Of note, the optimal methods to assess wasting are different from those used to assess lipodystrophy, with techniques to assess nonadipose tissue cellular mass or skeletal muscle mass being more important for protein-calorie malnutrition, whereas cross-sectional imaging

Table 1	
Levels of body composition analysis	
Level	**Components**
Atomic	Oxygen, carbon, hydrogen, nitrogen, potassium, sodium, phosphorus, chlorine, calcium, magnesium, sulfur, other atoms
Molecular	Water, lipid, protein, minerals, glycogen, and other molecules
Cellular	Body cell mass, adipocytes, extracellular fluid, extracellular solids
Tissue/organ	Skeletal muscle, adipose tissue, bone, viscera, other tissues
Whole body	Head, trunk, appendages

and DEXA are better at demonstrating alterations in body fat distribution in patients with HIV-associated lipodystrophy.

NUTRITIONAL ALTERATIONS IN THE PRE-HAART ERA

In 1987, the Centers for Disease Control and Prevention established HIV-associated wasting (defined as involuntary weight loss of greater than 10% from baseline plus either diarrhea or fever for 30 days or more) in the absence of a diagnosed concurrent illness as an AIDS-defining condition.[9,21,22] There have been no substantive changes in the definition since that time. However, many patients lose weight in the presence of a concurrent illness and also can be considered malnourished; clinical evaluation in others may be inadequate to detect the specific cause. The goal of the definition was to categorize patients as having AIDS, rather than HIV infection, both for reporting purposes as well as qualifying for medical and other entitlements. It provided no information about the cause or appropriate management.

Effects of HIV/AIDS on Macronutrient Status

The earliest nutritional studies were performed in severely ill, hospitalized patients with AIDS before the availability of any antiretroviral agents and demonstrated protein depletion (ie, transferrin, albumin) and muscle wasting (ie, midarm circumference).[22] In contrast, weight gain was often noted during hospitalization as a result of intravenous hydration in the presence of hypoalbuminemia. Although weight loss was often profound, the depletion of lean mass was even more striking; in contrast, body fat content was not severely depleted in many patients.[1] These studies were performed before the identification of HIV as the etiologic agent of AIDS and represent the natural history of tissue depletion at the start of the epidemic in New York City. Body composition studies performed in patients with wasting syndromes in the absence of nutritional support demonstrated that magnitude of weight loss and the severity of body cell mass depletion correlated with the timing of death.[3] Later studies demonstrated that depletion of lean mass occurs early in the disease course and may precede the development of weight loss.[23] The loss of lean mass is concentrated within the body cell mass, the metabolically active components of the muscles and visceral organs. The composition of weight loss differs in men and women, with men losing more lean mass and less body fat than do women.[24] However, clinical stability was associated with nutritional stability, indicating that wasting is not a universal phenomenon in HIV-infected individuals.[9] Weight loss from opportunistic infections is episodic and rapid, whereas weight loss related to malabsorption tends to be more chronic and slowly progressive.[25] Other factors, both behaviors and comorbidities, may also affect nutritional status, independent of HIV infection.

Effects of HIV/AIDS on Micronutrient Status

Many studies of micronutrients have been published but mostly in untreated patients. Low levels of several micronutrients have been reported, including vitamin B12, selenium, zinc, vitamin B6, other B vitamins, and fat-soluble vitamins, including vitamin A and vitamin D.[26] Vitamin A deficiency was associated with increased mortality in Africa and with an increased risk of maternal child transmission of HIV infection.[27] Selenium deficiency is recognized to occur commonly in HIV infection and was significantly associated with an increased relative risk of mortality.[28] Several studies have shown that HIV/AIDS is associated with enhanced oxidative stress. Antioxidant deficiency is potentially important because inflammatory mediators promote HIV replication.[29]

Nutrition and Wasting

Malnutrition is multifactorial in HIV infection, and the pathogenic mechanisms are similar in HIV and non-HIV infected people. Although some nutritional and metabolic alterations can be identified during the preclinical stage of disease, progressive malnutrition is limited to patients with a severe, chronic disease complication and, usually, severe immune depletion. The pathogenic processes underlying wasting involve alterations in caloric intake, nutrient absorption, or energy expenditure. Weight loss, ultimately, is a consequence of negative caloric balance, irrespective of cause. The relative roles of altered energy intake and expenditure have been examined. Grunfeld and colleagues[30] demonstrated that caloric intake was more important than resting energy expenditure in predicting short-term (1 month) change in body weight. Macallan and colleagues,[31] using the technique of doubly labeled water measurement, found that total energy expenditure was decreased in weight-losing patients and that the loss was confined to voluntary energy expenditure. However, caloric intake was decreased to a greater extent than was voluntary energy expenditure. Simply maintaining caloric intake by nonvolitional feeding does not necessarily replete lean mass (see later discussion).

There are several causes for reduced food intake, including local pathological conditions; focal or diffuse neurologic diseases; severe psychiatric disease; food insecurity because of psychosocial or economic factors; and anorexia caused by medications, malabsorption, systemic infections, or tumors (**Box 1**). Malabsorption in HIV/AIDS is usually related to small intestinal infections, usually protozoal, with partial villus atrophy and crypt hyperplasia (**Fig. 1**). Cryptosporidiosis is the most well known of these infections (**Fig. 2**). This organism causes a self-limited infection in immune-competent people and in most HIV-infected patients with peripheral blood CD4 lymphocyte counts greater than 200/mm^3 but it is progressive and ultimately fatal in the absence of HAART therapy. *Isospora belli*, microsporidia, and *Cyclospora cayetanensis* (**Figs. 3** and **4**) are other protozoa that localize in small intestinal mucosa. *Mycobacterium avium* complex infection (**Fig. 5**) of the small intestine promotes malabsorption, particularly of fats, because of lymphatic obstruction and exudative enteropathy. Patients with HIV/AIDS also develop a variety of systemic infections with fever, hypermetabolism, and anorexia.

Other metabolic alterations not necessarily associated with opportunistic infections include elevated resting energy expenditure, hypertriglyceridemia, and decreased serum cholesterol concentrations.[32] Hypertriglyceridemia is associated both with decreased clearance of chylomicrons as well as increased de novo fatty acid synthesis and elevated serum concentrations of bioactive interferon alpha.[33] Alterations of the hypophyseal pituitary adrenal and gonadal axes are common; deficiencies in testosterone and other endogenous anabolic factors may occur and promote protein depletion.

Box 1
Causes of poor food intake

Local pathologic conditions affecting chewing, swallowing, or gastrointestinal motility

Focal neurologic disease affecting food intake

Diffuse neurologic disease affecting the perception of hunger or ability to eat

Severe psychiatric disease

Food insecurity because of psychosocial or economic factors

Anorexia caused by medications, malabsorption, systemic infections, or tumors

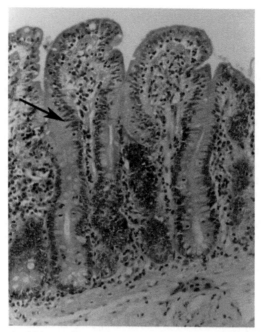

Fig. 1. A small intestinal biopsy demonstrating marked crypt hyperplasia and partial villus atrophy. The arrow is placed at the approximate level of the crypt/villus junction (hematoxylin and eosin, original magnification ×250).

Nutritional Management of Wasting

The rationale for nutritional therapy to patients with AIDS is straightforward: malnutrition has adverse consequences that can be prevented by improving nutritional status. Concepts guiding the decisions to provide nutritional support in HIV-infected patients are the same as in anyone with a chronic illness.

There are no data to support the standard use of oral supplements in HIV-infected individuals, in the presence or absence of wasting, though they often are prescribed in patients complaining of fatigue. There is little consensus about the use of

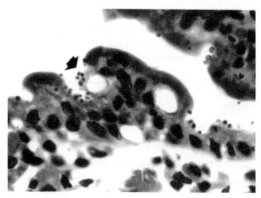

Fig. 2. A small intestinal biopsy from a patient with cryptosporidiosis, demonstrating the organisms (*arrow*) at the brush border level, where they invade and damage the apical portion of the enterocyte (acid fast stain, original magnification ×400).

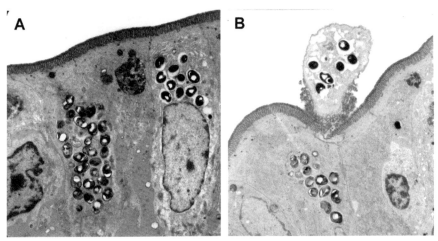

Fig. 3. (*A*) A small intestinal biopsy from a patient with microsporidiosis. Spores of *Entero-cytozoon bieneusi* are seen in the cytoplasm of epithelial cells. The organisms may be diffi-cult to detect on light microscopy. (*B*) A small intestinal biopsy from a patient with microsporidiosis. A dying cell containing spores of *E bieneusi* (electron micrograph, original magnification ×3500).

micronutrient supplements, such as antioxidant and vitamins, in the face of a nutritious diet. A study of vitamin A supplementation in African mothers with HIV/AIDS demon-strated a significant decline in vertical HIV transmission.[34] Micronutrient supplementa-tion has the greatest impact in patients with micronutrient deficiencies at baseline, even in the absence of antiretroviral therapy, though the effect may not be adequate if protein and caloric deficiencies persist.[35]

Several appetite stimulants have been studied or used in HIV-infected patients. The synthetic progestin, megestrol acetate, increases caloric intake and promotes weight gain and improved quality of life.[36] Dronabinol, a synthetic derivative of *Cannabis sativa* (marijuana), is approved for appetite stimulation in AIDS-related anorexia.

Several studies examined the effects of nonvolitional feeding on wasting. A pro-spective, open-label study in the pre-HAART era demonstrated gains in body cell

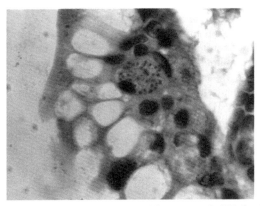

Fig. 4. A small intestinal biopsy from a patient with *Isospora belli* infection demonstrating the microgametocyte stage of infection (hematoxylin and eosin, original magnification ×1000).

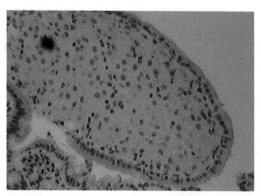

Fig. 5. A small intestinal biopsy from a patient with *Mycobacterium avium* complex infection. The villus is thickened and infiltrated with macrophages (foam cells) containing acid-fast bacilli. Of note, the patient has coexisting cryptosporidial infection (hematoxylin and eosin, original magnification ×250).

mass and body fat after percutaneous endoscopic gastrostomy (PEG) tube feeding.[37] Ockenga and colleagues[38] compared the clinical courses of patients with AIDS and non-AIDS patients who accepted or declined PEG feedings. Treatment was equally safe in both groups and led to nutritional benefits, but survival was not different in patients accepting or refusing PEG feedings. Total parenteral nutrition (TPN) was also studied in the pre-HAART era and promoted weight gain caused by an increase in body fat, without a change in lean mass.[39] However, patients with malabsorption syndromes or eating disorders responded well to TPN, with significant increases in body cell mass, whereas patients with systemic infections continued to lose body cell mass while gaining body fat. Thus, the response to TPN is related to the underlying condition rather than to the specific TPN formula. These results show that, although inadequate caloric intake is the most important promoter of weight loss, simply providing calories is not sufficient to reverse the loss of lean mass.

In a prospective randomized trial, TPN was compared with an oral, semielemental diet.[40] Although both the oral diet and TPN reversed weight loss in patients with AIDS with malabsorption, the caloric intake and weight change were both greater in the TPN group, whereas the quality of life was higher and health care costs lower in the oral-diet group. In a meta-analysis of nutritional therapy in patients with HIV, although energy and protein intake were increased in patients who had been supplemented with specific macronutrients, the outcomes were not different.[41]

A recurring theme in nutritional studies is that weight loss includes lean mass, especially skeletal muscle mass, although treatment-associated weight gain involves mainly body fat. For this reason, studies of anabolic agents were an area of active research in the pre-HAART era. Recombinant human growth hormone (rhGH) was shown to promote repletion of lean mass in studies performed both in the pre-HAART and HAART eras.[42,43] The increase in lean mass was associated with improvements in quality of life and physical performance. Anabolic steroids, including testosterone and its derivatives, were also studied in men and women and promoted lean mass repletion.[44,45] Because proinflammatory cytokines influence the wasting process, studies of cytokine inhibitors, antioxidants, omega-3 fatty acids, pentoxifylline (Trental), and thalidomide were performed, though with little evidence of benefit. However, resistance training exercise has been demonstrated to promote skeletal muscle repletion without systemic toxicity or potential for adverse interactions.[46]

THE LIPODYSTROPHY SYNDROME

Soon after the introduction of HAART, clinicians began to notice a constellation of metabolic and morphologic changes in treated patients.[47] A loss of subcutaneous adipose tissue, especially in the face, often associated with a gain in visceral and dorsocervical adipose tissue and no loss of lean mass, is common in HAART-treated patients.[48] The term *lipodystrophy* has been applied based on similarities to congenital or acquired conditions that include lipoatrophy and lipohypertrophy (**Fig. 6**) associated with dyslipidemia and insulin resistance, among other alterations.[7] Epidemiologic studies identified several risk factors (**Box 2**). Although the changes tend to cluster, they have some distinctive pathogenic pathways and may occur independently of one another.

The medical consequences of body fat redistribution have been known for more than one-half century since the French investigator, Jean Vague,[49] applied quantitative measures of body fat content in women with 2 different phenotypes, upper body and lower body obesity, which he termed android and gynoid, respectively. Upper body obesity was associated with adverse health outcomes, including diabetes mellitus and cardiovascular disease, whereas lower body obesity was not, despite having equivalent total body fat contents. The obvious conclusion, replicated many times since then, is that body fat distribution is more important than is total body fat in promoting adverse health outcomes. Initial observations suggested that lipoatrophy and lipohypertrophy in HIV/AIDS are closely linked, whereas epidemiologic studies suggest that these distinct compartments are affected differently by various influences (see later discussion). Premorbid body composition also strongly influences the clinical picture, with prior obesity associated with lipohypertrophy.

The major metabolic alterations seen in HAART-treated patients are similar to that seen in the general population, including dyslipidemia (elevated triglycerides and total cholesterol, decreased high-density lipoprotein [HDL] cholesterol) and insulin resistance. Generally, around 25% of treated patients with HIV fit the metabolic syndrome definition, similar to that of the normal population.[50] The incidence of hypertriglyceridemia varies by treatment regimen and is most common with certain protease

A   **B**

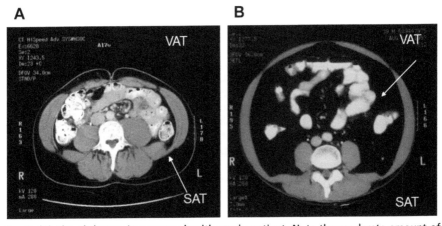

Fig. 6. (*A*) The abdomen in a young healthy male patient. Note the moderate amount of subcutaneous adipose tissue (SAT) (*black*) and very little visceral adipose tissue (VAT). (*B*) The abdomen in a patient with HIV-associated lipodystrophy. Note the virtual absence of subcutaneous adipose tissue (*black*) and the large amount of visceral adipose tissue. The *arrows* point to the correct compartment – SAT and VAT.

Box 2
Epidemiologic factors affecting the development of lipodystrophy

- Disease
  - Duration
  - Severity of immune deficiency
  - Magnitude of immune reconstitution
- Host
  - Age
  - Sex
  - Race
  - Family history, BMI
  - Diet
  - Exercise
  - Tobacco use
- Therapy
  - Specific agent
  - Duration of therapy

---

inhibitors. It is a direct effect of the drug as shown in a study of ritonavir administration to healthy HIV-seronegative volunteers.[51] In contrast to triglycerides, serum cholesterol concentrations are classically low in HIV-infected patients and increase during therapy, irrespective of the specific HAART regimen, as shown in an analysis of blood samples from a longitudinal cohort.[52] Seroconversion was associated with reductions in total, low-density lipoprotein (LDL), and HDL cholesterol concentrations. Total and LDL cholesterol levels increased during HAART, but LDL-cholesterol only increased to preinfection levels, which was interpreted as a return to prior health as opposed to drug toxicity. A similar argument has been made in the analysis of temporal trends in waist circumference.[53]

Alterations in glucose-metabolism first came to light with an alert from the Food and Drug Administration (FDA) about reports of diabetes mellitus associated with protease inhibitor use. Insulin resistance was found to occur in about one-half of protease inhibitor-treated patients compared with about one-quarter of patients on nucleoside analogue therapy in an early series.[54] Although asymptomatic, insulin resistance predicts a future risk of symptomatic atherosclerosis in non-HIV infected subjects.[55] Its genesis is multifactorial.[56] An acute, reversible effect of protease inhibitors on glucose transport into cells via glucose transporter type 4 (GLUT4) inhibition has been demonstrated.[57,58] Nucleoside reverse transcriptase inhibitors (NRTI) also promote insulin resistance, as shown in studies in healthy adults, an effect thought to be mediated by mitochondrial toxicity.[59] Other pathogenic factors include chronic inflammation, hepatitis C infection, elevations of free fatty acids caused by excess lipolysis, obesity with visceral fat accumulation, and others.

Pathogenesis

Several risk factors have been uncovered through epidemiologic investigations. Although most attention has been given to antiretroviral therapy, many host- and disease-related variables are important. Age, sex, race, premorbid weight and weight change, a personal or family history of the metabolic syndrome, diet, and exercise may all affect the diagnosis, as may the duration of disease, the severity of immune depletion, and the magnitude of the immune reconstitution during antiviral therapy (see **Box 2**). A genetic predisposition to the development of lipodystrophy was shown in a prospective study of HAART therapy using cluster analysis. Treated patients were classified by developing morphologic and metabolic abnormalities while on therapy, which were found to cluster. Studies of selected candidates revealed a polymorphism in the resistin gene, which strongly predicted the development of the changes.[60]

There is substantial clinical and experimental evidence for direct metabolic effects of antiretroviral agents. Initial observations associated the development of hyperlipidemia, insulin resistance, and body composition changes and linked them to protease inhibitor use.[47] Protease inhibitors may affect hepatic very-low-density lipoprotein secretion through an inhibition in intracellular apoprotein B and may also decrease glucose uptake through a reversible inhibition of the glucose transport molecule GLUT4.[57] However, lipoatrophy was shown to occur in patients not taking protease inhibitors and even before the application of HAART.[61,62]

The development of lipoatrophy is related to mitochondrial DNA (mtDNA) depletion within adipose tissue and muscle cells.[59,63] The development of liver failure as a consequence of mitochondrial toxicity from nucleoside analogue therapy first came to clinical attention during studies of a fluorinated uridine developed to treat chronic hepatitis B infection.[64] Several nucleoside reverse transcriptase inhibitors inhibit human mtDNA polymerase gamma, leading to mtDNA depletion. Intraclass differences among the NRTIs in the ability to cause mitochondrial dysfunction and local factors limit the complication to specific tissues. Mitochondrial toxicity may be covert or overt, implying a threshold for clinical sequelae. A large body of corroborating evidence from many experimental models, ranging from cell culture to clinical trials, has been published.

A consistent finding in antiretroviral treatment studies is that evidence of inflammation and immune activation may persist despite immune reconstitution and control of opportunistic conditions. There is a large body of literature linking inflammation and atherosclerosis in non-HIV situations and a growing body of information that suggests that a similar process occurs in HIV/AIDS. The field gained a strong impetus with the identification of microbial translocation and its association with immune activation.[65] Microbial translocation and immune activation have been associated with several long-term adverse outcomes beyond cardiovascular disease, including neurocognitive disorders, cancer, and frailty. Microbial translocation is now being sought and found in other diseases where its presence may affect outcomes.[66]

Diagnosis

Despite great interest and effort in understanding the nature of lipodystrophy, there has been little effort in deriving diagnostic criteria, leaving clinicians to manage the various alterations individually. Therefore, HIV medicine parallels the general practice of medicine; the HIV treater has had to become familiar with practice standards for general medicine. Identifying body composition alterations is especially difficult. Because there are no recognized normal values, the techniques for quantitating subcutaneous and visceral fat contents are not available for clinical use; surrogate measures, such as anthropometric analyses, are inaccurate.[67] In general, the diagnostic criteria for the metabolic alterations are the same as in the non-HIV population.

Consequences

Although there are many possible etiologic factors in the development of lipodystrophy, most are nonmodifiable, whereas drug therapy is modifiable. The recognition of lipodystrophy has fueled changes in HIV management, including reevaluation of the appropriate time to start therapy, switching therapy, stopping therapy, and providing consistent therapy. Not all of these changes have had a beneficial effect. For example, intermittent therapy was tested as a possible means to mitigate heart attack risk; but that study demonstrated an increase in myocardial infarction in patients who stopped and resumed therapy, which convinced the field that HIV infection itself should be considered as a cardiac risk factor.[68] Most importantly, the recognition of lipodystrophy and its adverse consequences has led to the development of new agents and new classes of agents that are largely free of mitochondrial toxicity and other adverse metabolic consequences.

Several aspects of the lipodystrophy syndrome are of clinical interest: cardiovascular disease,[69–71] cerebrovascular disease, diabetes mellitus,[72,73] neurocognitive dysfunction, bone disease,[74–77] and frailty. Frailty is a distinct clinical syndrome encompassing weight loss, weakness, exhaustion, and decreased activity; linkage to immune activation has been postulated in both HIV and aging.[78] Frailty is an increasingly recognized problem in clinical medicine and includes decreased muscle mass and function. Therefore, it may well be the future face of HIV-associated nutritional disorders.

Therapeutic Options

There are 4 possible responses to the development of lipodystrophy: do nothing, stop HAART, switch HAART, or treat the individual abnormalities. Advances in the field have led to the development of treatment regimens that are relatively free of mitochondrial and other metabolic toxicities, so that patients with these problems likely have them as a legacy of prior therapies. Unfortunately, lipoatrophy is not reversible to any significant extent. Most clinicians approach the metabolic complications as they would in non-HIV infected individuals, with some extra attention of possible drug-drug interactions. Complementary therapies (eg, weight control, smoking cessation) should be stressed in all cases, as they likely have a greater influence on the outcome than the individual antiretroviral agent.

Dietary modification has only a modest effect on serum lipid concentrations. Fibrates decrease serum triglyceride concentrations but do not significantly affect serum cholesterol concentrations, whereas the 3-hydroxy-3-methylglutaryl-coenzyme A reductase inhibitors (statins) decrease both serum cholesterol and, to a lesser extent, triglyceride concentrations.[79] However, the goals of clinical management of hyperlipidemia as defined by the National Cholesterol Education Program's criteria are often not reached in HIV-infected patients. The treatment of clinical diabetes mellitus is standard.[56] Most patients can be managed successfully with diet and oral agents. Diet and resistance training exercise are well known to affect total body and regional fat mass in non-HIV infected subjects and have similar effects in patients who are HIV+.[46,80] The FDA approved a growth hormone releasing factor to treat visceral fat accumulation in patients with HIV lipodystrophy.[81]

FUTURE CONSIDERATIONS/SUMMARY

Initially, HIV infection was seen as being different from other diseases. However, as clinical knowledge has grown, it has become clear that clinical alterations, including nutritional changes, in patients with HIV/AIDS occur by the same processes as in other diseases and that people who understand all of clinical medicine can understand HIV infection. Although wasting was the initial nutritional complication of HIV/AIDS to be recognized and lipodystrophy followed the initial application of HAART, sarcopenia and frailty may be the most important alteration in the near future. Further, some of the knowledge gained in studies of HIV/AIDS, such as microbial translocation, has been used to further our understanding of non-AIDS diseases.

REFERENCES

1. Kotler DP, Wang J, Pierson RN. Body composition studies in patients with the acquired immunodeficiency syndrome. Am J Clin Nutr 1985;42:1255–65.
2. Greene JB. Clinical approach to weight loss in the patient with HIV infection. Gastroenterol Clin North Am 1988;17:573–86.
3. Kotler DP, Tierney AR, Wang J, et al. Magnitude of body-cell-mass depletion and the timing of death from wasting in AIDS [key paper]. Am J Clin Nutr 1989;50:444–7.
4. Samji H, Cescon A, Hogg RS, et al. Closing the gap: increases in life expectancy among treated HIV-positive individuals in the United States and Canada. PLoS One 2013;8:e81355.
5. Friis-Moller N, Weber R, Reiss P, et al. Cardiovascular disease risk factors in HIV patients–association with antiretroviral therapy. Results from the DAD study. AIDS 2003;17:1179–93.
6. Engelson ES, Kotler DP, Tan Y, et al. Fat distribution in HIV-infected patients reporting truncal enlargement quantified by whole-body magnetic resonance imaging. Am J Clin Nutr 1999;69:1162–9.
7. Garg A. Clinical review#: lipodystrophies: genetic and acquired body fat disorders. J Clin Endocrinol Metab 2011;96:3313–25.
8. Singhania R, Kotler DP. Lipodystrophy in HIV patients: its challenges and management approaches. HIV AIDS (Auckl) 2011;3:135–43.
9. Kotler DP, Tierney AR, Brenner SK, et al. Preservation of short-term energy balance in clinically stable patients with AIDS. Am J Clin Nutr 1990;51:7–13.
10. Kotler DP, Reka S, Chow K, et al. Effects of enteric parasitoses and HIV infection upon small intestinal structure and function in patients with AIDS. J Clin Gastroenterol 1993;16:10–5.
11. Wang ZM, Pierson RN Jr, Heymsfield SB. The five-level model: a new approach to organizing body-composition research. Am J Clin Nutr 1992;56:19–28.
12. Jaffrin MY. Body composition determination by bioimpedance: an update. Curr Opin Clin Nutr Metab Care 2009;12:482–6. http://dx.doi.org/10.1097/MCO.0b013e32832da22c.
13. Freitas P, Carvalho D, Santos AC, et al. Assessment of body fat composition disturbances by bioimpedance analysis in HIV-infected adults. J Endocrinol Invest 2011;34:e321–9.
14. Perez-Matute P, Perez-Martinez L, Blanco JR, et al. Multiple frequency bioimpedance is an adequate tool to assess total and regional fat mass in HIV-positive patients but not to diagnose HIV-associated lipoatrophy: a pilot study. J Int AIDS Soc 2013;16:18609.
15. Thibault R, Cano N, Pichard C. Quantification of lean tissue losses during cancer and HIV infection/AIDS. Curr Opin Clin Nutr Metab Care 2011;14:261–7.
16. Durnin J, Womersley J. Body fat assessed from total body density and its estimation from skinfold thickness: measurements on 481 men and women aged from 16 to 72 years. Br J Nutr 1974;32:77–97.
17. Aghdassi E, Arendt B, Salit IE, et al. Estimation of body fat mass using dual-energy x-ray absorptiometry, bioelectric impedance analysis, and anthropometry in HIV-positive male subjects receiving highly active antiretroviral therapy. JPEN J Parenter Enteral Nutr 2007;31:135–41.

18. Mourtzakis M, Prado CM, Lieffers JR, et al. A practical and precise approach to quantification of body composition in cancer patients using computed tomography images acquired during routine care. Appl Physiol Nutr Metab 2008;33: 997–1006.

19. Scherzer R, Shen W, Bacchetti P, et al. Comparison of dual-energy X-ray absorptiometry and magnetic resonance imaging-measured adipose tissue depots in HIV-infected and control subjects. Am J Clin Nutr 2008;88:1088–96.

20. Macallan DC, Baldwin C, Mandalia S, et al. Treatment of altered body composition in HIV-associated lipodystrophy: comparison of rosiglitazone, pravastatin, and recombinant human growth hormone. HIV Clin Trials 2008;9:254–68.

21. Center for Diseases Control (CDC). Revision of the CDC surveillance case definition for acquired immunodeficiency syndrome. Council of State and Territorial Epidemiologists; AIDS Program, Center for Infectious Diseases. MMWR Morb Mortal Wkly Rep 1987;36(Suppl 1):1S–15S.

22. Kotler DP, Gaetz HP, Lange M, et al. Enteropathy associated with the acquired immunodeficiency syndrome. Ann Intern Med 1984;101:421–8.

23. Ott M, Lembcke B, Fischer H, et al. Early changes of body composition in human immunodeficiency virus-infected patients: tetrapolar body impedance analysis indicates significant malnutrition. Am J Clin Nutr 1993;57:15–9.

24. Kotler DP, Thea DM, Heo M, et al. Relative influences of sex, race, environment, and HIV infection on body composition in adults. Am J Clin Nutr 1999;69:432–9.

25. Macallan DC, Noble C, Baldwin C, et al. Prospective analysis of patterns of weight change in stage IV human immunodeficiency virus infection. Am J Clin Nutr 1993;58:417–24.

26. Baum MK. Role of micronutrients in HIV-infected intravenous drug users. J Acquir Immune Defic Syndr 2000;25(Suppl 1):S49–52.

27. Dreyfuss ML, Fawzi WW. Micronutrients and vertical transmission of HIV-1. Am J Clin Nutr 2002;75:959–70.

28. Baum MK, Shor-Posner G, Lai S, et al. High risk of HIV-related mortality is associated with selenium deficiency. J Acquir Immune Defic Syndr Hum Retrovirol 1997;15:370–4.

29. Folks TM, Justement J, Kinter A, et al. Cytokine-induced expression of HIV-1 in a chronically infected promonocyte cell line. Science 1987;238:800–2.

30. Grunfeld C, Pang M, Shimizu L, et al. Resting energy expenditure, caloric intake, and short-term weight change in human immunodeficiency virus infection and the acquired immunodeficiency syndrome. Am J Clin Nutr 1992;55: 455–60.

31. Macallan DC, Noble C, Baldwin C, et al. Energy expenditure and wasting in human immunodeficiency virus infection [key paper]. N Engl J Med 1995;333: 83–8.

32. Grunfeld C, Kotler DP, Hamadeh R, et al. Hypertriglyceridemia in the acquired immunodeficiency syndrome. Am J Med 1989;86:27–31.

33. Grunfeld C, Kotler DP, Shigenaga JK, et al. Circulating interferon-alpha levels and hypertriglyceridemia in the acquired immunodeficiency syndrome. Am J Med 1991;90:154–62.

34. Rahmathullah L, Underwood BA, Thulasiraj RD, et al. Reduced mortality among children in southern India receiving a small weekly dose of vitamin A. N Engl J Med 1990;323:929–35.

35. Baum MK, Campa A, Lai S, et al. Effect of micronutrient supplementation on disease progression in asymptomatic, antiretroviral-naive, HIV-infected adults in Botswana: a randomized clinical trial. J Am Med Assoc 2013;310:2154–63.

36. Von Roenn JH, Armstrong D, Kotler DP, et al. Megestrol acetate in patients with AIDS-related cachexia. Ann Intern Med 1994;121:393–9.
37. Kotler DP, Tierney AR, Ferraro R, et al. Enteral alimentation and repletion of body cell mass in malnourished patients with acquired immunodeficiency syndrome. Am J Clin Nutr 1991;53:149–54.
38. Ockenga J, Suttmann U, Selberg O, et al. Percutaneous endoscopic gastrostomy in AIDS and control patients: risks and outcome. Am J Gastroenterol 1996;91:1817–22.
39. Kotler DP, Tierney AR, Culpepper-Morgan JA, et al. Effect of home total parenteral nutrition on body composition in patients with acquired immunodeficiency syndrome. JPEN J Parenter Enteral Nutr 1990;14:454–8.
40. Kotler DP, Fogleman L, Tierney AR. Comparison of total parenteral nutrition and an oral, semielemental diet on body composition, physical function, and nutrition-related costs in patients with malabsorption due to acquired immunodeficiency syndrome. JPEN J Parenter Enteral Nutr 1998;22:120–6.
41. Grobler L, Siegfried N, Visser ME, et al. Nutritional interventions for reducing morbidity and mortality in people with HIV. Cochrane Database Syst Rev 2013;(2):CD004536.
42. Moyle GJ, Daar ES, Gertner JM, et al. Growth hormone improves lean body mass, physical performance, and quality of life in subjects with HIV-associated weight loss or wasting on highly active antiretroviral therapy. J Acquir Immune Defic Syndr 2004;35:367–75.
43. Schambelan M, Mulligan K, Grunfeld C, et al. Recombinant human growth hormone in patients with HIV-associated wasting. A randomized, placebo-controlled trial. Serostim Study Group. Ann Intern Med 1996;125:873–82.
44. Grinspoon S, Corcoran C, Askari H, et al. Effects of androgen administration in men with the AIDS wasting syndrome. A randomized, double-blind, placebo-controlled trial. Ann Intern Med 1998;129:18–26.
45. Miller K, Corcoran C, Armstrong C, et al. Transdermal testosterone administration in women with acquired immunodeficiency syndrome wasting: a pilot study. J Clin Endocrinol Metab 1998;83:2717–25.
46. Agin D, Gallagher D, Wang J, et al. Effects of whey protein and resistance exercise on body cell mass, muscle strength, and quality of life in women with HIV. AIDS 2001;15:2431–40.
47. Carr A, Samaras K, Burton S, et al. A syndrome of peripheral lipodystrophy, hyperlipidaemia and insulin resistance in patients receiving HIV protease inhibitors. AIDS 1998;12:F51–8.
48. Chen D, Misra A, Garg A. Clinical review 153: lipodystrophy in human immunodeficiency virus-infected patients. J Clin Endocrinol Metab 2002;87:4845–56.
49. Vague J. The degree of masculine differentiation of obesities: a factor determining predisposition to diabetes, atherosclerosis, gout, and uric calculous disease. Am J Clin Nutr 1956;4:20–34.
50. Mondy K, Overton ET, Grubb J, et al. Metabolic syndrome in HIV-infected patients from an urban, Midwestern US outpatient population. Clin Infect Dis 2007;44:726–34.
51. Purnell JQ, Zambon A, Knopp RH, et al. Effect of ritonavir on lipids and post-heparin lipase activities in normal subjects. AIDS 2000;14:51–7.
52. Riddler SA, Smit E, Cole SR, et al. Impact of HIV infection and HAART on serum lipids in men [key paper]. J Am Med Assoc 2003;289:2978–82.
53. Brown TT, Xu X, John M, et al. Fat distribution and longitudinal anthropometric changes in HIV-infected men with and without clinical evidence of lipodystrophy

and HIV-uninfected controls: a substudy of the Multicenter AIDS Cohort Study [key paper]. AIDS Res Ther 2009;6:8.

54. Walli R, Herfort O, Michl GM, et al. Treatment with protease inhibitors associated with peripheral insulin resistance and impaired oral glucose tolerance in HIV-1-infected patients. AIDS 1998;12:F167–73.

55. Fontbonne AM, Eschwege EM. Insulin and cardiovascular disease. Paris Prospective Study. Diabetes Care 1991;14:461–9.

56. Florescu D, Kotler DP. Insulin resistance, glucose intolerance and diabetes mellitus in HIV-infected patients. Antivir Ther 2007;12:149–62.

57. Murata H, Hruz PW, Mueckler M. The mechanism of insulin resistance caused by HIV protease inhibitor therapy. J Biol Chem 2000;275:20251–4.

58. Hresko RC, Hruz PW. HIV protease inhibitors act as competitive inhibitors of the cytoplasmic glucose binding site of GLUTs with differing affinities for GLUT1 and GLUT4 [key paper]. PLoS One 2011;6:e25237.

59. Fleischman A, Johnsen S, Systrom DM, et al. Effects of a nucleoside reverse transcriptase inhibitor, stavudine, on glucose disposal and mitochondrial function in muscle of healthy adults [key paper]. Am J Physiol Endocrinol Metab 2007;292:E1666–73.

60. Ranade K, Geese WJ, Noor M, et al. Genetic analysis implicates resistin in HIV lipodystrophy [key paper]. AIDS 2008;22:1561–8.

61. Saint-Marc T, Partisani M, Poizot-Martin I, et al. A syndrome of peripheral fat wasting (lipodystrophy) in patients receiving long-term nucleoside analogue therapy. AIDS 1999;13:1659–67.

62. Maia BS, Engelson ES, Wang J, et al. Antiretroviral therapy affects the composition of weight loss in HIV infection: implications for clinical nutrition. Clin Nutr 2005;24:971–8.

63. Mallon PW, Sedwell R, Rogers G, et al. Effect of rosiglitazone on peroxisome proliferator-activated receptor gamma gene expression in human adipose tissue is limited by antiretroviral drug-induced mitochondrial dysfunction [key paper]. J Infect Dis 2008;198:1794–803.

64. McKenzie R, Fried MW, Sallie R, et al. Hepatic failure and lactic acidosis due to fialuridine (FIAU), an investigational nucleoside analogue for chronic hepatitis B. N Engl J Med 1995;333:1099–105.

65. Brenchley JM, Price DA, Schacker TW, et al. Microbial translocation is a cause of systemic immune activation in chronic HIV infection [key paper]. Nat Med 2006;12:1365–71.

66. Wiest R, Lawson M, Geuking M. Pathological bacterial translocation in liver cirrhosis. J Hepatol 2014;60:197–209.

67. Falutz J, Rosenthall L, Kotler D, et al. Surrogate markers of visceral adipose tissue in treated HIV-infected patients: accuracy of waist circumference determination. HIV Med 2014;15:98–107.

68. El-Sadr WM, Lundgren J, Neaton JD, et al. CD4+ count-guided interruption of antiretroviral treatment. N Engl J Med 2006;355:2283–96.

69. Triant VA. HIV infection and coronary heart disease: an intersection of epidemics [key paper]. J Infect Dis 2012;205(Suppl 3):S355–61.

70. Subramanian S, Tawakol A, Burdo TH, et al. Arterial inflammation in patients with HIV. J Am Med Assoc 2012;308:379–86.

71. Sabin CA, Worm SW, Weber R, et al. Use of nucleoside reverse transcriptase inhibitors and risk of myocardial infarction in HIV-infected patients enrolled in the D:A:D study: a multi-cohort collaboration. Lancet 2008;371:1417–26.

72. Galli L, Salpietro S, Pellicciotta G, et al. Risk of type 2 diabetes among HIV-infected and healthy subjects in Italy. Eur J Epidemiol 2012;27:657–65.

73. Tien PC, Schneider MF, Cole SR, et al. Antiretroviral therapy exposure and incidence of diabetes mellitus in the Women's Interagency HIV Study. AIDS 2007; 21:1739–45.

74. Teichmann J, Stephan E, Lange U, et al. Osteopenia in HIV-infected women prior to highly active antiretroviral therapy. J Infect 2003;46:221–7.

75. Grund B, Peng G, Gibert CL, et al. Continuous antiretroviral therapy decreases bone mineral density. AIDS 2009;23:1519–29.

76. Bruera D, Luna N, David DO, et al. Decreased bone mineral density in HIV-infected patients is independent of antiretroviral therapy. AIDS 2003;17: 1917–23.

77. Duvivier C, Kolta S, Assoumou L, et al. Greater decrease in bone mineral density with protease inhibitor regimens compared with nonnucleoside reverse transcriptase inhibitor regimens in HIV-1 infected naive patients. AIDS 2009;23: 817–24.

78. Desquilbet L, Margolick JB, Fried LP, et al. Relationship between a frailty-related phenotype and progressive deterioration of the immune system in HIV-infected men. J Acquir Immune Defic Syndr 2009;50:299–306. http://dx.doi.org/10.1097/QAI.0b013e3181945eb0.

79. Aberg JA. Lipid management in patients who have HIV and are receiving HIV therapy. Endocrinol Metab Clin North Am 2009;38:207–22.

80. Driscoll SD, Meininger GE, Lareau MT, et al. Effects of exercise training and metformin on body composition and cardiovascular indices in HIV-infected patients. AIDS 2004;18:465–73.

81. Falutz J, Allas S, Blot K, et al. Metabolic effects of a growth hormone–releasing factor in patients with HIV. N Engl J Med 2007;357:2359–70.

Dyslipidemia and Cardiovascular Risk in Human Immunodeficiency Virus Infection

Theodoros Kelesidis, MD, PhD, Judith S. Currier, MD, MSc*

KEYWORDS

- Dyslipidemia • Cardiovascular risk • Human immunodeficiency virus
- Antiretroviral therapy

KEY POINTS

- Since the advent of effective antiretroviral therapy, cardiovascular disease has become a major cause of morbidity and mortality in the population with human immunodeficiency virus.
- The pathogenesis of atherosclerosis in human immunodeficiency virus–infected individuals is complex, and proatherogenic quantitative and qualitative changes in lipids have a major role in this process.
- HIV replication, chronic inflammation and immune activation, and exposure to antiretroviral drugs (either directly or through metabolic abnormalities) may contribute to development of dyslipidemia in human immunodeficiency virus infection.
- As we gain a better understanding of lipid abnormalities in human immunodeficiency virus–infected patients and their role in immune activation and cardiovascular disease, these findings must translate into interventions for clinical care.

INTRODUCTION

In the setting of highly active antiretroviral therapy (ART), cardiovascular disease (CVD), particularly coronary artery disease, is among the leading causes of mortality among human immunodeficiency virus (HIV)-infected subjects.[1] Several studies suggest that adults and children with HIV have an increased risk of CVD.[2–4] The full details of the pathogenesis of atherogenesis in HIV infection remain to be elucidated. Traditional risk prediction models to estimate cardiovascular risk do not include emerging

Disclosures: J.S. Currier: Received grant funds to UCLA from Merck. T. Kelesidis: None.
Division of Infectious Diseases, Department of Medicine, David Geffen School of Medicine, UCLA, 9911 W. Pico Boulevard, Suite 980, Los Angeles, CA 90035, USA
* Corresponding author. Center for Clinical AIDS Research and Education, David Geffen School of Medicine, UCLA, 9911 W. Pico Boulevard, Suite 980, Los Angeles, CA 90035.
E-mail address: jscurrier@mednet.ucla.edu

Endocrinol Metab Clin N Am 43 (2014) 665–684
http://dx.doi.org/10.1016/j.ecl.2014.06.003
0889-8529/14/$ – see front matter © 2014 Elsevier Inc. All rights reserved.

endo.theclinics.com

cardiovascular risk factors such as inflammation, coagulation disorders, immune activation, kidney disease, and HIV-1 RNA levels.[4–6] Understanding the pathophysiology of increased CVD in HIV infection will help us develop strategies to prevent and treat this leading cause of morbidity and mortality in HIV-infected subjects.

The prevalence of several traditional risk factors for CVD is higher in HIV-infected individuals than among age-matched controls.[2] Lipid changes may promote atherogenesis and may contribute to increased risk of CVD in HIV-infected subjects.[7] The patterns of dyslipidemia change during the course of HIV disease. In untreated disease, elevations in triglycerides and low high-density lipoprotein cholesterol (HDL-c) predominate. Dyslipidemia that occurs during treatment for HIV disease is characterized by a range of values of serum concentrations of total cholesterol (TC); triglycerides, depending on the ART used; very low-density lipoprotein (VLDL); low-density lipoprotein cholesterol (LDL-c); apolipoprotein B (apoB); and low levels of HDL-c.[7] In view of the high prevalence of dyslipidemia and the increased risk for CVD among patients with HIV, which is concerning for public health, this review aims to describe the changes in the lipid profile of HIV-infected patients and how these changes directly or indirectly contribute to the pathogenesis of atherosclerosis in HIV-infected subjects.[8] Although the exact mechanisms are incompletely understood,[9] we describe how host factors, HIV per se and ART, may contribute to lipid changes and how these atherogenic lipids may have a role in the development of atherosclerosis in HIV-infected patients.

FACTORS OTHER THAN DYSLIPIDEMIA MAY CONTRIBUTE TO ACCELERATED ATHEROSCLEROSIS IN HIV INFECTION

Cardiovascular risk factors have a major role in development of CVD disease. HIV-infected subjects have higher prevalence of established CVD risk factors, such as smoking, hypertension, insulin resistance, and dyslipidemia, compared with age-matched individuals.[9] Cocaine use, which is relatively common among some groups of HIV-infected patients, renal function, and albuminuria have also been associated with the risk for coronary artery disease in HIV-infected patients.[9,10] All of these risk factors are synergistic, and it is difficult to analyze the specific role of each. Recently, the Data Collection on Adverse Events of Anti-HIV Drugs (D:A:D) Study Group developed a risk assessment tool tailored to HIV-infected patients.[11]

HIV replication can directly promote atherogenesis. HIV replication increases chronic inflammation as a part of the immune response to the virus. These changes may, in turn, contribute to an increased risk for death.[4] HIV replication is associated with increased biomarkers of inflammation, including C-reactive protein (CRP). Elevated levels of CRP have been found to independently be associated with the risk of risk of myocardial infarction (MI) in adults, including those with HIV.[4] In HIV infection, high CRP levels predict HIV disease progression.[4] Increased concentrations of CRP, interleukin 6, and d-dimer have also been independently associated with CVD events in patients with HIV.[12] Identifying biomarkers of inflammation and cardiovascular disease in HIV-infected subjects on ART with suppressed viremia may help us develop new targets for therapeutic interventions.[13] The HIV virus can also cause increased endothelial injury caused by adhesion molecules and HIV Tat protein and may stimulate proliferation of vascular smooth muscle cells and induce coagulation disorders.[14] Collectively, these HIV-induced effects may directly increase atherogenesis.

Immune activation may promote atherosclerosis in the absence of residual viral replication. Several studies suggest that increased activation of innate immunity is associated with the presence of subclinical atherosclerosis in patients with HIV.[15–18] One potential mechanism that might trigger monocyte activation in HIV infection is microbial translocation across the gastrointestinal tract, which has been found to persist in treated HIV infection.[4,19] Markers of monocyte activation, such as high soluble CD14 and CD163, and bacterial translocation, such as endotoxin and soluble CD14, were independently associated with a faster rate of progression of subclinical atherosclerosis in several independent studies.[15–18] Collectively, these studies suggest that chronic monocyte activation could be an important marker of or target for future interventions to reduce CVD risk in treated patients with HIV. Further work is needed to determine contributing factors to immune activation and CVD and, importantly, whether atherogenic lipids may drive both immune activation and CVD in HIV infection.

DYSLIPIDEMIA AND CVD IN HIV INFECTION
Host Factors in HIV-Infected Subjects May Contribute to Dyslipidemia Development

HIV-infected subjects have increased prevalence of dyslipidemia; however, it is unclear to what extent this is associated with specific host factors. In the D:A:D study, 33.8% and 22.2% of a group of treated HIV-infected individuals had elevated levels of triglyceride and TC, respectively.[20] Longitudinal and cross-sectional studies have assessed the role of single-nucleotide polymorphisms on the incidence of dyslipidemia in HIV patients.[21] The Multicenter AIDS Cohort Study showed that biogeographical ancestry may contribute to development of ART-induced lipid changes.[22] In a study of the metabolome in HIV-infected patients on suppressive ART, the observed patterns of metabolites suggested decreased lipolysis and dysregulation of receptors controlling inflammation and lipid metabolism.[23] Overall, these data suggest that genetic and nongenetic host factors may contribute to the dyslipidemia in HIV-infected subjects.

The HIV Virus May Directly Induce Dyslipidemia

Mechanisms such as altered cytokine profile, decreased lipid clearance, and increased hepatic synthesis of VLDL, may explain how HIV infection, per se, might induce dyslipidemia and accelerate atherosclerosis based on data from in vitro, animal, and clinical studies.[6,9,24,25] The SMART (Strategies for Management of Antiretroviral Therapy) study compared the outcomes of HIV-infected patients who were randomly assigned to receive continuous or intermittent ART. This study confirmed an increased risk of CVD among patients who discontinued ART[6] and allowed comparison of lipid profiles between the treatment-interruption group and the continuous treatment group.[8] These findings suggested that HIV viremia may have a role in accelerated atherogenesis. More recently, data from a large cohort study of 27,000 HIV-infected adults in care suggested that immunodeficiency and ongoing viral replication both independently contributed to the risk of MI, further confirming the putative role of HIV in the pathogenesis of CVD.[26]

HIV viremia is associated with quantitative lipid abnormalities, including elevated serum concentrations of triglycerides and low levels of cholesterol. Several studies found the associations between uncontrolled HIV viremia and dyslipidemia and increased CVD risk. The impact of HIV infection on lipids was studied within the Multicenter AIDS Cohort Study, in which a significant reduction in TC, LDL, and HDL was found in a group of 50 HIV seroconverters comparing pre-HIV with post-HIV infection lipid levels.[27] In other studies, the levels of triglycerides were higher, and the levels of TC, LDL, and HDL were lower in HIV-infected patients receiving no ART when compared with uninfected controls.[28] Elevations in triglyceride levels during untreated HIV infection are thought to be caused by an increase in the levels of inflammatory cytokines (tumor necrosis factor–α, interleukins, interferon–α)[24] and steroid hormones.[28] HDL levels are also found to be low in both untreated and treated HIV-infected patients, regardless of the CD4+ T cell count.[27] The SMART study found that declines in HDL levels after stopping nonnucleoside reverse transcriptase inhibitor (NNRTI) treatment were associated with an increased risk of CVD, suggesting that the HDL-raising effects of this therapy had been cardioprotective.[29] Enkhmaa and colleagues[30] found that allele-specific apolipoprotein A (apoA) levels, which determine the amount of atherogenic small apoA related to a defined apoA allele size, were higher in individuals with low HIV viremia and high CD4 cell counts, indicating that HIV replication reduced allele-specific apoA levels. Therefore, HIV-infected individuals with immune reconstitution may have higher allele-specific apoA levels, which are related to progression of atherosclerosis.[30] Overall, these data suggest mechanisms that explain how the HIV virus, per se, may induce dyslipidemia.

HIV may induce qualitative changes in lipids such as HDL through effects on metabolism and function that lead to increased atherogenesis. HDL is generally accepted to have anti-inflammatory/antioxidant effects.[31] HIV may directly affect HDL metabolism by up-regulating the cholesteryl ester transfer protein activity, which enhances transfer of cholesterol to apoB lipoproteins that promote atherogenesis.[32] These effects on HDL metabolism in combination with HIV-related hypertriglyceridemia,[25] lead to an increased delivery of cholesterol to the arterial wall, where it is then taken up by macrophages, and atherogenic foam cells are formed. The capacity of HDL to increase cholesterol efflux from macrophages is an important function of HDL and may predict development of atherosclerosis.[33] The HIV Nef protein (which is abundant during untreated HIV) inhibits transporters important to cholesterol efflux in macrophages, and this may initiate atherogenesis in the arterial wall.[34] Intracellular cholesterol in monocytes in HIV-infected subjects is inversely associated with HDL-c levels; in contrast, in HIV-negative controls, cholesterol content in macrophages is correlated with LDL-c levels rather than with HDL-c.[35] In the SMART study, HDL-c, lipoprotein particle concentrations, and the apolipoproteins were better indices of CVD risk than LDL-c levels.[29] Consistent with these data, reduction in large lipoprotein particle concentrations after treatment with ART may indicate increased efflux of cholesterol from macrophages into smaller HDL particles.[8] Thus, HIV induces effects on HDL function and cholesterol transport that may contribute to increased rates of CVD in HIV- infected patients.

HIV replication may also modify HDL indirectly through increases in systemic inflammation. The inflammatory response observed during HIV infection may reduce HDL levels and compromise cholesterol efflux from macrophages.[31] Infections may induce nonspecific systemic inflammation that may at least partially modify HDL.[36] In the SMART trial, levels of biomarkers of inflammation were associated with changes in HDL levels independently of HIV RNA levels.[5,8] Finally, cytokines such as tumor necrosis factor-α and interleukin-6 appear to promote lipid peroxidation, and the production of reactive oxygen species,[37] and this may further contribute to formation of oxidized, modified lipoproteins such as oxidized HDL. However, it is unclear whether HIV-infected subjects have increased levels of oxidized LDL, a marker of oxidative stress associated with lipoproteins and an emerging CVD risk factor,[38] compared with uninfected subjects. The role of modified lipoproteins in CVD in HIV-infected subjects remains incompletely understood.

ART and Dyslipidemia

The introduction of ART led to substantial improvement in the prognosis of HIV patients,[39] but several of the drugs in the first generation of effective combination ART were associated with changes in lipid metabolism, abnormalities in fat (both lipohypertrophy and subcutaneous fat loss), insulin resistance, dyslipidemia, osteopenia, and lactic acidosis.[39] ART-associated dyslipidemia usually occurs within 3 months of starting treatment[9] and was first described in patients who used first-generation protease inhibitors (PIs) but was also observed in patients who received regimens consisting of nucleoside reverse-transcriptase inhibitors (NRTI) and NNRTIs. Studies with HIV-infected children and adolescents and HIV-infected older adults receiving effective ART found high rates of fat changes and dyslipidemia, therefore, high risk for cardiovascular diseases in all age groups of HIV-infected subjects.[9,39] A component of the initial changes in lipids has been ascribed to a return to health among patients with a chronic untreated illness who are undergoing effective treatment.[27]

Several studies investigated the potential effects of ART on risk of CVD and dyslipidemia. The specific effects of ART on dyslipidemia vary both within and across drug classes. Several randomized clinical trials have characterized changes in lipids after the initiation of ART. The AIDS Clinical Trials Group (ACTG) 5142 trial found important differences in metabolic outcomes in treatment-naive patients after the initiation of an NNRTI-sparing regimen (the boosted PI, lopinavir/ritonavir plus 2 NRTIs), PI-sparing regimen (NNRTI efavirenz [EFV] plus 2 NRTIs), or an NRTI-sparing regimen (lopinavir/ritonavir plus EFV).[40] Although the NRTI-sparing regimen (a combination that included lopinavir/ritonavir and EFV) had the lowest risk of lipoatrophy, it also had the greatest likelihood of lipid elevations and subsequent use of lipid-lowering agents. The SMART study helped put these changes into perspective by showing that interrupting therapy through a structured treatment interruption was associated with worse outcomes than remaining on treatment.[6] The D:A:D study, one of the most comprehensive surveys of CVD adverse events associated with ART, found a strong association between dyslipidemia and ART.[11,20] These studies highlighted common (owing to viral suppression) and differential (owing to ART) lipid effects on starting ART in ART-naive HIV-infected patients.

HIV-infected patients on ART have low levels HDL and modified lipoproteins compared with normolipemic subjects. HIV patients with dyslipidemia on ART have impaired plasma lipolytic activity that may lead to low HDL-c plasma concentration and triglyceride-rich LDL and HDL, which become less stable than HDL particles in normolipemic patients.[34] In addition, systemic inflammation may contribute to modification of HDL to a dysfunctional form that may increase the risk of CVD.[41] We previously found that HIV-infected subjects with suppressed viremia on ART have dysfunctional HDL.[42,43] In small study of HIV patients with low CVD risk profile, HDL function changed over time and was independently associated with obesity but not with subclinical atherosclerosis.[44] In another study, HIV-infected subjects had dysfunctional HDL compared with matched uninfected subjects with comparable HDL levels, and this modified HDL was associated with macrophage activation and with presence of noncalcified coronary plaque.[45] The role of HDL function in CVD in HIV-infected subjects with suppressed viremia remains to be determined.

Dyslipidemic effects of PIs

Patients, including children and pregnant women, with prolonged use of PIs often have hypertriglyceridemia, low levels of HDL-c and high levels of LDL-c, and apolipoproteins E and CIII; however, the effects vary by drugs within this class.[9,39] **Fig. 1** summarizes the mechanisms through which PIs may cause dyslipidemia.[46] **Table 1** summarizes the lipid effects of different drugs within the PI class.[20,47–51] Newer agents

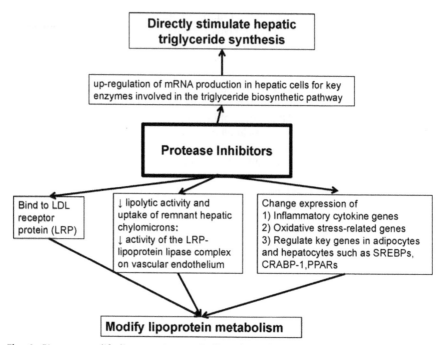

Fig. 1. PIs may modify lipoprotein metabolism through multiple mechanisms. PIs directly stimulate the biosynthesis of triglycerides in hepatic cells and may also directly modify the metabolism of lipoproteins by binding to cellular receptors, reducing lipolysis and by regulating expression of key genes involved in the regulation of metabolic pathways in adipocytes and hepatocytes. CRABP-1, cellular retinoic acid-binding protein 1; LRP, low-density lipoprotein receptor protein; PPARs, peroxisome proliferator-activated receptors; SREBPs, sterol regulatory element-binding proteins.

have less significant effects on lipids than the first drugs to be available within this class.[9,39,46] In the Data Collection on Adverse Events of Anti-HIV Drugs studies, within the PI class only cumulative exposure to lopinavir/ritonavir and indinavir were associated with increased risk of CVD, independently of lipid concentrations.[52] Overall, ritonavir-boosted atazanavir and darunavir have more favorable lipid effects and tolerability compared with other PIs (see **Table 1**). In view of the differences in metabolic effects of drugs within the PI class, future epidemiologic studies examining CVD risk in HIV need to consider the effects of individual PIs.

Dyslipidemic effects of NRTIs

Antiretroviral treatment regimens containing NRTIs have also been associated with metabolic alterations, particularly changes in serum triglyceride concentrations (**Table 2**).[9,39,52–61] Replacement of NRTIs such as stavudine with tenofovir is a strategy to reduce the cardiovascular risk and improve the lipid profile of patients with dyslipidemia.[9,39] Currently, the association between abacavir and excess CVD risk remains controversial. Several studies have found a consistent association[52,57]; however, others have not,[55,56] and the mechanism underlying this association remains unclear.[58] Switching from multidrug class-suppressive regimens to triple therapy containing 2 NRTIs showed increases in plasma lipids.[62] Overall, within the NRTI class, tenofovir and lamivudine/emtricitabine seem to be the drugs that are not associated with dyslipidemia.

Table 1
Main studies investigating the effects of PIs on lipids

PIs	Main Findings
Lopinavir/ritonavir and indinavir	D:A:D study: increased risk of MI with longer duration of treatment compared with other treatments.[20]
Lopinavir/ritonavir and ritonavir-boosted fosamprenavir	The French Hospital Database: increased risk of MI with longer duration of treatment compared with other treatments.
PI-treated patients switched to atazanavir-containing regimens	Several randomized trials: improvement of lipid parameters, while the immunologic and virologic efficacy of the regimen was maintained.[47]
Ritonavir-boosted atazanavir and darunavir	Different studies: pls recommended for the initial treatment of HIV infection because each has shown better lipid effects and overall tolerance than ritonavir-boosted lopinavir.[50,51]
Darunavir/ritonavir or atazanavir/ritonavir plus tenofovir-emtricitabine	Pilot study, Aberg and colleagues[48]: similar 48-wk lipid changes between darunavir and atazanavir.
Darunavir/ritonavir or atazanavir/ritonavir compared with raltegravir	Ofotokun and colleagues[49]: 96-wk trial found no difference in lipid profiles with atazanavir/ritonavir and darunavir/ritonavir. Raltegravir had more favorable lipid profile than both PIs.

Dyslipidemic effects of NNRTIs

In patients who have initiated NNRTIs as first-line therapy, increases in the serum concentrations of TC, HDL, LDL, and triglycerides have been observed (**Table 3**).[11,63–70] Many studies have reported that NNRTI may induce greater increases in HDL levels compared with PIs, hence, balancing out the overall lipid risk profile.[70] Patients treated with efavirenz had increases of TC (at least 3% mean relative increase in levels) and triglyceride (at least 10% mean relative increase in levels) concentrations.[63] Switching from a PI to efavirenz may improve the lipid profile, depending on the specific PI used.[71] With regard to other agents, the newer NNRTIs, rilpivirine and etravirine, have more favorable lipid profiles than efavirenz.[72]

Dyslipidemic effects of integrase inhibitors and C-C chemokine receptor type 5 antagonists

The integrase inhibitors, raltegravir, elvitegravir, and dolutegravir, and the C-C chemokine receptor type 5 (CCR5) receptor antagonist, maraviroc, appear to have little or no impact on lipid parameters, even in long-term use.[73,74] Switching to these agents in patients who are well suppressed on first-line therapy may benefit many HIV-infected patients by improving their lipid profiles (**Table 4**).[74–85] Preliminary studies support the beneficial lipid profile of unboosted integrase inhibitors.[79] Recent data suggest that elvitegravir-cobicistat-tenofovir-emtricitabine induced similar changes in lipids compared with atazanavir/ritonavir and had less prominent effects on total and LDL cholesterol compared with efavirenz.[83,84] Data from 2 independent studies confirms that the boosted PIs, atazanavir and darunavir, are associated with greater increases in TC and triglycerides compared with raltegravir.[48,49]

Table 2
Studies investigating the effects of different NRTIs on lipids

NRTIs	Comments
Stavudine	Stavudine is still used in some developing countries and at full doses induces significant metabolic abnormalities compared with other ART such as tenofovir.[53]
	No association between stavudine use and risk of MI was found in the D:A:D study.[57]
Tenofovir	Regimens containing tenofovir are associated with lower serum concentrations of LDL-c, TC, and triglycerides compared with regimens using other NRTIs, suggesting a lipid-lowering action of tenofovir, which differs from that of other NRTIs.[54]
	No association between tenofovir use and risk of MI was found in the D:A:D study.[52]
	Several studies[100] found maintained virologic suppression and improved cholesterol concentrations in patients with increased lipid concentrations on ritonavir-boosted, PI-based regimens that included abacavir who were switched to tenofovir.
Abacavir and didanosine	The use of the NRTIs abacavir and didanosine was found to be an independent risk factor for myocardial infarction in the D:A:D study.[52,57]
	Several analyses with conflicting results have been performed in an attempt to better understand the association between abacavir and, to a lesser extent, didanosine and CVD events.[55,56]
	In a meta-analysis based on 52 clinical trials and a total 14,174 HIV-infected adults who received abacavir (n = 9502) or not (n = 4672), baseline demographics and HIV disease characteristics, including lipids values, MI rates were similar.[58]
	Further data are needed to evaluate any association between abacavir and increased risk of MI.
Tenofovir-emtricitabine vs abacavir-lamivudine	In the ACTG 5202 study, changes in lipid concentrations were generally greater with abacavir-lamivudine than tenofovir-emtricitabine (when combined with either efavirenz or atazanavir/ritonavir); however, researchers found no differences in the TC:HDL-c ratios.[59]
	In a study examining lipid subfractions, a more atherogenic LDL profile was noted in patients switched to abacavir-lamivudine compared with tenofovir-emtricitabine, including a decrease in LDL level in the abacavir group.[60]
	Of note, in the SPIRAL study,[61] no significant differences in lipid concentrations were identified between the tenofovir and abacavir recipients who switched from a ritonavir-boosted PI to raltegravir, suggesting that the combination of a ritonavir-boosted PI and abacavir might have distinct lipid effects.

LIPID CHANGES DURING TREATED HIV DISEASE MAY CONTRIBUTE TO IMMUNE ACTIVATION IN HIV INFECTION

A hallmark of HIV infection is activation of the immune system, which persists to some degree even after the initiation of effective ART.[19] Although the exact mechanisms that drive this immune activation are unclear, residual HIV replication, microbial translocation, and inflammatory lipids are potential contributors. Modified lipoproteins such as oxidized LDL carry oxidized lipids and may regulate immunity.[86] We recently showed that HIV-infected subjects have dysfunctional HDL that is associated with biomarkers of T-cell activation.[87] We also showed that among HIV-infected subjects but not controls that dysfunctional HDL was significantly associated with circulating levels of the macrophage activation marker, soluble CD163.[45] The temporal relationship between these observations remains unclear. Among HIV-infected patients, studies suggest that after the initiation of ART, salutary changes to HDL structure occur, possibly caused by improvements in immune activation.[8] Data suggesting that oxidized forms of LDL are present in atherosclerotic lesions and constitute major epitopes for natural antibodies show that these lipids may be a stimulus for monocytes from HIV-infected subjects.[38,88,89] Modified lipoproteins may also directly activate immune cells such as macrophages and T cells.[90] Further studies are needed to elucidate the interplay between immune activation, ART, HDL structure/function of modified lipoproteins, and CVD risk in HIV.

MANAGEMENT OF LIPID DISORDERS
Diagnosis of Lipid Disorders in the Context of CVD

Current HIV treatment recommendations emphasize the importance of CVD risk screening in all patients starting ART and throughout the course of treatment.[91,92] Fasting lipid levels should be obtained at initiation of care for HIV-infected subjects and before and within 1 to 3 months after starting ART.[91] In addition, screening for other metabolic abnormalities should also be performed. For example, fasting blood glucose or hemoglobin A1c should be obtained before and within 1 to 3 months after starting ART.[91,92] When triglycerides are greater than 500 mg/dL, the measurements of non–HDL-c, apoB, or both may be useful because measurement of LDL-c may underestimate the CVD risk.[9,41] However, although fasting lipid levels determine well-established quantitative lipid abnormalities, there are no established diagnostic methods to determine qualitative abnormalities of lipids and lipoproteins.

Treatment of Dyslipidemia in HIV Infection

Management of dyslipidemia in patients with HIV follows recommendations for the general population according to the National Cholesterol Education Program Guidelines **(Table 5)**.[9,39,91–94]

Lifestyle changes are the initial step in management of dyslipidemia and CVD risk in HIV-infected subjects. Lifestyle modifications including diet, exercise, and smoking cessation should be the first step in management, whereas lipid-lowering therapy and ART changes should be considered for patients at high risk of CVD.[91] Diet and exercise improved lipid profile in patients on ART with hypertriglyceridemia[95]; however, a recent meta-analysis of dietary intervention studies in patients with HIV reported only slight effects on triglyceride concentrations.[96]

Lipid-lowering therapy should be prescribed with caution in HIV-infected patients. There are significant drug interactions between lipid-lowering agents and PIs most notably among the statin drugs simvastatin and lovastatin.[9] HIV guidelines recommend the use of statins that have fewer interactions with ART, such as pravastatin and atorvastatin,[91] whereas use of newer statins such as pitavastatin may further reduce these interactions.[91] Treating hypertriglyceridemia may be challenging in HIV-infected patients. In a recent study, fibrates were more effective than fish oil or atorvastatin at lowering plasma triglycerides in HIV-infected patients with hypertriglyceridemia,[93] suggesting that fibrates should be the first choice.

Switch strategies that deploy newer antiretrovirals with more favorable lipid profile (integrase inhibitors, second-generation NNRTIs, and newer PIs) are increasingly used as an intervention for ART-related dyslipidemia. Improvements in lipids have been seen when patients with dyslipidemia on ritonavir-boosted PIs were switched from abacavir to tenofovir[97] or when the PI was switched to another agent.[98] The

Table 3	
Studies investigating the effects of different NNRTIs on lipids	
NNRTIs	**Comments**
Efavirenz	Patients treated with efavirenz presented a significant increase of TC and triglyceride concentrations[63] compared with baseline.
	In the ACTG study 5202[64] participants randomly assigned to efavirenz had statistically significantly greater increases in TC and LDL-c concentrations but not in TC:HDL-c ratios compared with participants receiving atazanavir/ritonavir (each in combination with abacavir-lamivudine or tenofovir-emtricitabine).
	A recent meta-analysis compared the effects of the NNRTI, efavirenz, and various ritonavir-boosted PIs (including darunavir/ritonavir) on lipid levels using data from 15 clinical trials of first-line antiretroviral therapy in which standardized 48-wk lipids data were reported (n = 6368).[65] In this study, efavirenz and the more recently introduced PIs, such as DRV and atazanavir, had only a modest impact on serum lipids and their pattern of effect differed.
	In a substudy of a trial in 91 antiretroviral-naïve patients randomly assigned to tenofovir + emtricitabine + atazanavir/ritonavir or EFV (patients assigned to EFV had greater increases in TC, LDL-c, and HDL-c and in large HDL particles, but not in TC:HDL-c ratio or indication for lipid-lowering interventions relative to patients assigned to atazanavir and ritonavir.[66]
Nevirapine	ART regimens containing nevirapine are associated with a favorable lipid profile, mainly because they provide higher serum concentrations of HDL-c.[63]
Etravirine	Switching from efavirenz or ritonavir-boosted PIs to etravirine led to a significant improvement of lipids irrespective of the presence of previous hyperlipidemia and type of ART.[67]
Rilpivirine	Two phase 3 trials (ECHO[68] and THRIVE[69]) of similar design, with the exception of the background NRTI regimen, compared rilpivirine with efavirenz in ART-naive patients with HIV. After 48 wk, TC, HDL-c, LDL-c and triglyceride concentrations were significantly greater in the patients randomly assigned to efavirenz than those receiving rilpivirine; however, the TC:HDL-c ratio did not change significantly between the treatment groups because of a greater HDL increase in the patients given efavirenz.

SWITCHMRK study[98] found that switch from a lopinavir/ritonavir-based regimen to a raltegravir-based regimen had favorable effects on the lipid profile in patients. However, clinicians should consider prior treatment history before switching antiretrovirals, as higher rates of virologic failure have been noted among those with prior failure who were switched from a boosted PI to a raltegravir based regimen.

Strategies to increase HDL cholesterol levels and HDL function in HIV-infected individuals should be investigated. Although there are available therapies for elevated LDL-c levels, therapeutic strategies to increase HDL levels are limited and of unclear clinical significance.[99] In general, treatment with NNRTI-based regimens appears to increase HDL levels more so than therapy with other classes of drugs. The clinical significance of this effect is unclear. Thus, therapies that may also improve HDL function in HIV infection need further study as a CVD prevention strategy.

SUMMARY

As the HIV population ages, it is important to prevent development of long-term comorbidities such as CVD. The mechanisms of atherosclerosis in HIV remain to be fully elucidated. Host, virus, immune deficiency, and ART factors have a major role in the increased risk for CVD in HIV and lipid changes may both be a consequence and a driver of these interactions (**Fig. 2**). During untreated HIV infection, lipid

Table 4
Studies investigating the effects of different NNRTIs on lipids

New Antivirals	Comments
Maraviroc	In a mouse model of genetic dyslipidemia, maraviroc reduced atherosclerotic progression by interfering with inflammatory cell recruitment into plaques and by reversing the proinflammatory profile.[75]
	Switching from PIs or NNRTIs to maraviroc, decreased TC and triglycerides in a small, randomized, clinical trial.[76]
	MacInnes and colleagues[74] investigated treatment-naive patients randomly assigned to receive either maraviroc or efavirenz in combination with zidovudine-lamivudine for up to 96 wk. The investigators reported that of the patients with baseline TC and LDL-c less than the National Cholesterol Education Programme treatment thresholds, more patients receiving efavirenz than those treated with maraviroc exceeded the thresholds for TC and LDL-c. Additionally, among participants with baseline lipid concentrations exceeding National Cholesterol Education Programme thresholds, 84% of patients on efavirenz vs 50% of those on maraviroc still exceeded the thresholds at 96 wk.
Raltegravir	In the STARTMRK trial, Rockstroh and colleagues[77] compared raltegravir with efavirenz in treatment-naive adults, and identified that 240-wk increases in fasting triglycerides and TC, LDL-c, and HDL-c were significantly greater in those receiving efavirenz than raltegravir. Additionally, 9% of adults given raltegravir vs 34% given efavirenz needed initiation of lipid-lowering treatment during follow-up.
	Switching from different class-suppressive regimens to raltegravir and tenofovir and emtricitabine or abacavir and lamivudine led to improvements in plasma lipids after 48 wk.[78]
	In virologically suppressed aging HIV-positive patients, there are promising results from small, short-term studies assessing dual therapy with raltegravir and a nonnucleoside reverse inhibitor such as etravirine or nevirapine.[79,80]
Dolutegravir	Dolutegravir is a once-daily integrase inhibitor that does not need a boosting drug. In the SPRING-2 trial,[81] a 96-wk, phase 3, randomized, double-blind, noninferiority study comparing dolutegravir with raltegravir in treatment-naive patients, no significant changes in lipid measures were shown in either treatment group.
Elvitegravir-cobicistat-emtricitabine-tenofovir DF	The fixed-dose combination of elvitegravir-cobicistat-emtricitabine-tenofovir DF, has been compared with efavirenz-tenofovir-emtricitabine and ritonavir plus atazanavir plus emtricitabine-tenofovir DF in treatment-naive adults, and statistically similar overall changes in lipid profiles among the 3 regimens were found.[82]
	Rockstroh and colleagues[83] compared elvitegravir-cobicistat with atazanavir/ritonavir in treatment-naive patients and reported that after 96 wk, changes in TC were greater with elvitegravir-cobicistat, but triglyceride increases were greater with atazanavir/ritonavir, and no difference in the TC:HDL-c ratio was noted between the 2 treatment groups.
	Sax and colleagues[84] compared treatment of efavirenz-tenofovir DF-emtricitabine with elvitegravir-cobicistat-emtricitabine and showed that mean changes in TC, HDL-c, and LDL-c were greater in the efavirenz than elvitegravir-cobicistat group, whereas the TC:HDL-c ratio was the same in both groups. In another study, Elion and colleagues[85] randomly assigned treated patients to either elvitegravir or raltegravir combination with a ritonavir-boosted PI and a third active drug. No differences in lipid concentrations were reported between the 2 treatment groups.
	Collectively, these results suggest that elvitegravir-cobicistat-tenofovir DF-emtricitabine has a similar lipid profile to ritonavir-atazanavir, and has less severe TC and LDL-c perturbations (but also less HDL improvement) than does efavirenz.

Table 5
Treatment of dyslipidemia in the context of CVD in HIV infection

Therapeutic Intervention	Comments
Lifestyle modifications	Diet, exercise, and smoking cessation.
Lipid-lowering therapy	
Statins that have minimal interactions with ART	PIs and ritonavir mainly inhibit cytochrome P and could increase the toxicity of some statins. NNRTIs (eg, efavirenz) are inducers of cytochrome P and could reduce statin efficacy. In the HIV-infected patient taking a PI, statins with a low risk for interaction with PIs should be preferred, such as pravastatin, fluvastatin, low-dose atorvastatin, or low-dose rosuvastatin.[9,91,92]
Fibrates	Fibrates should be prescribed when the triglyceride concentration is >500 mg/d.[9]
Fish oil	Limited evidence on the role of omega-3 fatty acids on the management and prevention of the metabolic abnormalities in HIV-infected patients but randomized, controlled clinical trials have not shown a clear benefit.[93]
Switch strategies	
Switch PI to an NNRTI or to a new drug such as integrase or CCR5 inhibitors	See evidence presented in **Tables 1–4**.
Switch first-generation NRTIs (eg, stavudine) to second-generation NRTIs (eg, tenofovir)	See evidence presented in **Table 2**.
Switch first-generation NNRTIs (eg, efavirenz) to new NNRTI (eg, etravirine, rilpivirine)	See evidence presented in **Table 3**.
Switch first-generation NNRTIs (eg, efavirenz) to a new drug such as integrase inhibitors (eg, raltegravir)	See evidence presented in **Tables 2** and **4**.
Manage other comorbidities that may contribute to CVD	Regarding hypertension, blockers of the rennin-angiotensin system should be the first therapy because of their protective effects on the vasculature, kidney function, and favorable metabolic effects.[9] Telmisartan is being evaluated for favorable effects on visceral adiposity in HIV-infected subjects.[39] Antiplatelet drugs such as aspirin, clopidogrel, prasugrel, and ticagrelor should be given according to the guidelines for the general population.[9] Diabetes and insulin resistance should be managed according to the guidelines for the general population and HIV-infected subjects.[91,92]

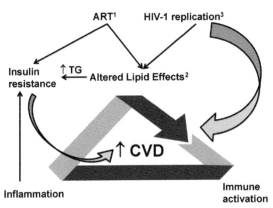

Fig. 2. Factoring influencing dyslipidemia and CVD risk in HIV. ART directly alters lipid metabolism and may increase the risk of insulin resistance (1). The lipid effects of ART include elevated triglycerides and for some agents elevations in TC. The elevations in triglycerides may also contribute to insulin resistance and to CVD risk (2). HIV replication per se increases immune activation and may have a direct effect on CVD risk (3). In addition HIV replication may indirectly alter HDL function via indirect effects on inflammation. These altered lipids may have direct and indirect immunoregulatory effects and induce further activation of immune cells (T cells and monocytes/macrophages), which may further increase systemic inflammation. Inflammation also contributes to insulin resistance, which, in turn, may increase CVD risk. Thus, there are complex interactions between these pathophysiologic processes that are at least partially driven by altered lipids that are formed during HIV infection and that may directly or indirectly contribute to increased CVD in HIV-infected subjects. TG, triglycerides.

alterations are associated with the virus and its effects on the immune system. These are characterized by a decrease of TC, LDL-c, and HDL-c and by an increase of triglyceride levels. In contrast, ART regimens promoted distinct alterations in the lipid metabolism of these patients and vary by individual agents. Thus, it is critical to address traditional risk factors for CVD, such as dyslipidemia, in the HIV-infected population. Clinicians need to focus on improved methods for screening and treatment of lipid disorders while taking into consideration potential drug-drug interactions, particularly with statins and ART. Newer HIV drugs, such as etravirine, rilpivirine, raltegravir, dolutegravir, and elvitegravir, are metabolically well-tolerated drug options and may be particularly useful for aging HIV-infected patients. As our understanding of genetic predisposition to dyslipidemia in HIV-infected patients improves, these findings should translate from research to clinical care. Further research is needed to fully elucidate the pathophysiology of dyslipidemia in HIV-infected patients, with particular emphasis on defining the roles of lipids in inflammation, immune activation, and CVD.

REFERENCES

1. Sackoff JE, Hanna DB, Pfeiffer MR, et al. Causes of death among persons with AIDS in the era of highly active antiretroviral therapy: New York City. Ann Intern Med 2006;145(6):397–406.
2. Currier JS, Lundgren JD, Carr A, et al. Epidemiological evidence for cardiovascular disease in HIV-infected patients and relationship to highly active antiretroviral therapy. Circulation 2008;118(2):e29–35.
3. Triant VA, Lee H, Hadigan C, et al. Increased acute myocardial infarction rates and cardiovascular risk factors among patients with human immunodeficiency virus disease. J Clin Endocrinol Metab 2007;92(7):2506–12.

4. Triant VA, Meigs JB, Grinspoon SK. Association of C-reactive protein and HIV infection with acute myocardial infarction. J Acquir Immune Defic Syndr 2009; 51(3):268–73.
5. Baker JV, Neuhaus J, Duprez D, et al. Changes in inflammatory and coagulation biomarkers: a randomized comparison of immediate versus deferred antiretroviral therapy in patients with HIV infection. J Acquir Immune Defic Syndr 2011;56(1):36–43.
6. El-Sadr WM, Lundgren J, Neaton JD, et al. CD4+ count-guided interruption of antiretroviral treatment. N Engl J Med 2006;355(22):2283–96.
7. Grunfeld C, Delaney JA, Wanke C, et al. Preclinical atherosclerosis due to HIV infection: carotid intima-medial thickness measurements from the FRAM study. AIDS 2009;23(14):1841–9.
8. Baker JV, Neuhaus J, Duprez D, et al. Inflammation predicts changes in high-density lipoprotein particles and apolipoprotein A1 following initiation of antiretroviral therapy. AIDS 2011;25(17):2133–42.
9. Boccara F, Lang S, Meuleman C, et al. HIV and coronary heart disease: time for a better understanding. J Am Coll Cardiol 2013;61(5):511–23.
10. Choi AI, Li Y, Deeks SG, et al. Association between kidney function and albuminuria with cardiovascular events in HIV-infected persons. Circulation 2010;121(5): 651–8.
11. Friis-Moller N, Thiebaut R, Reiss P, et al. Predicting the risk of cardiovascular disease in HIV-infected patients: the data collection on adverse effects of anti-HIV drugs study. Eur J Cardiovasc Prev Rehabil 2010;17(5):491–501.
12. Duprez DA, Neuhaus J, Kuller LH, et al. Inflammation, coagulation and cardiovascular disease in HIV-infected individuals. PLoS One 2012;7(9):e44454 [Important reference for key points].
13. Kaplan RC, Landay AL, Hodis HN, et al. Potential cardiovascular disease risk markers among HIV-infected women initiating antiretroviral treatment. J Acquir Immune Defic Syndr 2012;60(4):359–68.
14. Gresele P, Falcinelli E, Sebastiano M, et al. Endothelial and platelet function alterations in HIV-infected patients. Thromb Res 2012;9(3):301–8.
15. Kelesidis T, Kendall MA, Yang OO, et al. Biomarkers of microbial translocation and macrophage activation: association with progression of subclinical atherosclerosis in HIV-1 infection. J Infect Dis 2012;206(10):1558–67.
16. Burdo TH, Lo J, Abbara S, et al. Soluble CD163, a novel marker of activated macrophages, is elevated and associated with noncalcified coronary plaque in HIV-infected patients. J Infect Dis 2011;204(8):1227–36.
17. Subramanian S, Tawakol A, Burdo TH, et al. Arterial inflammation in patients with HIV. JAMA 2012;308(4):379–86.
18. Blodget E, Shen C, Aldrovandi G, et al. Relationship between microbial translocation and endothelial function in HIV infected patients. PLoS One 2012;7(8): e42624.
19. Brenchley JM, Price DA, Schacker TW, et al. Microbial translocation is a cause of systemic immune activation in chronic HIV infection. Nat Med 2006;12(12): 1365–71.
20. Friis-Moller N, Weber R, Reiss P, et al. Cardiovascular disease risk factors in HIV patients–association with antiretroviral therapy. Results from the DAD study. AIDS 2003;17(8):1179–93.
21. Egana-Gorrono L, Martinez E, Cormand B, et al. Impact of genetic factors on dyslipidemia in HIV-infected patients starting antiretroviral therapy. AIDS 2013; 27(4):529–38.

22. Nicholaou MJ, Martinson JJ, Abraham AG, et al. HAART-associated dyslipidemia varies by biogeographical ancestry in the multicenter AIDS cohort study. AIDS Res Hum Retroviruses 2013;29(6):871–9 [Important reference for key points].

23. Cassol E, Misra V, Holman A, et al. Plasma metabolomics identifies lipid abnormalities linked to markers of inflammation, microbial translocation, and hepatic function in HIV patients receiving protease inhibitors. BMC Infect Dis 2013;13:203.

24. Grunfeld C, Feingold KR. The role of the cytokines, interferon alpha and tumor necrosis factor in the hypertriglyceridemia and wasting of AIDs. J Nutr 1992; 122(3 Suppl):749–53.

25. Grunfeld C, Pang M, Doerrler W, et al. Lipids, lipoproteins, triglyceride clearance, and cytokines in human immunodeficiency virus infection and the acquired immunodeficiency syndrome. J Clin Endocrinol Metab 1992;74(5): 1045–52 [Important reference for key points].

26. Drozd DR, Nance RM, Delaney JA. et al. Lower CD4 Count and Higher Viral Load Are Associated With Increased Risk of Myocardial Infarction. Centers for AIDS Research Network of Integrated Clinical Systems (CNICS) Cohort. 21st Conference on Retroviruses and Opportunistic Infections. Boston (MA), March 3–6, 2014. [abstract: 739].

27. Riddler SA, Smit E, Cole SR, et al. Impact of HIV infection and HAART on serum lipids in men. JAMA 2003;289(22):2978–82 [Important reference for key points].

28. Grunfeld C, Kotler DP, Hamadeh R, et al. Hypertriglyceridemia in the acquired immunodeficiency syndrome. Am J Med 1989;86(1):27–31.

29. Duprez DA, Kuller LH, Tracy R, et al. Lipoprotein particle subclasses, cardiovascular disease and HIV infection. Atherosclerosis 2009;207(2):524–9.

30. Enkhmaa B, Anuurad E, Zhang W, et al. HIV disease activity as a modulator of lipoprotein(a) and allele-specific apolipoprotein(a) levels. Arterioscler Thromb Vasc Biol 2013;33(2):387–92.

31. Khovidhunkit W, Memon RA, Feingold KR, et al. Infection and inflammation-induced proatherogenic changes of lipoproteins. J Infect Dis 2000;181(Suppl 3): S462–72.

32. Rose H, Hoy J, Woolley I, et al. HIV infection and high density lipoprotein metabolism. Atherosclerosis 2008;199(1):79–86.

33. Khera AV, Cuchel M, Llera-Moya M, et al. Cholesterol efflux capacity, high-density lipoprotein function, and atherosclerosis. N Engl J Med 2011;364(2): 127–35.

34. Mujawar Z, Rose H, Morrow MP, et al. Human immunodeficiency virus impairs reverse cholesterol transport from macrophages. PLoS Biol 2006;4(11):e365 [Important reference for key points].

35. Feeney ER, McAuley N, O'Halloran JA, et al. The expression of cholesterol metabolism genes in monocytes from HIV-infected subjects suggests intracellular cholesterol accumulation. J Infect Dis 2013;207(4):628–37.

36. Van Lenten BJ, Hama SY, de Beer FC, et al. Anti-inflammatory HDL becomes pro-inflammatory during the acute phase response. Loss of protective effect of HDL against LDL oxidation in aortic wall cell cocultures. J Clin Invest 1995; 96(6):2758–67.

37. Grinspoon S, Carr A. Cardiovascular risk and body-fat abnormalities in HIV-infected adults. N Engl J Med 2005;352(1):48–62.

38. Holvoet P, Lee DH, Steffes M, et al. Association between circulating oxidized low-density lipoprotein and incidence of the metabolic syndrome. JAMA 2008; 299(19):2287–93.

39. Lake JE, Currier JS. Metabolic disease in HIV infection. Lancet Infect Dis 2013; 13(11):964–75.
40. Haubrich RH, Riddler SA, DiRienzo AG, et al. Metabolic outcomes in a randomized trial of nucleoside, nonnucleoside and protease inhibitor-sparing regimens for initial HIV treatment. AIDS 2009;23(9):1109–18 [Important reference for key points].
41. Navab M, Reddy ST, Van Lenten BJ, et al. HDL and cardiovascular disease: atherogenic and atheroprotective mechanisms. Nat Rev Cardiol 2011;8(4): 222–32.
42. Kelesidis T, Currier JS, Huynh D, et al. A biochemical fluorometric method for assessing the oxidative properties of HDL. J Lipid Res 2011;52(12):2341–51.
43. Kelesidis T, Yang OO, Currier JS, et al. HIV-1 infected patients with suppressed plasma viremia on treatment have pro-inflammatory HDL. Lipids Health Dis 2011;10:35.
44. Kelesidis T, Yang OO, Kendall MA, et al. Dysfunctional HDL and progression of atherosclerosis in HIV-1-infected and -uninfected adults. Lipids Health Dis 2013; 12:23.
45. Zanni MV, Kelesidis T, Fitzgerald ML, et al. HDL redox activity is increased in HIV-infected men in association with macrophage activation and noncalcified coronary atherosclerotic plaque. Antivir Ther, in press.
46. Carr A, Samaras K, Chisholm DJ, et al. Pathogenesis of HIV-1-protease inhibitor-associated peripheral lipodystrophy, hyperlipidaemia, and insulin resistance. Lancet 1998;351(9119):1881–3 [Important reference for key points].
47. Lang S, Mary-Krause M, Cotte L, et al. Increased risk of myocardial infarction in HIV-infected patients in France, relative to the general population. AIDS 2010; 24(8):1228–30.
48. Aberg JA, Tebas P, Overton ET, et al. Metabolic effects of darunavir/ritonavir versus atazanavir/ritonavir in treatment-naive, HIV type 1-infected subjects over 48 weeks. AIDS Res Hum Retroviruses 2012;28(10):1184–95.
49. Ofotokun I, Ribaudo H, Na L, et al. Darunavir or atazanavir vs raltegravir lipid changes are unliked to ritonavir exposure: ACTG 5257. Presented at the 21st Conference on Retroviruses and Opportunistic Infections. Boston (MA), March 3–6, 2014. [abstract: #746].
50. Mobius U, Lubach-Ruitman M, Castro-Frenzel B, et al. Switching to atazanavir improves metabolic disorders in antiretroviral-experienced patients with severe hyperlipidemia. J Acquir Immune Defic Syndr 2005;39(2):174–80.
51. Mills AM, Nelson M, Jayaweera D, et al. Once-daily darunavir/ritonavir vs. lopinavir/ritonavir in treatment-naive, HIV-1-infected patients: 96-week analysis. AIDS 2009;23(13):1679–88.
52. Worm SW, Sabin C, Weber R, et al. Risk of myocardial infarction in patients with HIV infection exposed to specific individual antiretroviral drugs from the 3 major drug classes: the data collection on adverse events of anti-HIV drugs (D: A:D) study. J Infect Dis 2010;201(3):318–30 [Important reference for key points].
53. Menezes CN, Crowther NJ, Duarte R, et al. A randomized clinical trial comparing metabolic parameters after 48 weeks of standard- and low-dose stavudine therapy and tenofovir disoproxil fumarate therapy in HIV-infected South African patients. HIV Med 2014;15(1):3–12.
54. Crane HM, Grunfeld C, Willig JH, et al. Impact of NRTIs on lipid levels among a large HIV-infected cohort initiating antiretroviral therapy in clinical care. AIDS 2011;25(2):185–95.

55. Ribaudo HJ, Benson CA, Zheng Y, et al. No risk of myocardial infarction associated with initial antiretroviral treatment containing abacavir: short and long-term results from ACTG A5001/ALLRT. Clin Infect Dis 2011;52(7):929–40.

56. Lang S, Mary-Krause M, Cotte L, et al. Impact of individual antiretroviral drugs on the risk of myocardial infarction in human immunodeficiency virus-infected patients: a case-control study nested within the French Hospital Database on HIV ANRS cohort CO4. Arch Intern Med 2010;170(14):1228–38.

57. Sabin CA, Worm SW, Weber R, et al. Use of nucleoside reverse transcriptase inhibitors and risk of myocardial infarction in HIV-infected patients enrolled in the D: A:D study: a multi-cohort collaboration. Lancet 2008;371(9622): 1417–26.

58. Brothers CH, Hernandez JE, Cutrell AG, et al. Risk of myocardial infarction and abacavir therapy: no increased risk across 52 GlaxoSmithKline-sponsored clinical trials in adult subjects. J Acquir Immune Defic Syndr 2009;51(1):20–8.

59. Sax PE, Tierney C, Collier AC, et al. Abacavir/lamivudine versus tenofovir DF/emtricitabine as part of combination regimens for initial treatment of HIV: final results. J Infect Dis 2011;204(8):1191–201.

60. Saumoy M, Ordonez-Llanos J, Martinez E, et al. Low-density lipoprotein size and lipoprotein-associated phospholipase A2 in HIV-infected patients switching to abacavir or tenofovir. Antivir Ther 2011;16(4):459–68.

61. Martinez E, d'Albuquerque PM, Perez I, et al. Abacavir/lamivudine versus tenofovir/emtricitabine in virologically suppressed patients switching from ritonavir-boosted protease inhibitors to raltegravir. AIDS Res Hum Retroviruses 2013; 29(2):235–41.

62. Guaraldi G, Zona S, Cossarizza A, et al. Randomized trial to evaluate cardiometabolic and endothelial function in patients with plasma HIV-1 RNA suppression switching to darunavir/ritonavir with or without nucleoside analogues. HIV Clin Trials 2013;14(4):140–8.

63. Williams P, Wu J, Cohn S, et al. Improvement in lipid profiles over 6 years of follow-up in adults with AIDS and immune reconstitution. HIV Med 2009;10(5): 290–301.

64. Daar ES, Tierney C, Fischl MA, et al. Atazanavir plus ritonavir or efavirenz as part of a 3-drug regimen for initial treatment of HIV-1. Ann Intern Med 2011;154(7): 445–56.

65. Hill A, Sawyer W, Gazzard B. Effects of first-line use of nucleoside analogues, efavirenz, and ritonavir-boosted protease inhibitors on lipid levels. HIV Clin Trials 2009;10(1):1–12.

66. Gotti D, Cesana BM, Albini L, et al. Increase in standard cholesterol and large HDL particle subclasses in antiretroviral-naive patients prescribed efavirenz compared to atazanavir/ritonavir. HIV Clin Trials 2012;13(5):245–55.

67. Casado JL, de los Santos I, Del Palacio M, et al. Lipid-lowering effect and efficacy after switching to etravirine in HIV-infected patients with intolerance to suppressive HAART. HIV Clin Trials 2013;14(1):1–9.

68. Molina JM, Cahn P, Grinsztejn B, et al. Rilpivirine versus efavirenz with tenofovir and emtricitabine in treatment-naive adults infected with HIV-1 (ECHO): a phase 3 randomised double-blind active-controlled trial. Lancet 2011;378(9787): 238–46.

69. Cohen CJ, Andrade-Villanueva J, Clotet B, et al. Rilpivirine versus efavirenz with two background nucleoside or nucleotide reverse transcriptase inhibitors in treatment-naive adults infected with HIV-1 (THRIVE): a phase 3, randomised, non-inferiority trial. Lancet 2011;378(9787):229–37.

70. van der Valk M, Kastelein JJ, Murphy RL, et al. Nevirapine-containing antiretroviral therapy in HIV-1 infected patients results in an anti-atherogenic lipid profile. AIDS 2001;15(18):2407–14.

71. Vigano A, Aldrovandi GM, Giacomet V, et al. Improvement in dyslipidaemia after switching stavudine to tenofovir and replacing protease inhibitors with efavirenz in HIV-infected children. Antivir Ther 2005;10(8):917–24.

72. Fatkenheuer G, Duvivier C, Rieger A, et al. Lipid profiles for etravirine versus efavirenz in treatment-naive patients in the randomized, double-blind SENSE trial. J Antimicrob Chemother 2012;67(3):685–90.

73. Rockstroh JK, Lennox JL, DeJesus E, et al. Long-term treatment with raltegravir or efavirenz combined with tenofovir/emtricitabine for treatment-naive human immunodeficiency virus-1-infected patients: 156-week results from STARTMRK. Clin Infect Dis 2011;53(8):807–16.

74. MacInnes A, Lazzarin A, Di Perri G, et al. Maraviroc can improve lipid profiles in dyslipidemic patients with HIV: results from the MERIT trial. HIV Clin Trials 2011; 12(1):24–36.

75. Cipriani S, Francisci D, Mencarelli A, et al. Efficacy of the CCR5 antagonist maraviroc in reducing early, ritonavir-induced atherogenesis and advanced plaque progression in mice. Circulation 2013;127(21):2114–24.

76. Bonjoch A, Pou C, Perez-Alvarez N, et al. Switching the third drug of antiretroviral therapy to maraviroc in aviraemic subjects: a pilot, prospective, randomized clinical trial. J Antimicrob Chemother 2013;68(6):1382–7.

77. Rockstroh JK, DeJesus E, Lennox JL, et al. Durable efficacy and safety of raltegravir versus efavirenz when combined with tenofovir/emtricitabine in treatment-naive HIV-1-infected patients: final 5-year results from STARTMRK. J Acquir Immune Defic Syndr 2013;63(1):77–85.

78. Fabbiani M, Mondi A, Colafigli M, et al. Safety and efficacy of treatment switch to raltegravir plus tenofovir/emtricitabine or abacavir/lamivudine in patients with optimal virological control: 48-week results from a randomized pilot study (Raltegravir Switch for Toxicity or Adverse Events, RASTA Study). Scand J Infect Dis 2014;46(1):34–45.

79. Monteiro P, Perez I, Laguno M, et al. Dual therapy with etravirine plus raltegravir for virologically suppressed HIV-infected patients: a pilot study. J Antimicrob Chemother 2014;69(3):742–8.

80. Reliquet V, Chirouze C, Allavena C, et al. Nevirapine-raltegravir combination, an NRTI and PI/r sparing regimen, as maintenance antiretroviral therapy in virologically suppressed HIV-1-infected patients. Antivir Ther 2014;19(1):117–23.

81. Raffi F, Rachlis A, Stellbrink HJ, et al. Once-daily dolutegravir versus raltegravir in antiretroviral-naive adults with HIV-1 infection: 48 week results from the randomised, double-blind, non-inferiority SPRING-2 study. Lancet 2013;381(9868):735–43.

82. FDA notifications. Ongoing safety review of abacavir, possible MI risk. AIDS Alert 2011;26(5):58–9.

83. Rockstroh JK, DeJesus E, Henry K, et al. A randomized, double-blind comparison of coformulated elvitegravir/cobicistat/emtricitabine/tenofovir DF vs ritonavir-boosted atazanavir plus coformulated emtricitabine and tenofovir DF for initial treatment of HIV-1 infection: analysis of week 96 results. J Acquir Immune Defic Syndr 2013;62(5):483–6.

84. Sax PE, DeJesus E, Mills A, et al. Co-formulated elvitegravir, cobicistat, emtricitabine, and tenofovir versus co-formulated efavirenz, emtricitabine, and tenofovir for initial treatment of HIV-1 infection: a randomised, double-blind, phase 3 trial, analysis of results after 48 weeks. Lancet 2012;379(9835):2439–48.

85. Elion R, Molina JM, Ramon Arribas LJ, et al. A randomized phase 3 study comparing once-daily elvitegravir with twice-daily raltegravir in treatment-experienced subjects with HIV-1 infection: 96-week results. J Acquir Immune Defic Syndr 2013;63(4):494–7.

86. Tsimikas S, Miller YI. Oxidative modification of lipoproteins: mechanisms, role in inflammation and potential clinical applications in cardiovascular disease. Curr Pharm Des 2011;17(1):27–37.

87. Kelesidis T, Flores M, Tseng CH, et al. HIV-infected adults with suppressed viremia on antiretroviral therapy have dysfunctional HDL that is associated with T cell activation. Abstract 662; Presented at IDWeek 2012. San Diego (CA), October 17–21, 2012.

88. Bjorkbacka H, Fredrikson GN, Nilsson J. Emerging biomarkers and intervention targets for immune-modulation of atherosclerosis - a review of the experimental evidence. Atherosclerosis 2013;227(1):9–17.

89. Yilmaz A, Jennbacken K, Fogelstrand L. Reduced IgM levels and elevated IgG levels against oxidized low-density lipoproteins in HIV-1 infection. BMC Infect Dis 2014;14:143.

90. Graham LS, Parhami F, Tintut Y, et al. Oxidized lipids enhance RANKL production by T lymphocytes: implications for lipid-induced bone loss. Clin Immunol 2009;133(2):265–75.

91. Aberg JA, Gallant JE, Ghanem KG, et al. Primary care guidelines for the management of persons infected with HIV: 2013 update by the HIV Medicine Association of the Infectious Diseases Society of America. Clin Infect Dis 2014;58(1):1–10 [Important reference for key points].

92. Lundgren JD, Battegay M, Behrens G, et al. European AIDS Clinical Society (EACS) guidelines on the prevention and management of metabolic diseases in HIV. HIV Med 2008;9(2):72–81.

93. Munoz MA, Liu W, Delaney JA, et al. Comparative effectiveness of fish oil versus fenofibrate, gemfibrozil, and atorvastatin on lowering triglyceride levels among HIV-infected patients in routine clinical care. J Acquir Immune Defic Syndr 2013;64(3):254–60.

94. Grinspoon SK, Grunfeld C, Kotler DP, et al. State of the science conference: Initiative to decrease cardiovascular risk and increase quality of care for patients living with HIV/AIDS: executive summary. Circulation 2008;118(2):198–210.

95. Wooten JS, Nambi P, Gillard BK, et al. Intensive lifestyle modification reduces Lp-PLA2 in dyslipidemic HIV/HAART patients. Med Sci Sports Exerc 2013;45(6):1043–50.

96. Stradling C, Chen YF, Russell T, et al. The effects of dietary intervention on HIV dyslipidaemia: a systematic review and meta-analysis. PLoS One 2012;7(6):e38121.

97. Campo R, DeJesus E, Bredeek UF, et al. SWIFT: prospective 48-week study to evaluate efficacy and safety of switching to emtricitabine/tenofovir from lamivudine/abacavir in virologically suppressed HIV-1 infected patients on a boosted protease inhibitor containing antiretroviral regimen. Clin Infect Dis 2013;56(11):1637–45.

98. Eron JJ, Young B, Cooper DA, et al. Switch to a raltegravir-based regimen versus continuation of a lopinavir-ritonavir-based regimen in stable HIV-infected patients with suppressed viraemia (SWITCHMRK 1 and 2): two multicentre, double-blind, randomised controlled trials. Lancet 2010;375(9712):396–407 [Important reference for key points].

99. Singh IM, Shishehbor MH, Ansell BJ. High-density lipoprotein as a therapeutic target: a systematic review. JAMA 2007;298(7):786–98.
100. Behrens G, Maserati R, Rieger A, et al. Switching to tenofovir/emtricitabine from abacavir/lamivudine in HIV-infected adults with raised cholesterol: effect on lipid profiles. Antivir Ther 2012;17(6):1011–20.

Diabetes Mellitus Type 2 and Abnormal Glucose Metabolism in the Setting of Human Immunodeficiency Virus

Colleen Hadigan, MD, MPH[a],*, Sarah Kattakuzhy, MD[b]

KEYWORDS

- Diabetes • Human immunodeficiency virus • Disorders of glucose metabolism
- Combination antiretroviral therapy • Cardiovascular disease

KEY POINTS

- HIV cohort studies estimate the prevalence of diabetes at 3% to 4% among HIV-infected individuals, although this is likely to be conservative given study populations utilized.
- The etiology of DM in the HIV infected population is related to traditional risk factors as well as disease specific mechanisms such as medications, drug effects, and associated conditions.
- The diagnosis of diabetes in HIV can be made using both fasting blood glucose and HbA1c, as current studies do not favor a specific diagnostic strategy.
- HIV-infected patients with diabetes demonstrate increased rates of and worsened clinical outcomes for multiple high-risk conditions including cardiovascular, liver, and chronic kidney disease.
- There are currently no studies comparing diabetes treatment strategies in the setting of HIV and, as such, current ADA guidelines serve as the guiding tool for treatment.

Disclosures: The authors have no potential conflicts of interest to report.
Support: This review was prepared with support from the Intramural Research Program of the National Institute of Allergy and Infectious Diseases at the National Institutes of Health. This project has been funded in whole or in part with federal funds from the National Cancer Institute, National Institutes of Health, under Contract No: HHSN261200800001E. The content of this publication does not necessarily reflect the views or policies of the Department of Health and Human Services, nor does mention of trade names, commercial products, or organizations imply endorsement by the US Government.

[a] Laboratory of Immunoregulation, National Institute of Allergy and Infectious Diseases, NIH, 10 Center Drive, Bethesda, MD 20892, USA; [b] Laboratory of Immunoregulation, Leidos Biomedical Research, Inc., Frederick National Laboratory for Cancer Research, 5705 Industry Lane, Frederick, MD 21702, USA
* Corresponding author.
E-mail address: hadiganc@niaid.nih.gov

Endocrinol Metab Clin N Am 43 (2014) 685–696
http://dx.doi.org/10.1016/j.ecl.2014.05.003
0889-8529/14/$ – see front matter Published by Elsevier Inc.
endo.theclinics.com

The landscape of human immunodeficiency virus (HIV) care has changed dramatically in the last 10 years. While the advent of combination antiretroviral therapy (cART) has saved an estimated 14 million life-years in low-income and middle-income countries, it has also altered the natural history of HIV infection. Numerous studies have demonstrated that as HIV patients gain control of the disease (as measured by viral load below the limit of detection and rising CD4 count), there is a parallel increase in chronic medical illness.[1] A recent study by Kim and colleagues[2] observed that two-thirds of a treated HIV-infected cohort had the presence of multimorbidity or the clustering of 2 or more chronic medical illnesses. These diseases, including cardiovascular disease and diabetes, are not benign, and collectively contribute to the decreased life expectancy of HIV-infected patients on treatment.

Diabetes mellitus (DM) and disorders of glucose metabolism are increasingly common in the United States and affect morbidity and cardiovascular disease in all populations, including persons living with HIV. In 2011 the American Diabetes Association (ADA) estimated that 25.8 million, or 8.5% of the United States population, carry a diagnosis of type 2 DM. Prediabetes, defined by a fasting glucose of 100 to 126 mg/dL or a hemoglobin A1c (HbA_{1c}) level of 5.7% to 6.4%, affects an additional 79 million Americans. Although lifestyle-associated risk factors are thought to be the main progenitor of this epidemic, HIV-infected patients with disorders of glucose metabolism have established a divergent and multifactorial pathogenesis in comparison with their noninfected counterparts. In addition to traditional risk factors such as obesity, both direct and indirect effects of cART medication, HIV-associated conditions such as hepatitis C and opiate drug use, and the HIV virus itself have been proposed as mechanisms of hyperglycemia and diabetes in this context (**Fig. 1**).

DM is a systemic disease, and carries risk for HIV-infected patients beyond cardiovascular disease. Disorders of glucose metabolism in this population have been associated with increased prevalence and worsened outcomes in a diverse array of conditions ranging from neurocognitive changes to renal impairment and albuminuria. Hence, the diagnosis and treatment of this condition represents a potential wide impact on general health.

Diabetes is an emerging issue in the HIV-infected population that is important to characterize as the clinical course of HIV changes. This review discusses: (1) the epidemiology of DM in HIV; (2) the proposed mechanisms of glucose intolerance; (3) challenges in diagnosis; (4) associated health risks; and (5) current treatment strategies.

EPIDEMIOLOGY

As the use of cART spread in the late 1990s, there was early recognition that disorders of glucose metabolism were linked to cART. Initial studies evaluated this in the context of specific medications such as protease inhibitors (PIs) and emerging conditions such as lipodystrophy.

Calza and colleagues[3] evaluated the prevalence of DM and metabolic syndrome in an observational cohort of 775 HIV-infected patients on cART seen in an Italian clinic between July and September 2009. Diabetes was diagnosed through one-time fasting blood glucose greater than 126 mg/dL, random glucose greater than 200 mg/dL, or history of hypoglycemic medications. The prevalence of DM was 4.5%, impaired fasting glucose 9.4%, hyperinsulinemia 11.9%, and metabolic syndrome 9.1%. There were no significant differences found in type of cART, presence of liver disease, cholesterol levels, or blood pressure measurements between diabetic and nondiabetic patients.

Similarly, Galli and colleagues[4] conducted a cross-sectional investigation of 4249 HIV-infected patients and 9148 healthy controls. Diabetes was diagnosed using fasting blood glucose greater than 126 mg/dL, reported history of DM, or prescription of

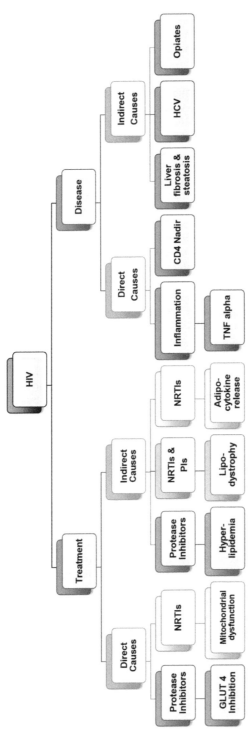

Fig. 1. The multifactorial human immunodeficiency virus (HIV)-specific mechanisms responsible for insulin resistance and diabetes in persons with HIV infection. GLUT 4, glucose transporter type 4; HCV, hepatitis C virus; NRTI, nucleoside reverse transcriptase inhibitor; PI, protease inhibitor; TNF, tumor necrosis factor.

hypoglycemic medication. The prevalence of DM was 4%, compared with 2.5% within the non–HIV-infected population.

In 1999 a large, multinational cohort was established to prospectively evaluate potential adverse effects of cART. The Data Collection on Adverse Events of Anti-HIV Drugs (D:A:D) cohort of 33,389 HIV-infected patients found the prevalence of diabetes, defined by fasting blood glucose greater than 126 mg/dL on 2 separate readings, physician record, or antidiabetic therapy, was 2.85% at entry to the study.[5]

Taken together, a conservative evaluation from largely European cohort data estimates the prevalence of diabetes among HIV-infected patients at 3% to 4%. It should be noted that these study populations were overwhelmingly male and relatively young, with limited ethnic and racial diversity. Previous data from the Multicenter AIDS Cohort Study (MACS), which evaluated 533 HIV-infected men and contemporary uninfected controls from multiple United States cities between 1999 and 2003, found an overall prevalence of DM of 14% in HIV compared with 5% in the noninfected control group.[6] The higher prevalence may be related to the definition of diabetes, which included fasting glucose greater than 126 mg/dL in addition to self-report, and the higher body mass index (BMI) compared to other cohorts. Numerous demographic and social factors that contribute to DM prevalence should be taken into account, but in the studies that included matched uninfected subjects as a comparator group the prevalence of diabetes was greater among those with HIV.

Of note, Capeau and colleagues[7] determined the incidence of DM in a cohort of 1046 HIV-infected patients prospectively followed between 1999 and 2009 as they started cART. The overall incidence was 14.1 cases per 1000 person-years, although there was a trend for the incidence of DM to decline over time. For example, in the period between 1999 and 2000, the incidence was 23.2 per 1000 person-years, whereas it was as low as 2.7 cases per 1000 person-years in the period of 2005 to 2006. Elements of cART, in addition to traditional risk factors such as age, BMI, and waist-to-hip ratio, were associated with incident DM, but the decline in incidence over time may reflect changes in cART practices and the development of less toxic cART alternatives.

In the United States, diabetes is known to disproportionately affect those of African American, Hispanic, and Native American descent. Within the HIV-infected diabetic population, data on the influence of race and ethnicity are limited. The aforementioned studies of prevalence consist largely of white men, limiting the power to evaluate an association with a minority race. Adeyemi and colleagues[8] used data from the Women's Interagency HIV Study, a prospective study of predominantly African American and Hispanic HIV-infected and matched HIV-uninfected women from multiple United States cities, to evaluate factors related to insulin resistance. In this report of nondiabetic women (754 HIV-infected and 328 uninfected), there was a higher rate of insulin resistance as measured by homeostasis model assessment of insulin resistance (HOMA-IR) among Hispanic women, but no difference in insulin resistance by HIV status. Hispanic race remained a significant associated risk factor for HOMA-IR score of 2.6 or more after adjusting for age, BMI, hepatitis C infection, and PI use. Further studies are necessary to further outline the impact of race and ethnicity on the prevalence of diabetes in the HIV-infected population.

MECHANISMS

Despite the contribution of several mechanisms of pathogenesis unique to HIV, traditional risk factors play a significant role in the development of diabetes in the HIV-infected population. Although studies have demonstrated a lower BMI in HIV-infected patients with diabetes when compared with noninfected matched cohorts,[9] the association between DM and obesity persists in HIV. For example, Galli and colleagues[4] found that the prevalence of DM in those with normal BMI was 3.2% in HIV-infected patients and 1.1% in those uninfected. However, in the overweight and obese categories, DM prevalence increased to 3.9% and 12.7% among HIV-infected patients compared with 3.1% and 7.8%, respectively, in HIV-uninfected patients. Similarly, the D:A:D cohort demonstrated an increase in relative rate of new-onset DM with increasing weight category.[10] Obesity in HIV is discussed elsewhere in this issue by Mankal and colleagues, but the association between obesity and diabetes, as in noninfected patients, is strong.

Similarly, genetics appear to contribute to the development of diabetes in HIV. Recent genomic studies have established several common single-nucleotide polymorphisms (SNPs) associated with diabetes in the general population. Rotger and colleagues[11] evaluated 22 SNPs associated with the development of DM in 94 patients with diabetes in the Swiss HIV Cohort and in 550 HIV-infected nondiabetic controls. Four common SNPs were found to influence DM risk, and this association became stronger as the number of risk alleles increased. Furthermore, the relative contribution of genetic variation and other risk factors to the development of diabetes was assessed; SNPs accounted for 14% of DM risk variability, whereas cART exposure accounted for 3% and age 19% of the variability in DM. This emerging area of research highlights the importance of non-HIV risk factors in the pathogenesis of DM in HIV.

Various studies investigated ART-naïve populations to assess any inherent connection between the HIV virus and development of glucose disorders. Unfortunately, the available data do not suggest a clear answer. Brown and colleagues[12] evaluated cumulative exposure to cART and markers of insulin resistance in 533 HIV-positive men of the MACS cohort, and found that ART-naïve patients demonstrated a lower QUICKI (Quantitative Insulin Sensitivity Check Index) score (-0.04; 95% confidence interval [CI] -0.07–0.01) and higher odds of fasting hyperinsulinemia (odds ratio 1.08; 95% CI 1.02–1.13). However, this relationship was not borne out in subsequent studies. Galli and colleagues[4] found that HIV-infected patients who were ART-naïve had a lower prevalence of diabetes (0.8%) compared with HIV-infected patients on therapy (4%) or an uninfected comparison cohort (2.5%).

One proposed pathway for the influence of HIV on diabetes and glucose is through generalized inflammation, with upregulation of chemokines involved in insulin regulation. For example, Brown and colleagues[13] found that higher markers of tumor necrosis factor–α activation after 48 weeks of cART was associated with increased odds of subsequent diabetes after adjustment for age, BMI, CD4 count, and type of cART. However, conflicting data provide no definitive conclusion to this hypothesis. More studies have focused on the relative contribution of cART to the incidence of diabetes in HIV.

In the D:A:D cohort, De Wit and colleagues[5] found that cumulative exposure to cART carried an adjusted relative risk (RR) of 1.11 per year (95% CI 1.07–1.15; $P = .0001$). Exposure to the specific nucleoside reverse transcriptase inhibitor (NRTI) stavudine was associated with an increased risk of diabetes (RR 1.19 per year exposure; 95% CI 1.15–1.25; $P = .0001$), as were didanosine and zidovudine, but to a lesser extent. In another large prospective trial, Capeau and colleagues[7] found that stavudine use was associated with a significant increase in hazard ratio for DM, peaking in the second year of use (hazard ratio 2.81, 95% CI 1.4–5.64; $P = .004$). The protease inhibitor indinavir was also associated with an increased hazard ratio of 2.55 (95% CI 1.36–4.79), although this declined in the subsequent years of use. Using the MACS Cohort, Brown and colleagues[12] also found that stavudine exposure was associated with a significantly lower QUICKI value and increased risk of hyperinsulinemia; lamivudine and indinavir exposure demonstrated similar results. The Women's Interagency HIV Study (WIHS)[14] found that NRTI exposure was associated with a higher median HOMA score compared with no NRTI in a cohort of HIV-infected women and uninfected controls. Each additional year of NRTI use was associated with a 2% increase in median HOMA. Median HOMA increased 6% per year of stavudine exposure. No significant relationship between markers of insulin resistance and exposure to lamivudine, zidovudine, abacavir, and tenofovir was identified, nor did they find any significant relationship with PIs or non-NRTIs as classes of antiretroviral therapy.

Overall, data support an increased prevalence of diabetes among HIV-infected patients treated with stavudine, with mixed data regarding indinavir and other agents. Observed discrepancies may be attributed to changes in cART-prescribing practices over time, with more recent studies reporting less use of first-generation PIs and thymidine analogues. For initiation of HIV therapy, current treatment guidelines do not include the described agents implicated in diabetes and insulin resistance. However, observations regarding risk associated with agents such as stavudine remain applicable, as it continues to be used in resource-limited settings globally. Future studies will need to reevaluate the influence of contemporary antiretroviral treatment practices on diabetes and glucose metabolism in the modern era of antiretroviral therapy.

Side effects of cART such as lipodystrophy and hyperlipidemia play an important role in the association between diabetes and HIV, and are addressed directly in other sections of this review. Other conditions known to occur with increased frequency in HIV-infected patients have also been found to influence the development of disordered glucose metabolism. For example, opioid use is common in HIV-infected patients, and has been linked to aberrant glucose metabolism in animal studies. In an investigation of women with or at risk of HIV by Howard and colleagues,[15] opiate use was associated with increased prevalence of DM among both past (18% vs 9%) and current opioid users (15% vs 10%), independent of multiple factors including hepatitis C infection. Opiate use in the cohort was also associated with an increased incidence of diabetes during the period from 2000 to 2006.

This study also found a higher prevalence of diabetes among hepatitis C coinfected patients (16% vs 10% among those without hepatitis C), a finding identified in other studies of both HIV-infected and HIV-uninfected populations. This condition is thought to be mediated by hepatic steatosis and liver fibrosis, with resultant insulin resistance. In a cross-sectional study of 432 HIV-monoinfected patients, DallaPiazza and colleagues[16] identified liver fibrosis estimated by aspartate aminotransferase to platelet ratio index (APRI) (where a score of >1.5 is predictive of significant liver fibrosis) in association with diabetes. The overall prevalence of DM was 8%, but this increased to 17% in patients with APRI greater than 1.5. Although the design and sample size cannot establish causality, diabetes was the most significant risk factor associated with fibrosis. The investigators suggest that liver fibrosis, independent of viral hepatitis, may be prevalent in HIV-monoinfected patients, with important implications in the risk of diabetes.

Taken together, these data demonstrate the wide array of pathogenesis in the development of insulin resistance and diabetes in HIV. Though multifactorial, the disease is related to known demographic risk factors, in particular age, obesity, and genetic variants, but specific medications such as stavudine and associated conditions such as lipodystrophy, opiate use, and liver fibrosis are also contributory for many patients.

DIAGNOSTICS

The definition of DM in the aforementioned studies demonstrates the variability of diagnostic criteria available today, and may underlie the differences in prevalence and incidence among various cohorts. The current ADA guidelines underscore that either fasting blood glucose, HbA$_{1c}$, oral glucose tolerance test (OGTT), or random glucose with classic symptoms of hyperglycemia can be performed to diagnose diabetes.[17] For the first 3 strategies, outside of unequivocal hyperglycemia, repeat testing should occur for confirmation. Interval testing is recommended to occur every 3 years. The only group of distinction remains pregnant women, for whom OGTT is the diagnostic test of choice. Studies have evaluated the performance of diagnostic strategies in the setting of HIV, but optimal diabetes screening guidelines have not been established specifically for HIV-infected patients.

One study determined the proportion of incident DM cases among 377 HIV-infected or at-risk adults using fasting and OGTT 120-minute glucose levels tested 18 months apart.[18] Of those diagnosed with DM during the study, 44% were detected only by a fasting plasma glucose, 31% were detected only by the 120-minute plasma glucose level on OGTT, and 25% were detected by both tests, with no difference between infected and noninfected patients. A similar pattern of detection was found for the diagnosis of prediabetes. The investigators conclude that given one-third of diabetes cases were detected only by use of OGTT, performing fasting glucose testing alone may miss a significant number of individuals with diabetes.

Recently, Tien and colleagues[19] also explored the effect of definition on case detection of DM, using the WIHS cohort. The researchers used 3 definitions of diabetes: (1) the measures (fasting blood glucose >126 mg/dL, reported DM diagnosis or medications for hyperglycemia) used by most of the large cohort studies, (2) including a second confirmatory fasting blood glucose, and (3) including an HbA$_{1c}$ of greater than 6.5%. The results demonstrated the highest case detection for definition (1), with an incidence rate of 2.44 per 100 person-years in the HIV-infected population and 1.89 per 100 person-years in the uninfected comparison, a difference of 1.2 fold. Although the greatest prevalence in both infected and noninfected patients was seen with single fasting glucose greater than 126 mg/dL, the addition of confirmatory testing or an HbA$_{1c}$ level increased the accuracy of diagnosis and only slightly attenuated the association between DM and HIV.

In a retrospective chart review of 395 HIV-infected, primarily black and Hispanic men, Eckhardt and colleagues[20] compared elevated fasting blood glucose with HbA$_{1c}$. Using fasting blood glucose as the gold standard, investigators found that the sensitivity of HbA$_{1c}$ was poor at 40.9%, but specificity high at 97.5%; peak sensitivity and specificity was found at an HbA$_{1c}$ cutoff of 5.8%. This investigation and others have noted that elevations of mean corpuscular volume (MCV) in patients with HIV tend to underestimate glycemia when using HbA$_{1c}$.[9] Despite these observations, HbA$_{1c}$ can be used in conjunction with fasting blood glucose for clinical decision making.

Overall, there are no specific recommendations for diabetes surveillance or testing in the context of HIV infection. For practical purposes, most investigations conclude that fasting blood glucose and HbA$_{1c}$ are the diagnostic tests of choice, and that there is not enough evidence in the HIV population to recommend for or against either strategy. The recently updated Infectious Disease Society of America (IDSA) primary care guidelines recommend fasting glucose and/or HbA$_{1c}$, and suggest consideration of a 5.8% HbA$_{1c}$ threshold cutoff.[21] The IDSA guidelines also recommend testing every 6 to 12 months in HIV-infected patients, which does deviate from the ADA recommendations for the general population to be screened every 3 years. At present there is insufficient evidence to recommend an ideal time interval, especially as the only study to address this used the OGTT. However, given the prevalence of diabetes in HIV, this additional guidance can be used in conjunction with clinical evaluation.

EFFECTS

Diabetes is a systemic illness with well-established, targeted end-organ effects. In the setting of HIV, strong data support the association between diabetes and the risk of cardiovascular disease. In a study using the D:A:D cohort, Worm and colleagues[22] investigated the predictive value of preexisting DM and heart disease for subsequent cardiac events in the context of HIV infection. Among the 33,347 patients enrolled, the prevalence of diabetes was 2.9% and the prevalence of heart disease was 1.1%. There were 698 incident cardiac events (incidence of 4.4 per 1000 person-years). These events were divided into 4 risk categories: previous heart disease alone, diabetes alone, both prior coronary heart disease and DM, and neither diagnosis. Although previous cardiac disease had a stronger RR (9.04; 95% CI 7.1–11.49) than diabetes (RR 3.03, 95% CI 2.34–3.93) for incident cardiac events, their combined effect was substantial (RR 11.66, 95% CI 7.42–18.3). In this cohort of mainly 30- to 40-year-old adults, the average length of diabetes diagnosis was only 5 years, which may be insufficient time for resultant vascular damage to occur. In a subanalysis, the risk of heart disease increased with longer duration of diabetes, highlighting the potential for a stronger relationship with extended clinical follow-up. In addition, the study noted the high prevalence of cardiac risk factors such as tobacco use, which is often overrepresented among HIV-infected populations. A study by Calvo-Sanchez and colleagues[23] further illustrates these findings. This retrospective chart review used 2 parallel case-control studies to evaluate the rate of acute coronary syndrome (ACS) in HIV, with matched populations of HIV-infected patients without ACS, HIV-uninfected patients with ACS, and healthy volunteers. Whereas the population-attributable risk (PAR) of diabetes was 6.57 (95% CI −8.87–16.96), smoking held the largest fraction, with a PAR of 54.35 (95% CI 29.33–70.51), which was significantly larger than that observed in the HIV-uninfected population.

The effects of diabetes in cardiovascular health potentially extend beyond incidence of cardiac events. In a study by Lorgis and colleagues,[24] data from a French database of 277,303 patients with acute myocardial infarction (MI) was separated into parallel cohorts of HIV-infected and uninfected patients. After 1 year of follow-up, multiple post-MI complications were followed including hospitalizations, heart failure, and recurrent MI. A diagnosis of diabetes was associated with an increased risk of heart failure, with an odds ratio of 5.34 (95% CI 2.39–11.9) within this period. Similarly, in the HIV-HEART study, Reinsch and colleagues[25] investigated the prevalence of diastolic dysfunction, a potential early marker of coronary artery disease, in a cross-sectional cohort of 698 HIV-infected patients. Patients with diabetes were found to be 4 times as likely to have diastolic dysfunction, despite a prevalence of only 2% in the study population.

Although cardiac disease is an important contributor to mortality in persons living with HIV, liver disease also disproportionately affects this population. Much of this is related to coinfection with hepatitis C and B. However, significant liver abnormalities have also been found in HIV-monoinfected patients, and diabetes may play a role in their modulation. As noted previously, DallaPiazza and colleagues[16] showed that HIV-infected patients with a diagnosis of diabetes were 3 times more likely to have an APRI score indicating liver fibrosis in comparison with those without diabetes. Although data were not collected on potential confounders such as cART and other hepatotoxic medications, this study sheds light on important interplay between diabetes and liver disease in HIV.

Renal disease is also a significant risk in the HIV-infected population, and the presence of diabetes seems to have an additive effect. To assess the interaction between diabetes and development of chronic kidney disease (CKD), Medapalli and colleagues[26] measured progression to a glomerular filtration rate of less than 45 mL/min/1.73 m² using data from the large Veterans Aging Cohort Study. The presence of both HIV and DM was associated with a hazard ratio of 4.47 (95% CI 3.87–5.17) for development of CKD. In a subgroup of 7328 patients with HIV infection, excluding those with acute or chronic renal injury, the incidence of progression to CKD was 9.7%, and diabetes was associated with a hazard ratio of 1.78 (95% CI 1.49–2.12), representing a stronger association with development of CKD than with use of cART, HIV RNA, or CD4 count. The additive effect of DM and HIV is also seen in earlier measures of renal disease, such as albuminuria. In a cross-sectional study of HIV-infected patients with and without diabetes, and matched uninfected controls with diabetes, Kim and colleagues[27] identified a high prevalence of albuminuria in HIV-infected diabetics (34% HIV/DM vs 13% HIV vs 16% DM). The association with HIV and DM remained significant when a multivariate model controlled for multiple potential confounders including age, race, blood pressure, gender, BMI, and use of angiotensin-converting enzyme inhibitors or angiotensin II receptor blockers. These studies demonstrate that the untoward effects of DM in the context of HIV infection may contribute to renal dysfunction and CKD.

One of the most common complications of uncontrolled DM in the general population is peripheral neuropathy. In the HIV population, this relationship is confounded by the independent risk of HIV-mediated and cART-mediated neuropathy. In an AIDS Clinical Trials Group study of neuropathy,[28] 2141 patients who initiated cART from 2000 to 2007 were followed to determine the prevalence and risk factors for peripheral neuropathy in HIV. Throughout the evolution of treatment before, during, and after discontinuation of neurotoxic cART, diabetes remained positively associated with symptomatic and asymptomatic neuropathy. These investigators subsequently showed that the use of glucose-lowering therapies was protective against neuropathy and its progression in HIV-infected patients.[29] The impact of diabetes and insulin resistance on the nervous system may also apply to the brain and cognition. To examine the relationship between HIV neurocognitive disorder and metabolic variables, McCutchan and colleagues[30] completed a cross-sectional substudy of 130 HIV-infected patients. In the population older than 55 years, those with neurocognitive impairment (defined as a global deficiency score of >0.5) were more likely to have a concomitant diagnosis of DM (52.4% vs 29.9%; $P = .05$).

The aforementioned studies support the idea that diabetes is a significant risk factor for organ system dysfunction in the context of HIV. However, the implications of diabetes in the HIV-infected population may also extend to psychosocial factors. A study by Dray-Spira and colleagues[31] evaluated the risk of work cessation in a cohort of persons living with chronic HIV infection. One-third of patients stopped working within 5 years of their HIV diagnosis. Regarding multiple risk factors, diabetes was associated with a hazard ratio of 5.6 (95% CI 1.5–18.5; $P<.005$), whereas HIV disease severity and HIV discrimination had no significant relationship with work cessation. The investigators concluded that comorbid conditions such as DM constitute a major barrier to retained employment in French HIV-infected patients.

Taken together, these studies demonstrate the widespread impact of diabetes as a risk factor for multiple pathways of morbidity and mortality in the HIV-infected population.

TREATMENT

At present there are no randomized controlled trials of diabetes treatment specific to patients with HIV infection. Multiple studies have analyzed the use of thiazolidinedione (TZD) medication in the setting of lipodystrophy, with improvements seen in measures of insulin resistance. However, given the declining prevalence of lipodystrophy along with the proposed increase in cardiac risk associated with the use of TZD, application beyond this clinical setting is not currently recommended. Similarly, switching classes or specific combinations of antiretroviral therapy in the absence of hyperglycemia induced by stavudine or indinavir has not been shown to improve measures of insulin resistance.

Despite the lack of clinical data regarding various treatment options, several studies have looked at the efficacy of overall diabetes treatment and management in the HIV-infected population. Satlin and colleagues[32] completed a retrospective cross-sectional study of 142 HIV-infected adults with type 2 DM. The investigators found that one-third of patients had inadequate glycemic control, as defined by HbA_{1c} level higher than 7.5 for more than 6 months over the year. Although most uncontrolled patients were on insulin (60% vs 20%; $P<.001$), this may simply reflect that insulin initiation is in part triggered by measures of HbA_{1c}. The overall frequency that ADA clinical goals were achieved was poor, with approximately 30% who met high-density lipoprotein and triglyceride goals, and 40% who met blood pressure goals. A study set in a Malawi diabetes clinic discovered similar findings. Cohen and colleagues[33] analyzed 620 patients, separating outcomes between HIV-infected and HIV-uninfected patients. HIV diabetes patients had poor control to an extent similar to that of their noninfected counterparts, with an average HbA_{1c} of 9.0% versus 9.5%, respectively. In short, HIV-infected patients appear to have a disease-control profile similar to that of their noninfected counterparts. However, it should be noted that this is a poor level of control which, given the additive effects of diabetes in the setting of HIV, carries an additional layer of risk.

As such, the current ADA guidelines serve as the basis for ongoing management of DM in the HIV-infected population. Further studies are needed to assess the issue of optimal therapeutics.

SUMMARY

Successful screening, diagnosis, treatment, and management of diabetes have emerged as an important component of HIV care. HIV cohort studies estimate the prevalence of diabetes at 3% to 4% among HIV-infected individuals. Studies on the impact of ethnicity and race on this prevalence are limited.

As in the general population, traditional risk factors such as age, BMI, and genetics play a significant role in the development of diabetes in persons living with HIV. However, multiple other mechanisms contribute to the pathogenesis of DM in HIV-infected patients. Antiretroviral agents, in addition to drug effects such as hyperlipidemia and lipodystrophy, have been associated with increased incidence of diabetes. HIV is a risk factor for other conditions such as opiate use, liver fibrosis, and steatosis; in these groups diabetes is found in increased prevalence.

The diagnosis of diabetes in HIV can be made using both fasting blood glucose and HbA_{1c}, as current studies do not favor a specific diagnostic strategy. Recognition and diagnosis is necessary, however, given the far-ranging health effects associated with diabetes in this population. Increased rates of cardiovascular disease and cardiac complications have been found in HIV-infected patients with diabetes. Diabetes in HIV has also been associated with worsened liver disease, measures of CKD, and increased rates of unemployment.

There are currently no studies comparing diabetes treatment strategies in the setting of HIV and, as such, current ADA guidelines serve as the guiding tool for treatment. Future research should address this knowledge gap and address specific subpopulations related to HIV, such as those with advanced liver disease. In addition, the recently updated HIV treatment guidelines demonstrate the rapidity of turnover in cART recommendations. As HIV treatment practices evolve, recurrent studies of diabetes prevalence are necessary to recalibrate the scope of this issue.

REFERENCES

1. Hasse B, Ledergerber B, Furrer H, et al. Morbidity and aging in HIV-infected persons: the Swiss HIV cohort study. Clin Infect Dis 2011;53(11):1130–9.
2. Kim DJ, Westfall AO, Chamot E, et al. Multimorbidity patterns in HIV-infected patients: the role of obesity in chronic disease clustering. J Acquir Immune Defic Syndr 2012;61(5):600–5.
3. Calza L, Masetti G, Piergentili B, et al. Prevalence of diabetes mellitus, hyperinsulinaemia and metabolic syndrome among 755 adult patients with HIV-1 infection. Int J STD AIDS 2011;22(1):43–5.
4. Galli L, Salpietro S, Pellicciotta G, et al. Risk of type 2 diabetes among HIV-infected and healthy subjects in Italy. Eur J Epidemiol 2012;27(8):657–65.
5. De Wit S, Sabin CA, Weber R, et al. Incidence and risk factors for new-onset diabetes in HIV-infected patients: the Data Collection on Adverse Events of Anti-HIV Drugs (D: A:D) study. Diabetes Care 2008;31(6):1224–9.
6. Brown TT, Cole SR, Li X, et al. Antiretroviral therapy and the prevalence and incidence of diabetes mellitus in the multicenter AIDS cohort study. Arch Intern Med 2005;165(10):1179–84.
7. Capeau J, Bouteloup V, Katlama C, et al. Ten-year diabetes incidence in 1046 HIV-infected patients started on a combination antiretroviral treatment. AIDS 2012;26(3):303–14.
8. Adeyemi OM, Livak B, Orsi J, et al. Vitamin D and insulin resistance in non-diabetic women's interagency HIV study participants. AIDS Patient Care STDS 2013;27(6):320–5.
9. Kim PS, Woods C, Georgoff P, et al. A1C underestimates glycemia in HIV infection. Diabetes Care 2009;32(9):1591–3.
10. Petoumenos K, Worm SW, Fontas E, et al. Predicting the short-term risk of diabetes in HIV-positive patients: the Data Collection on Adverse Events of Anti-HIV Drugs (D: A:D) study. J Int AIDS Soc 2012;15(2):17426.
11. Rotger M, Gsponer T, Martinez R, et al. Impact of single nucleotide polymorphisms and of clinical risk factors on new-onset diabetes mellitus in HIV-infected individuals. Clin Infect Dis 2010;51(9):1090–8.
12. Brown TT, Li X, Cole SR, et al. Cumulative exposure to nucleoside analogue reverse transcriptase inhibitors is associated with insulin resistance markers in the Multicenter AIDS Cohort Study. AIDS 2005;19(13):1375–83.
13. Brown TT, Tassiopoulos K, Bosch RJ, et al. Association between systemic inflammation and incident diabetes in HIV-infected patients after initiation of antiretroviral therapy. Diabetes Care 2010;33(10):2244–9.
14. Tien PC, Schneider MF, Cole SR, et al. Antiretroviral therapy exposure and insulin resistance in the Women's Interagency HIV study. J Acquir Immune Defic Syndr 2008;49(4):369–76.
15. Howard AA, Hoover DR, Anastos K, et al. The effects of opiate use and hepatitis C virus infection on risk of diabetes mellitus in the Women's Interagency HIV Study. J Acquir Immune Defic Syndr 2010;54(2):152–9.
16. DallaPiazza M, Amorosa VK, Localio R, et al. Prevalence and risk factors for significant liver fibrosis among HIV-monoinfected patients. BMC Infect Dis 2010;10:116.

17. American Diabetes Association. Diagnosis and classification of diabetes mellitus. Diabetes Care 2014;37(Suppl 1):S81–90.
18. Polsky S, Floris-Moore M, Schoenbaum EE, et al. Incident hyperglycaemia among older adults with or at-risk for HIV infection. Antivir Ther 2011;16(2):181–8.
19. Tien PC, Schneider MF, Cox C, et al. Association of HIV infection with incident diabetes mellitus: impact of using hemoglobin A1C as a criterion for diabetes. J Acquir Immune Defic Syndr 2012;61(3):334–40.
20. Eckhardt BJ, Holzman RS, Kwan CK, et al. Glycated hemoglobin A(1c) as screening for diabetes mellitus in HIV-infected individuals. AIDS Patient Care STDS 2012;26(4):197–201.
21. Aberg JA, Gallant JE, Ghanem KG, et al. Primary care guidelines for the management of persons infected with HIV: 2013 update by the HIV medicine association of the Infectious Diseases Society of America. Clin Infect Dis 2014;58(1):e1–34.
22. Worm SW, De Wit S, Weber R, et al. Diabetes mellitus, preexisting coronary heart disease, and the risk of subsequent coronary heart disease events in patients infected with human immunodeficiency virus: the Data Collection on Adverse Events of Anti-HIV Drugs (D: A:D Study). Circulation 2009;119(6):805–11.
23. Calvo-Sanchez M, Perello R, Perez I, et al. Differences between HIV-infected and uninfected adults in the contributions of smoking, diabetes and hypertension to acute coronary syndrome: two parallel case-control studies. HIV Med 2013; 14(1):40–8.
24. Lorgis L, Cottenet J, Molins G, et al. Outcomes after acute myocardial infarction in HIV-infected patients: analysis of data from a French nationwide hospital medical information database. Circulation 2013;127(17):1767–74.
25. Reinsch N, Neuhaus K, Esser S, et al. Prevalence of cardiac diastolic dysfunction in HIV-infected patients: results of the HIV-HEART study. HIV Clin Trials 2010; 11(3):156–62.
26. Medapalli RK, Parikh CR, Gordon K, et al. Comorbid diabetes and the risk of progressive chronic kidney disease in HIV-infected adults: data from the Veterans Aging Cohort Study. J Acquir Immune Defic Syndr 2012;60(4):393–9.
27. Kim PS, Woods C, Dutcher L, et al. Increased prevalence of albuminuria in HIV-infected adults with diabetes. PLoS One 2011;6(9):e24610.
28. Evans SR, Ellis RJ, Chen H, et al. Peripheral neuropathy in HIV: prevalence and risk factors. AIDS 2011;25(7):919–28.
29. Evans SR, Lee AJ, Ellis RJ, et al. HIV peripheral neuropathy progression: protection with glucose-lowering drugs? J Neurovirol 2012;18(5):428–33.
30. McCutchan JA, Marquie-Beck JA, Fitzsimons CA, et al. Role of obesity, metabolic variables, and diabetes in HIV-associated neurocognitive disorder. Neurology 2012;78(7):485–92.
31. Dray-Spira R, Legeai C, Le Den M, et al. Burden of HIV disease and comorbidities on the chances of maintaining employment in the era of sustained combined antiretroviral therapies use. AIDS 2012;26(2):207–15.
32. Satlin MJ, Hoover DR, Glesby MJ. Glycemic control in HIV-infected patients with diabetes mellitus and rates of meeting American Diabetes Association management guidelines. AIDS Patient Care STDS 2011;25(1):5–12.
33. Cohen DB, Allain TJ, Glover S, et al. A survey of the management, control, and complications of diabetes mellitus in patients attending a diabetes clinic in Blantyre, Malawi, an area of high HIV prevalence. Am J Trop Med Hyg 2010;83(3): 575–81.

Alteration in Pancreatic Islet Function in Human Immunodeficiency Virus

Steen B. Haugaard, MD, DMSc

KEYWORDS

- Insulin secretion • Prehepatic • Proinsulin • Lipodystrophy • Antiretroviral therapy
- Nonglucose insulin secretagogues • Insulin-like growth factors • Incretins

KEY POINTS

- Nonglucose secretagogues, fat redistribution, and insulin resistance of beta cells them-selves are among the mechanisms impairing insulin secretion in patients on modern anti-human immunodeficiency virus (anti-HIV) therapy.
- Protease inhibitors are thought to directly impair insulin processing and secretion, but recent in vivo data challenge this view; thus, controlled trials are warranted.
- Hepatic extraction of insulin and insulin-like growths factors, which exhibit insulin effects, exerts influence on the demand on insulin secretion in HIV-infected patients.
- Although proinsulin processing may not be influenced directly by protease inhibitors and nucleoside analogues, the lipodystrophy syndrome they promote is highly associated with defective proinsulin secretion.
- Although the incretins are essential for normal insulin secretion, the data on how modern anti-HIV therapy influences incretin secretion and effect are sparse.

THE BETA CELL, INSULIN RESISTANCE, AND HUMAN IMMUNODEFICIENCY VIRUS-ASSOCIATED LIPODYSTROPHY SYNDROME

The function of the beta cell in the pancreatic islets of Langerhans is decisive in facil-itating a normal glucose homeostasis. The primary drive force of an increased insulin secretion of the individual is the prevalent insulin resistance of various organ systems, in particular liver, muscle, and adipose tissue. The mechanisms and prevalence of in-sulin resistance in human immunodeficiency virus (HIV) infection and its association with antiretroviral therapy are the focus of another article by Hadigan and colleagues

Disclosure: The Clinical Research Center, Copenhagen University Hospital, Hvidovre, Copenha-gen, Denmark, has supported this paper by a working grant.
Department of Internal Medicine and the Clinical Research Centre, University of Copenhagen Amager Hvidovre Hospitals, Italiensvej 1, DK-2300 Copenhagen S, Denmark
E-mail address: sbhau@dadlnet.dk

Endocrinol Metab Clin N Am 43 (2014) 697–708
http://dx.doi.org/10.1016/j.ecl.2014.06.004
0889-8529/14/$ – see front matter © 2014 Elsevier Inc. All rights reserved.

in this issue. As long as the beta cell can secrete sufficient insulin to overcome insulin resistance, plasma glucose excursions are kept within normal range. But if the insulin production and secretory machinery cannot match the required output, hyperglycemia and type 2 diabetes develop. In the case of severe insulin resistance, the call for adequate insulin secretion to keep a normoglycemic state may exceed tenfold that which is necessary if organ systems exhibit normal insulin sensitivity. The HIV-associated lipodystrophy syndrome (HALS) encompasses the phenotype of HIV-infected patients who loose subcutaneous adipose tissue in limps and face and accumulate intra-abdominal visceral adipose tissue.[1] HALS was seen after the introduction of combined antiretroviral therapy of nucleoside reverse transcriptase inhibitors (NRTIs) and protease inhibitors (PIs) almost 20 years ago.[2] HALS is related to insulin resistance through different mechanism, which, among several mechanisms includes alteration in insulin signaling in muscle tissue.[3] While HALS was observed in approximately half of those HIV-infected patients treated with first-generation PIs and first-generation NRTIs (in particular thymidine analogues), the incidence has decreased with introduction of new generations of antiretroviral drug combinations. Of interest, a recent cohort study has shown that newer antiretroviral regimes may not ameliorate HALS,[4] and this fact may have great impact on those patients who already exhibit HALS, because they may benefit little from a change in anti-HIV therapy. This interpretation of HALS being partially refractory to the newer less mitochondrial toxic NRTIs and newer less metabolic deteriorating PI regimens, however, must await further cohort studies. The fact that HIV-infected patients without prevalent comorbidities caused by modern antiretroviral therapy exhibit better prognosis than most well treated non-HIV infected type 2 diabetes patients in terms of life expectancy and quality of life should highlight the importance of the long-term metabolic impact of modern antiretroviral therapy.[5]

FIRST PHASE INSULIN SECRETION, PREHEPATIC INSULIN SECRETION, AND ITS REGULATION

An impaired first-phase insulin release after intravenous glucose may be an early sign of a defect in beta cell function.[6] An impaired first-phase insulin release in relation to the prevalent insulin sensitivity (ie, a reduction in disposition index [the product of first-phase insulin release and insulin sensitivity]) of approximately 50% was demonstrated in normoglycemic HALS patients compared with normoglycemic non-HALS patients.[7]

The first-pass extraction of insulin in HIV-infected patients is related to the prevalent insulin resistance and may vary from 30% to 80% of the amount of insulin secreted from the pancreatic islet cells.[8] C-peptide is secreted in equimolar amount to insulin and does not show-first pass extraction by the liver. Therefore, prehepatic insulin secretion rates can be calculated from plasma C-peptide measurements (eg, by use of the ISEC [Insulin SECretion]) computer program.[9] ISEC has been validated to calculate insulin secretion rates (ISRs) during an intravenous glucose tolerance test (IVGTT)[10,11] and has been applied to calculate ISR during a meal tolerance test, under a hyperinsulinemic euglycemic clamp, and during basal conditions.[9] The author and colleagues observed that an increased prehepatic insulin secretion in normoglycemic HALS patients was not down-regulated during a hyperinsulinemic clamp, which was preceded by an intravenous glucose bolus to stimulate endogenous insulin secretion.[12] By contrast, a control group of HIV-negative subjects, matched for insulin secretion and sensitivity to the HALS patients, showed a significant reduction in basal insulin secretion in that setting. Of interest, HALS patients showed a paradoxical positive correlation between the plasma insulin and prehepatic insulin secretion during the clamp, the latter correlating strongly with the nonglucose secretagogues in plasma (ie, triglyceride, alanine, and glucagon, respectively).[12] In a subsequent study, the author and colleagues could demonstrate that the nonglucose secretagogues plasma triglyceride, alanine, glucagon, lactate, and tumor necrosis factor alpha (TNF-α) were associated with alterations in the first-phase prehepatic insulin secretion response to intravenous glucose in normoglycemic HALS patients.[13] These data suggest a combination of dysregulation and insulin resistance of the insulin secreting beta cells in those patients with sustained increased prehepatic insulin secretion during exogenous insulin infusion. The data also highlight the potential role of nonglucose insulin secretagogues in dysregulation of insulin secretion in HIV-infected patients.

During an oral glucose tolerance test (OGTT), a group of HALS patients showed increased prehepatic insulin secretion, decreased insulin clearance, and insulin resistance compared with a control group of nonlipodystrophic HIV-infected patients on highly active antiretroviral therapy (HAART).[14] Because insulin responsiveness (ie, the change in insulin secretion per unit change in plasma glucose) was not increased in insulin-resistant HALS patients compared with their more insulin-sensitive nonlipodystrophic counterparts, HALS patients displayed an increased prevalence of glucose intolerance and diabetes.[14] That is, the product of insulin responsiveness to glucose (named B_{total}) and insulin sensitivity derived from an OGTT ($ISI_{composite}$) ie, the disposition index ([Di]), was significantly reduced in HALS patients compared with control subjects in that study.[14] In fact, the author and colleagues were able to demonstrate a significant hyperbolic correlation between B_{total} and $ISI_{composite}$ in those patients with normal glucose tolerance and a left shift in relation to the fitted curve of the patients with impaired glucose tolerance and diabetes mellitus.[14]

HEPATIC INSULIN EXTRACTION AND BETA CELL PROTECTION

In HIV-negative subjects, reduction of hepatic insulin extraction has been observed in insulin-resistant states.[15–17] By combining previously validated methods,[9,18–20] the author and colleagues were able to calculate hepatic extraction of insulin and posthepatic insulin clearance using data of prehepatic insulin secretion during fasting and during the steady state of a hyperinsulinemic clamp.[8] The author and colleagues showed that normoglycemic HALS patients display attenuated hepatic insulin extraction and posthepatic clearance rates in proportion to insulin resistance, which may be considered a beta-cell protective mechanism.[8] In accordance, by using prehepatic first-phase insulin release, estimated from the C-peptide concentration instead of plasma insulin concentrations, to calculate the Di as previously suggested,[21] the median of the Di in the previously mentioned study[7] was estimated to be decreased by 75% ($P<.01$) in HALS-patients compared with the control group of HIV-infected patients without lipodystrophy. This indicates that the beta cell cannot compensate for the concomitant insulin resistance in HALS patients. It may also be realized that a reduction in hepatic and systemic insulin clearance may contribute to the hyperinsulinemia of normoglycemic HALS patients.

DYSREGULATION OF INSULIN SECRETION IN HIV INFECTION AND ITS RELATION TO THE HALS PHENOTYPE

Dysregulation of insulin secretion in HALS patients may be of particular clinical significance for the insulin resistance and phenotype of these patients. First, increasing plasma insulin concentrations slightly throughout 3 days produced insulin resistance in HIV-negative healthy subjects.[22] Second, it was shown that hyperinsulinemia ($\sim$800 pM) in the setting of a hyperinsulinemic euglycemic clamp could increase TNF-α expression in subcutaneous fat, which was found to be significant within 2 hours of the onset of hyperinsulinemia.[23] HALS patients, and in particular those with impaired glucose tolerance, are likely to increase plasma insulin to this level (~800 pM) during an oral glucose tolerance test, reflecting a postprandial state.[24] It may be hypothesized that a dysregulation of insulin secretion, mediated in part by high levels of plasma triglyceride and other nonglucose insulin secretagogues,[12] would increase insulin resistance and postprandial insulin levels, resulting in an increase in expression of TNF-α from subcutaneous adipose tissue in HIV-infected patients receiving HAART. An increased TNF-α expression and increased local TNF-α production may suppress adiponectin[25] and peroxisome proliferator-activated receptor (PPAR)-γ[26] expression and production in this fat compartment, thereby promoting apoptosis. Thus, a vicious cycle would be established in such patients, leading to a lipodystrophic phenotype (**Fig. 1**).

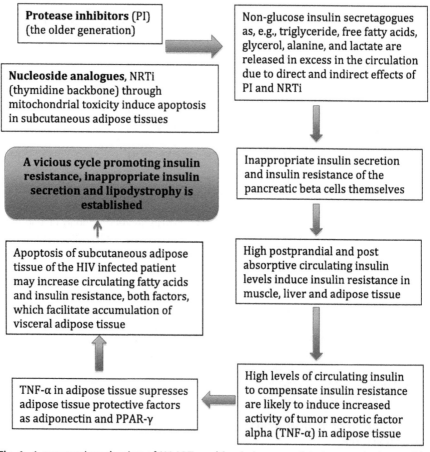

Fig. 1. A proposed mechanism of HAART resulting in inappropriate increased release of insulin, which may affect negatively on insulin sensitivity and adipose tissue distribution. It is postulated that excess release of nonglucose insulin secretagogues play a decisive role in dysregulation of insulin secretion, inducing insulin resistance in HIV-infected patients and promoting a phenotype of subcutaneous loss of adipose tissue and central visceral accumulation of adipose tissue, defining HALS.

EFFECT OF PIS AND NUCLEOSIDE ANALOGUES ON BETA CELL FUNCTION

In vitro experiments have shown that the PIs ritonavir, indinavir, amprenavir, and nelfinavir may directly reduce insulin secretion at the level of the beta cell.[27] This has also been demonstrated in vivo, where increased insulin resistance has not been met by increased insulin secretion due to PI therapy.[21,28] However, in a more recent study, ritonavir/lopinavir was not associated with increased insulin resistance or alteration in insulin secretion by using sensitive measures as the hyperinsulinemic hyperglycemic clamp technique.[29] It could be argued that this study only included 8 healthy volunteers, and the study duration was only 4 weeks; additionally, no control group was included. Of interest, the study showed a doubling of triglyceride level, and as triglyceride is a strong nonglucose insulin secretagogue, a defect in insulin secretion could have been masked by the insulin secretory stimulation effect of triglyceride. The level at which PIs may induce defects in the beta cell processing machinery has not been fully elucidated, but potassium and anion channels were inhibited by nelfinavir and ritonavir in an in vitro beta cell model.[30] In accordance with the author's in vivo data of insulin resistance of the beta cell itself, PIs may inhibit insulin signaling on the beta cell in vitro.[31] Chronic exposure to PIs, at least in vitro, may lead to apoptosis of beta cells.[32] In a clinical perspective, the reduction of insulin secretion by PIs may implicate increased demand and strain on beta cells, and cause an early perturbation in beta cell function and increased risk of impaired glucose tolerance.

The data on how different NRTIs may influence beta cell function in HIV-infected patients are indirect. Thus, the thymidine analogues stavudine and zidovudine are thought to be toxic to the mitochondrion in several tissues including muscle tissue[33] and adipose tissue,[34] where they may impose insulin resistance and apoptosis and increase risk of development of HALS. Apoptosis of adipose tissue secondary to thymidine analogues may increase lipolysis and circulating free fatty acids and glycerol, themselves nonglucose insulin secretagogues, leading to inappropriate insulin secretion. Also, increased lipolysis is associated with insulin resistance through several mechanisms, resulting in increased demand on the beta cell. Newer antiretroviral regimes avoiding thymidine analogues seem to be less toxic and may thus potentially improve beta cell function of HIV-infected patients compared with the older regimes.[35]

PROINSULIN PROCESSING AND SECRETION DEFECTS IN HIV

Normal function of the insulin-processing machinery in pancreatic beta cells is important for glucose homeostasis, because it facilitates an appropriate release of insulin.[36,37] Type 2 diabetes patients secrete an increased amount of intact proinsulin (IP) and 32–33 split proinsulin (SP), and the ratio of total proinsulin to insulin is increased, reflecting a defect in insulin processing.[38,39] In nondiabetic individuals, greater concentrations of IP and SP have been shown to be associated with an increased risk of developing type 2 diabetes.[40,41] Accordingly, insulin precursors are secreted in increased quantities in various states of insulin resistance.[42–44] Behrens and colleagues observed increased fasting total proinsulin and a disproportionally increased early release of total proinsulin relative to insulin during an OGTT in PI-treated compared with PI-naïve HIV-infected patients,[45] suggesting that PIs may cause hyperproinsulinemia. By contrast, Woerle and colleagues,[21] who examined HIV-infected patients before and following 12 weeks on PI therapy, found that PI treatment increased plasma insulin, whereas total proinsulin remained unchanged, consistent with the in vitro observation that PIs per se do not alter proinsulin processing in beta-cells.[46] The author and colleagues have found increased IP and SP in insulin-resistant normoglycemic HALS patients on HAART compared with their insulin-sensitive counterparts. They noted an inverse correlation between the SP/insulin ratio versus insulin sensitivity and the incremental total proinsulin/insulin ratio versus Di. Both of these observations may argue for a subtle beta cell dysfunction in normoglycemic HIV-infected patients on HAART with IR and low Di in that study.[47] This picture was reproduced during an oral glucose tolerance test, in which the ratio of total proinsulin to C-peptide was increased both during the early and late phases of the test in the normoglycemic insulin-resistant lipodystrophic HIV-infected patients compared with their normoglycemic insulin-sensitive nonlipodystrophic counterparts (**Fig. 2**).[48] These data are valid, because plasma C-peptide may be only weakly associated with insulin sensitivity of the individual.[10] Kinetics are linear over a wide range of plasma concentrations similar to that of proinsulin, and C-peptide and proinsulin do not show first-pass clearance in the liver.[49] The effect of PIs upon proinsulin

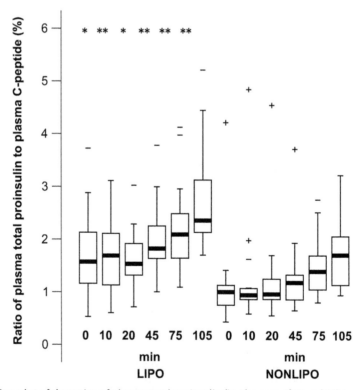

Fig. 2. Box-plot of the ratios of plasma total proinsulin (ie, the sum of IP and SP) to plasma C-peptide indicated for each time point during an OGTT, when these values were measured. Note that lipodystrophic patients (LIPO) are presented at the left side and nonlipodystrophic patients (NONLIPO) are presented at the right side of the panel. "−" indicates cases with values between 1.5 and 3 box lengths from the upper or lower edge of the box, whereas "+" indicates cases with values exceeding 3 box lengths. The box length is the interquartile range. * indicates P<.05, and ** indicates P<.01 for comparison between LIPO and NONLIPO. At each time point, the LIPO exhibit increased ratio of proinsulin compared with NONLIPO, indicative of defective insulin processing in the pancreatic beta cell during prandial stimulation of the beta cell in LIPO. (*From* Haugaard SB, Andersen O, Halsall I, et al. Impaired proinsulin secretion before and during oral glucose stimulation in HIV-infected patients who display fat redistribution. Metabolism 2007;56:943; with permission.)

processing, if any, is, most likely, indirect (ie, mediated through the metabolic pertur-bations induced by these drugs, eg, insulin resistance and dyslipidemia).[2,50]

INSULIN-LIKE GROWTH FACTORS, THEIR GLUCOSE REGULATORY ROLE, AND THEIR BETA CELL PROTECTIVE ACTION

The-insulin like growth factors IGF-I and IGF-II exhibit insulin-like effects and support insulin in improving glucose homeostasis.[51,52] Studies in HIV-infected patients on HAART have revealed that total IGF-I is similar in patients with and without lipodystro-phy,[53–55] despite reduced growth hormone (GH) secretion during night[55] and reduced GH rebound after a glucose challenge in lipodystrophic patients.[56] The author and col-leagues have observed that the correlation between total and free IGF-I is strong in HIV-infected patients on HAART,[53] which was also found during treatment with growth hormone (0.7 mg/d) of such patients.[57] Taken together, total IGF-I may be a strong marker for free IGF-I in HIV-infected patients on HAART. On a molar basis, the potency of free IGF-I and free IGF-II on glucose disposal is approximately 6% of that of insu-lin.[51,58] Because serum concentrations of free IGF-I plus free IGF-II ranged from 200 to 350 pmol/L in both lipodystrophic and nonlipodystrophic HIV-infected patients on HAART, this would be equivalent to insulin concentrations of 12 to 21 pmol/L, which corresponds to approximately 15% to 25% of the fasting plasma insulin concentration of the insulin-resistant lipodystrophic patients in that study.[53] These data are in sup-port of a glucose homeostatic role for IGF-I and IGF-II, at least during fasting. More-over, IGF binding proteins 1 and 2 were reduced in insulin-resistant HIV-infected (lipodystrophic) patients.[53] This might be a physiologic regulator mechanism to pro-vide higher levels of free IGF-I and free IGF-II. Indeed, the author and colleagues found that both IGF binding proteins 1 and 2 correlated positively with insulin sensitivity in that study,[53] which may be considered consistent with the hypothesis that these IGF binding proteins are gluco-regulators.[59] Finally, it was observed in that study that IGF binding protein 3 protease was not increased in insulin-resistant HALS pa-tients compared with nonlipodystrophic HIV-infected patients on HAART and healthy control subjects.[53] However, IGF binding protein 3 protease was inversely correlated with IGF binding protein 3, the main binding protein for IGF-I. By controlling for strong covariates for free IGF-I (ie, IGF binding protein 3 and total IGF-I), it was found that IGF binding protein 3 protease correlated positively with free IGF-I in HALS patients. This would suggest that this protease may play a role for the relative amount of free IGF-I in these patients, which is in agreement with the general opinion of the physiologic significance of IGF binding protein 3 protease.[60]

INCRETIN HORMONES

To the author's knowledge, only 1 study has addressed the issue of incretin hormone secretion and action in HIV-infected patients on HAART.[61] This is surprising, inasmuch as the incretin hormones, glucagon-like peptide-1 (GLP-1), and glucose-dependent insulinotropic polypeptide (GIP) are responsible for as much as half of meal-induced insulin release in healthy subjects[62] and therefore play important roles in glucose ho-meostasis in people. GLP-1 analogues are used as therapeutics in type 2 diabetes where they improve beta cell function and reduce insulin resistance through several pathways.[63] Glucose-intolerant HIV-infected patients on HAART were found to display a more pronounced GLP-1 response to an oral glucose challenge (75 g) compared with their counterparts with normal glucose tolerance; this could represent a compen-satory mechanism.[61] Moreover, in that study, the number of lipodystrophic patients was greater in the group with impaired glucose tolerance, which may indicate that

HIV lipodystrophy per se does not produce impairment in GLP-1 release. GIP secretion did not differ between patients with normal and impaired glucose tolerance.[61] However, GIP secretion was positively correlated with insulin secretion, which was found to be independent of plasma glucose during the OGTT,[61] and it was hypothesized that GIP may improve insulin secretion in HIV-infected patients on HAART, because GIP has been shown to stimulate insulin secretion and lead to cellular proliferation of insulin-producing cells.[61,64] It remains to be examined whether specific antiretroviral drugs may impact acutely on incretin hormone release, thereby influencing insulin release through this pathway.

In therapeutic terms, the incretin hormones are likely to restore a number of the beta cell pathophysiological perturbations of HIV-infected patients. At least the GLP-1 analogues deserve clinical trials to address their possible therapeutic option on metabolic complications related to modern anti-HIV therapy. Until now, only casuistic observations exist on their use in HIV-infected patients with type 2 diabetes.[65,66] A safety trial on the dipeptidyl 4 inhibitor sitagliptin, a facilitator of endogenous incretins, showed that this drug improved glucose tolerance and was safe in respect to viral suppression and CD4+ T lymphocyte number.[67] In that study, however, no data were provided on the effects of sitagliptin on insulin secretion and prehepatic insulin secretion in relation to insulin sensitivity. Also, no data on the effect of sitagliptin on lipid metabolism were obtained in that study.

CONCLUSIVE REMARKS

Impaired regulation of insulin secretion may in part explain hyperinsulinemia in HIV patients on HAART and in particular those who exhibit HALS. Dysregulation of insulin secretion in these patients could be a direct effect of the PIs but also a product of an inappropriate increased concentration of the nonglucose secretagogues (eg, circulating triglyceride, TNF-α, alanine, and lactate, associated with HALS and PI therapy). Apoptosis of adipose tissue secondary to toxic effect of thymidine NRTI may also contribute to increasing nonglucose secretagogues. Evidence of insulin resistance at the level of the beta cell itself has been demonstrated in patients with HALS. Defects in the insulin processing machinery are early findings in HALS patients, already observed in those with a normal glucose tolerance. Although hepatic extraction of insulin and metabolic clearance of insulin seem to correlate to insulin sensitivity in HIV-infected patients, this may indirectly lead to hyperinsulinemia and insulin resistance. Insulin-like growth-factors may contribute as much as 25% to the insulin effect in the fasting state in HIV-infected patients and the regulation of their associated binding proteins appears to work appropriately. The incretin system and its regulation in HIV-infected patients have been sparsely studied. Given the importance of incretins in glucose homeostasis and insulin secretion, it should be an area of future research.

ACKNOWLEDGMENTS

I'm indebted to Professor Sten Madsbad and Associate Professor, Research Director Ove Andersen for strong support through the years, including fruitful discussions on metabolic research, HIV-associated lipodystrophy syndrome, and clinical trials.

REFERENCES

1. Carr A, Emery S, Law M, et al. An objective case definition of lipodystrophy in HIV-infected adults: a case–control study. Lancet 2003;361:726–35.

2. Carr A, Samaras K, Burton S, et al. A syndrome of peripheral lipodystrophy, hyperlipidaemia and insulin resistance in patients receiving HIV protease inhibitors. AIDS 1998;12:F51–8.
3. Haugaard SB, Andersen O, Madsbad S, et al. Skeletal muscle insulin signaling defects downstream of phosphatidylinositol 3-kinase at the level of Akt are associated with impaired nonoxidative glucose disposal in HIV lipodystrophy. Diabetes 2005;54:3474–83.
4. Guaraldi G, Stentarelli C, Zona S, et al. The natural history of HIV-associated lipodystrophy in the changing scenario of HIV infection. HIV Med 2014. [Epub ahead of print].
5. Obel N, Omland LH, Kronborg G, et al. Impact of non-HIV and HIV risk factors on survival in HIV-infected patients on HAART: a population-based nationwide cohort study. PLoS One 2011;6:e22698.
6. Kahn SE, Prigeon RL, McCulloch DK, et al. Quantification of the relationship between insulin sensitivity and beta- cell function in human subjects. Evidence for a hyperbolic function. Diabetes 1993;42:1663–72.
7. Haugaard SB, Andersen O, Dela F, et al. Defective glucose and lipid metabolism in human immunodeficiency virus-infected patients with lipodystrophy involve liver, muscle tissue and pancreatic beta-cells. Eur J Endocrinol 2005;152:103–12.
8. Haugaard SB, Andersen O, Hansen BR, et al. In nondiabetic, human immunodeficiency virus-infected patients with lipodystrophy, hepatic insulin extraction and posthepatic insulin clearance rate are decreased in proportion to insulin resistance. Metabolism 2005;54:171–9.
9. Hovorka R, Soons PA, Young MA. ISEC: a program to calculate insulin secretion. Comput Methods Programs Biomed 1996;50:253–64.
10. Hovorka R, Koukkou E, Southerden D, et al. Measuring pre-hepatic insulin secretion using a population model of C- peptide kinetics: accuracy and required sampling schedule. Diabetologia 1998;41:548–54.
11. Kjems LL, Volund A, Madsbad S. Quantification of beta-cell function during IVGTT in type II and non- diabetic subjects: assessment of insulin secretion by mathematical methods. Diabetologia 2001;44:1339–48.
12. Haugaard SB, Andersen O, Storgaard H, et al. Insulin secretion in lipodystrophic HIV-infected patients is associated with high levels of nonglucose secretagogues and insulin resistance of beta-cells. Am J Physiol Endocrinol Metab 2004;287:E677–85.
13. Haugaard SB, Andersen O, Pedersen SB, et al. Glucose-stimulated prehepatic insulin secretion is associated with circulating alanine, triglyceride, glucagon, lactate and TNF-alpha in patients with HIV-lipodystrophy. HIV Med 2006;7:163–72.
14. Haugaard SB, Andersen O, Volund A, et al. Beta-cell dysfunction and low insulin clearance in insulin-resistant human immunodeficiency virus (HIV)-infected patients with lipodystrophy. Clin Endocrinol (Oxf) 2005;62:354–61.
15. Faber OK, Christensen K, Kehlet H, et al. Decreased insulin removal contributes to hyperinsulinemia in obesity. J Clin Endocrinol Metab 1981;53:618–21.
16. Peiris AN, Mueller RA, Smith GA, et al. Splanchnic insulin metabolism in obesity. Influence of body fat distribution. J Clin Invest 1986;78:1648–57.
17. Rossell R, Gomis R, Casamitjana R, et al. Reduced hepatic insulin extraction in obesity: relationship with plasma insulin levels. J Clin Endocrinol Metab 1983;56:608–11.
18. Iozzo P, Beck-Nielsen H, Laakso M, et al. Independent influence of age on basal insulin secretion in nondiabetic humans. European Group for the Study of Insulin Resistance. J Clin Endocrinol Metab 1999;84:863–8.

19. Polonsky KS, Given BD, Hirsch L, et al. Quantitative study of insulin secretion and clearance in normal and obese subjects. J Clin Invest 1988;81:435–41.

20. Van Cauter E, Mestrez F, Sturis J, et al. Estimation of insulin secretion rates from C-peptide levels. Comparison of individual and standard kinetic parameters for C-peptide clearance. Diabetes 1992;41:368–77.

21. Woerle HJ, Mariuz PR, Meyer C, et al. Mechanisms for the deterioration in glucose tolerance associated with HIV protease inhibitor regimens. Diabetes 2003;52:918–25.

22. Iozzo P, Pratipanawatr T, Pijl H, et al. Physiological hyperinsulinemia impairs insulin-stimulated glycogen synthase activity and glycogen synthesis. Am J Physiol Endocrinol Metab 2001;280:E712–9.

23. Krogh-Madsen R, Plomgaard P, Keller P, et al. Insulin stimulates interleukin-6 and tumor necrosis factor-alpha gene expression in human subcutaneous adipose tissue. Am J Physiol Endocrinol Metab 2004;286:E234–8.

24. Haugaard SB. Toxic metabolic syndrome associated with HAART. Expert Opin Drug Metab Toxicol 2006;2:429–45.

25. Lihn AS, Richelsen B, Pedersen SB, et al. Increased expression of TNF-{alpha}, IL-6, and IL-8 in HALS: implications for reduced adiponectin expression and plasma levels. Am J Physiol Endocrinol Metab 2003;285:E1072–80.

26. Bastard JP, Caron M, Vidal H, et al. Association between altered expression of adipogenic factor SREBP1 in lipoatrophic adipose tissue from HIV-1-infected patients and abnormal adipocyte differentiation and insulin resistance. Lancet 2002;359:1026–31.

27. Koster JC, Remedi MS, Qiu H, et al. HIV protease inhibitors acutely impair glucose-stimulated insulin release. Diabetes 2003;52:1695–700.

28. Dube MP, Edmondson-Melancon H, Qian D, et al. Prospective evaluation of the effect of initiating indinavir-based therapy on insulin sensitivity and B-cell function in HIV-infected patients. J Acquir Immune Defic Syndr 2001;27:130–4.

29. Pao VY, Lee GA, Taylor S, et al. The protease inhibitor combination lopinavir/ritonavir does not decrease insulin secretion in healthy, HIV-seronegative volunteers. AIDS 2010;24:265–70.

30. Neye Y, Dufer M, Drews G, et al. HIV protease inhibitors: suppression of insulin secretion by inhibition of voltage-dependent K+ currents and anion currents. J Pharmacol Exp Ther 2006;316:106–12.

31. Schutt M, Zhou J, Meier M, et al. Long-term effects of HIV-1 protease inhibitors on insulin secretion and insulin signaling in INS-1 beta cells. J Endocrinol 2004; 183:445–54.

32. Zhang S, Carper MJ, Lei X, et al. Protease inhibitors used in the treatment of HIV+ induce beta-cell apoptosis via the mitochondrial pathway and compromise insulin secretion. Am J Physiol Endocrinol Metab 2009;296:E925–35.

33. Haugaard SB, Andersen O, Pedersen SB, et al. Depleted skeletal muscle mitochondrial DNA, hyperlactatemia, and decreased oxidative capacity in HIV-infected patients on highly active antiretroviral therapy. J Med Virol 2005;77: 29–38.

34. Lagathu C, Eustace B, Prot M, et al. Some HIV antiretrovirals increase oxidative stress and alter chemokine, cytokine or adiponectin production in human adipocytes and macrophages. Antivir Ther 2007;12:489–500.

35. Curran A, Ribera E. From old to new nucleoside reverse transcriptase inhibitors: changes in body fat composition, metabolic parameters and mitochondrial toxicity after the switch from thymidine analogs to tenofovir or abacavir. Expert Opin Drug Saf 2011;10:389–406.

36. Halban PA. Proinsulin processing in the regulated and the constitutive secretory pathway. Diabetologia 1994;37(Suppl 2):S65–72.
37. Hales CN. The pathogenesis of NIDDM. Diabetologia 1994;37(Suppl 2):S162–8.
38. Kahn SE, Halban PA. Release of incompletely processed proinsulin is the cause of the disproportionate proinsulinemia of NIDDM. Diabetes 1997;46:1725–32.
39. Ostrega D, Polonsky K, Nagi D, et al. Measurement of proinsulin and intermediates. Validation of immunoassay methods by high-performance liquid chromatography. Diabetes 1995;44:437–40.
40. Wareham NJ, Byrne CD, Williams R, et al. Fasting proinsulin concentrations predict the development of type 2 diabetes. Diabetes Care 1999;22:262–70.
41. Zethelius B, Byberg L, Hales CN, et al. Proinsulin and acute insulin response independently predict type 2 diabetes mellitus in men—report from 27 years of follow-up study. Diabetologia 2003;46:20–6.
42. Heaton DA, Millward BA, Gray IP, et al. Increased proinsulin levels as an early indicator of B-cell dysfunction in non-diabetic twins of type 1 (insulin-dependent) diabetic patients. Diabetologia 1988;31:182–4.
43. Kahn SE, Horber FF, Prigeon RL, et al. Effect of glucocorticoid and growth hormone treatment on proinsulin levels in humans. Diabetes 1993;42:1082–5.
44. Ward WK, LaCava EC, Paquette TL, et al. Disproportionate elevation of immunoreactive proinsulin in type 2 (non-insulin-dependent) diabetes mellitus and in experimental insulin resistance. Diabetologia 1987;30:698–702.
45. Behrens G, Dejam A, Schmidt H, et al. Impaired glucose tolerance, beta cell function and lipid metabolism in HIV patients under treatment with protease inhibitors. AIDS 1999;13:F63–70.
46. Danoff A, Ling WL. Protease inhibitors do not interfere with prohormone processing. Ann Intern Med 2000;132:330.
47. Haugaard SB, Andersen O, Hales CN, et al. Hyperproinsulinaemia in normoglycaemic lipodystrophic HIV-infected patients. Eur J Clin Invest 2006;36:436–45.
48. Haugaard SB, Andersen O, Halsall I, et al. Impaired proinsulin secretion before and during oral glucose stimulation in HIV-infected patients who display fat redistribution. Metabolism 2007;56:939–46.
49. Tillil H, Frank BH, Pekar AH, et al. Hypoglycemic potency and metabolic clearance rate of intravenously administered human proinsulin and metabolites. Endocrinology 1990;127:2418–22.
50. Saves M, Raffi F, Capeau J, et al. Factors related to lipodystrophy and metabolic alterations in patients with human immunodeficiency virus infection receiving highly active antiretroviral therapy. Clin Infect Dis 2002;34:1396–405.
51. Guler HP, Zapf J, Froesch ER. Short-term metabolic effects of recombinant human insulin-like growth factor I in healthy adults. N Engl J Med 1987;317:137–40.
52. Zierath JR, Bang P, Galuska D, et al. Insulin-like growth factor II stimulates glucose transport in human skeletal muscle. FEBS Lett 1992;307:379–82.
53. Haugaard SB, Andersen O, Hansen BR, et al. Insulin-like growth factors, insulin-like growth factor-binding proteins, insulin-like growth factor-binding protein-3 protease, and growth hormone-binding protein in lipodystrophic human immunodeficiency virus-infected patients. Metabolism 2004;53:1565–73.
54. Koutkia P, Meininger G, Canavan B, et al. Metabolic regulation of growth hormone by free fatty acids, somatostatin, and ghrelin in HIV-lipodystrophy. Am J Physiol Endocrinol Metab 2004;286:E296–303.
55. Rietschel P, Hadigan C, Corcoran C, et al. Assessment of growth hormone dynamics in human immunodeficiency virus-related lipodystrophy. J Clin Endocrinol Metab 2001;86:504–10.

56. Andersen O, Haugaard SB, Hansen BR, et al. Different growth hormone sensitivity of target tissues and growth hormone response to glucose in HIV-infected patients with and without lipodystrophy. Scand J Infect Dis 2004;36:832–9.

57. Haugaard SB, Andersen O, Flyvbjerg A, et al. Growth factors, glucose and insulin kinetics after low dose growth hormone therapy in HIV-lipodystrophy. J Infect 2005;52(6):389–98.

58. Frystyk J, Vestbo E, Skjaerbaek C, et al. Free insulin-like growth factors in human obesity. Metabolism 1995;44:37–44.

59. Baxter RC. Insulin-like growth factor binding proteins as glucoregulators. Metabolism 1995;44:12–7.

60. Skjaerbaek C, Frystyk J, Orskov H, et al. Differential changes in free and total insulin-like growth factor I after major, elective abdominal surgery: the possible role of insulin-like growth factor-binding protein-3 proteolysis. J Clin Endocrinol Metab 1998;83:2445–9.

61. Andersen O, Haugaard SB, Holst JJ, et al. Enhanced glucagon-like peptide-1 (GLP-1) response to oral glucose in glucose-intolerant HIV-infected patients on antiretroviral therapy. HIV Med 2005;6:91–8.

62. Nauck MA, Bartels E, Orskov C, et al. Additive insulinotropic effects of exogenous synthetic human gastric inhibitory polypeptide and glucagon-like peptide-1-(7-36) amide infused at near-physiological insulinotropic hormone and glucose concentrations. J Clin Endocrinol Metab 1993;76:912–7.

63. Mudaliar S, Henry RR. Effects of incretin hormones on beta-cell mass and function, body weight, and hepatic and myocardial function. Am J Med 2010;123: S19–27.

64. Trumper A, Trumper K, Trusheim H, et al. Glucose-dependent insulinotropic polypeptide is a growth factor for beta (INS-1) cells by pleiotropic signaling. Mol Endocrinol 2001;15:1559–70.

65. Diamant M, van AM. Liraglutide treatment in a patient with HIV and uncontrolled insulin-treated type 2 diabetes. Diabetes Care 2012;35:e34.

66. Oriot P, Hermans MP, Selvais P, et al. Exenatide improves weight loss insulin sensitivity and beta-cell function following administration to a type 2 diabetic HIV patient on antiretroviral therapy. Ann Endocrinol (Paris) 2011;72:244–6.

67. Goodwin SR, Reeds DN, Royal M, et al. Dipeptidyl peptidase IV inhibition does not adversely affect immune or virological status in HIV infected men and women: a pilot safety study. J Clin Endocrinol Metab 2013;98:743–51.

Hypogonadism in the HIV-Infected Man

Vincenzo Rochira, MD, PhD[a,b,*], Giovanni Guaraldi, MD, PhD[c]

KEYWORDS

- Androgen deficiency • Testosterone • LH • Gonadotropins • Premature aging
- Antiretroviral therapy • SHBG • Health status

KEY POINTS

- Hypogonadism is common and occurs prematurely in human immunodeficiency virus (HIV)-infected men, the prevalence being around 25% in young to middle-aged men with HIV.
- Hypogonadotropic hypogonadism due to hypothalamic-pituitary dysfunction is more frequent than primary hypergonadotropic hypogonadism in HIV-infected men.
- Signs and symptoms of hypogonadism become less specific in men with HIV because of the overlap with signs and symptoms of the HIV infection and do not help in ruling out the diagnosis.
- Total testosterone (T), luteinizing hormone (LH), sex hormone–binding globulin (SHBG) for calculated free T are the best assays for the detection of T deficiency.
- HIV-infected men with severe serum T deficiency and those with mild hypogonadism coupled with signs and symptoms of T deficiency may benefit from T replacement treatment.

INTRODUCTION

Since the first cases of HIV infection and AIDS were described, reports have been made of male hypogonadism among these patients.[1,2] With the increasing burden of the HIV epidemic, male hypogonadism[2] and adrenal insufficiency[3] became the most common endocrine diseases diagnosed and managed in the AIDS clinics.

Disclosure: The authors have nothing to disclose.
[a] Unit of Endocrinology, Department of Biomedical, Metabolic and Neural Sciences, University of Modena and Reggio Emilia, Modena, Italy; [b] Azienda USL of Modena, Modena, Italy; [c] Infectious and Tropical Disease Unit, Department of Medical and Surgical Sciences of Mother, Child and Adult, Metabolic Clinic, University of Modena and Reggio Emilia, Via del Pozzo 71, Modena 41124, Italy
* Corresponding author. Unit of Endocrinology, NOCSAE, Via P. Giardini 1355, Modena 41126, Italy.
E-mail address: rochira.vincenzo@unimore.it

Endocrinol Metab Clin N Am 43 (2014) 709–730
http://dx.doi.org/10.1016/j.ecl.2014.06.005
endo.theclinics.com

Hence, T treatment started to be offered to HIV-infected men, especially those with AIDS wasting syndrome.[4]

In the mid-1990s, the debut of highly active antiretroviral therapy (HAART) led to a stop of disease progression to AIDS and a marked reduction of HIV-associated mortality.[5,6] Notwithstanding the changes observed in the natural history of the disease, T deficiency continues to be diagnosed in HIV-infected men.

EPIDEMIOLOGY

The reported prevalence of hypogonadism among HIV-infected men varies depending on both the definition and the type of T measurement used and study dates. Since the introduction of HAART, HIV-infected men are living longer and their health status has improved in accordance with the changed spectrum of comorbidities.[5,6] For that reason, prevalence data of male hypogonadism are reported here according to the pre-HAART and post-HAART periods.

Prevalence of Male Hypogonadism in the Pre-HAART Era

Several studies investigated the prevalence of male hypogonadism among HIV-infected men,[2,7–13] with differing results (**Table 1**). These differences are likely due to heterogeneous methods used for the diagnosis of male hypogonadism, such as the use of arbitrary diagnostic criteria or different cutoff ranges of serum total T (270–400 ng/dL) (see **Table 1**).[2,9–13] At that time, specific cutoff values for the diagnosis of male hypogonadism were not available even in the general population. Based on all published data, the prevalence of hypogonadism in men with HIV infection was about 30% to 40% based on the result of an a posteriori estimate (see **Table 1**).

Other methodological aspects, such as blood sampling outside of standard early morning testing[2,7,10,12] or the small patient sample size,[7,8,12] may also have contributed to such a wide variance of prevalence rates (see **Table 1**).

The studies that investigated serum circulating gonadotropins found inappropriately normal LH serum levels despite low T (hypogonadotropic hypogonadism)[2,9,11,13] or elevated serum LH levels (hypergonadotropic hypogonadism).[7,12,14]

High frequency of male hypogonadism was almost always associated with the progression of HIV infection to AIDS.[9,12]

Finally, only one study reported higher serum T levels in HIV-infected men than in HIV-uninfected men.[15]

Prevalence of Male Hypogonadism in the HAART Era

The benefits of HAART treatment on the health status of men living with HIV resulted in a clear reduction of the occurrence of hypogonadism (**Table 2**). In the past, AIDS led to poor general clinical conditions because of wasting syndrome, a severe clinical condition, and opportunistic infections.[16] It is not possible to establish with certainty whether there has been a true decline in disease prevalence because data available from the pre-HAART and HAART period are not fully comparable. Several larger studies on male hypogonadism in HIV became available in the last 2 decades (see **Table 2**). Furthermore, more accurate methods for the measurement of androgens became available,[17] and guidelines provided criteria for the diagnosis of hypogonadism based on serum T levels (see following paragraphs for details).[18]

Current estimates of the prevalence of male hypogonadism in HIV-infected men generally range from 13% to 40% according to different study settings,[19–30] with a few studies reporting lower (3%–6%)[31,32] or higher (about 60%) prevalence rates (see **Table 2**).[33–35] The persistent elevation in the percentage of men with low serum

Table 1
Prevalence of hypogonadism in HIV-infected men in the pre-HAART era according to data available in the literature

Authors, Year	Number of HIV Patients	Age Range (y)	Mean Age (y)	Prevalence of Hypogonadism (%)	Diagnostic Criteria of Hypogonadism			Journal
					Serum T	LH	Morning T	
Dobs et al,[2] 1988[a]	70	NA	37	38	Total T<360 ng/dL	Yes	No	Am J Med
Croxson et al,[7] 1989[a]	59	21–44	33[b]	~65	Total T < mean total T in HIV-uninfected controls	Yes	No	JCE&M
Villette et al,[8] 1990[a]	13	21–54	30	NA	Total T < mean total T in HIV-uninfected controls	No	Yes	JCE&M
Raffi et al,[9] 1991[a]	67	NA	NA	14	Total T<300 ng/dL	Yes	Yes	AIDS
Wagner et al,[10] 1995[a]	234	22–67	40	38	Total T<400 ng/dL	No	NA	J Acquir Immune Defic Syndr Hum Retrovirol
Grinspoon et al,[11] 1996[a]	77	NA	39	26 (49) [25]	Total T<270 ng/dL (free T<12 pg/mL) [Total T<270 ng/dL & free T<12 pg/mL]	Yes	Yes	JCE&M
Salehian et al,[12] 1999[a]	56	NA	34	43	Total T<350 ng/dL	Yes	NA	Endocr Pract
Arver et al,[13] 1999[a]	148	23–66	40	32	Total T<275 ng/dL	Yes	NA	J Androl

Abbreviation: NA, data not available.
[a] Prospective studies.
[b] Median.
Data from Refs.[2,7–13]

Table 2
Prevalence of hypogonadism in HIV-infected men treated with HAART according to data available in the literature

Authors, Year	Number of Patients	Age Range (y)	Mean Age (y)	Prevalence of Hypogonadism (%)	Serum T	LH	Morning T	Journal
Berger et al,[19] 1998[a]	127	21–54	37	17	Total T<194 ng/dL and/or free T<34 pg/mL[b]	No	Not known	12th World AIDS Conference Abstracts
Rietschel et al,[20] 2000[c]	90	NA	~40	21	free T<12 pg/mL[b]	No	Not known	Clin Infect Dis
Fisher et al,[21] 2000[a]	88	21–63	40	20	free T<12 pg/mL[b]	No	Not known	Int. Conference on AIDS 2000 Abstracts
Klein et al,[33] 2005[c]	275	49–74	~54	54	Total T<300 ng/dL	Yes	No	Clin Infect Dis
Dubè et al,[31] 2007[c]	213	32–44	37[d]	6	Total T<260 ng/dL	No	Not in all patients	Clin Infect Dis
Crum-Cianflone et al,[22] 2007[c]	296	19–72	39	17	Total T<300 ng/dL	Not in all	Yes	Aids Patient Care STDs
Wunder et al,[34] 2008[c]	97	35–45	~40[d]	60	Free T within the age-adjusted normal range[b]	Yes	No	HIV Med
Collazos et al,[32] 2009[e]	188	33.5–38.6	35.8[d]	3	Total T<260 ng/dL	Yes	No	JIAPAC
Moreno-Perez et al,[23] 2010[c]	90	25–68	42	13	Calculated free T<63.6 pg/mL	Yes	Yes	J Sex Med

					Definition of hypogonadism			Journal
Rochira et al,[24] 2011[c]	1325	20–69	45[d]	16 (30)	Total T<300 ng/dL (including patients with Total T≥300 ng/dL, but elevated LH)	Yes	Yes	PLoS One
Pepe et al,[25] 2012[c]	50	40–69	48	26	Calculated free T<64.8 pg/mL	Yes	Yes	Clin Endocrinol
Amini Lari et al,[35] 2012[c]	237	22–63	37	68	free T<4.5 pg/mL[b]	Yes	Yes	AIDS Behav
Monroe et al,[26] 2012[f]	175	18–65	44	25	free T<52 pg[g]	No	Not known	J Mens Health
Sunchatawirul et al,[27] 2012[c]	491	34–44	37[d]	25	Calculated free T<64.8 pg/mL	No	Yes	Int J STD AIDS
De Ryck et al,[28] 2013[c]	49[h]	41–54	49	37	Calculated free T<64.8 pg/mL	No	Yes	J Sex Med
Blick 2013 et al,[29] 2013[c]	401	43–53	48	41	Total T<300 ng/dL or Calculated free T<50 pg/mL plus 1 or more symptoms of hypogonadism	No	NA	Postgrad Med
Monroe et al,[30] 2014[c]	364	NA	48[d]	24	Total T<300 ng/dL or calculated free T<50 pg/mL	No	Yes	AIDS Res Ther

Abbreviation: NA, data not available.
[a] Retrospective studies based on chart review.
[b] Direct free T measurement with commercially available kits.
[c] Prospective studies.
[d] Median.
[e] Retrospective studies.
[f] Type of study not clear.
[g] Free T measured by equilibrium dialysis.
[h] A subset of patients all with erectile dysfunction.
Data from Refs.[19–35]

T levels is even more pronounced when compared with data obtained from HIV-uninfected subjects, especially in consideration of the young age of some men with HIV and hypogonadism.[24] Hypogonadism in HIV-uninfected men is generally a disease occurring later in life. The 20% to 30% prevalence of hypogonadism in HIV-uninfected men older than 50 years is similar to that found in younger HIV-infected men.[36–38] In the presence of HIV infection, hypogonadism is common in young to middle-aged men, occurring even in men aged 20 to 40 years, as evident by the mean age of all the cohorts studied both in the pre-HAART (see **Table 1**) and HAART (see **Table 2**) eras.[24] Conversely, hypogonadism is a rare disease before the age of 40 years in HIV-uninfected men.[39]

In general, most of the studies on hypogonadism in men living with HIV have several limitations related to sample size or methods used. In particular, the overall prevalence of hypogonadism in men with HIV is known, but little is known about its stratification in antiretroviral-naive patients or in patients administered with different HAART schemes. In HAART-naive patients, the prevalence of male hypogonadism remains absolutely controversial, ranging from 6%[31] to 71%[34] in 213 and 97 HIV-infected men, respectively (see **Table 2**).

The small number of subjects ($n<100$) enrolled in some studies does not allow precise determination of the true prevalence rate.[20,21,23,25,28,34] At present, only 4 studies were performed on more than 300 HIV-infected patients,[24,27,29,30] and all fixed a prevalence of hypogonadism around 25%. These 4 studies did not suffer from bias due to blood sampling timing, hormonal assays, and retrospective design of the study (see **Table 2**). Conversely, several pitfalls, such as blood sampling not drawn at early morning,[19–21,26,28,31–34] the use of highly inaccurate assays for direct measurement of free serum T level alone[20,21,34,35] or absolutely arbitrary thresholds,[34,35] and the retrospective analysis of data,[21,32] make the result less reliable in most of the studies and support the idea that a researcher expert in male hypogonadism had been not involved in designing the study, as also confirmed by the publication of the results mainly in journals of the infectious disease area (see **Table 2**).

PATHOGENESIS OF MALE HYPOGONADISM IN MEN WITH HIV

The pathogenesis of hypogonadism in HIV-infected men remains unclear. Hypothesis on the underlying causes and mechanisms have been provided based on some well-recognized pathophysiologic phenomena, but their cause-effect relationships need to be substantiated by further evidence.[40] The authors provide the state of the art on known risk factors and predictor of T deficiency, as well as on pathophysiologic issues that contribute the genesis of hypogonadism in men with HIV infection.

Risk Factors and Predictors of T Deficiency

Among the classical factors correlated with hypogonadism in HIV-uninfected men, most, such as age, body mass index, weight, indexes of visceral adiposity, alcohol consumption, cigarette smoking, and sedentary lifestyle, were only weakly[22–24,26,27,33] or not[19] associated with low serum T levels (**Box 1**). Even diabetes, prediabetes, serum circulating lipids, hypertension,[26,27,41] and several indexes of subclinical cardiovascular diseases such as coronary artery calcification and carotid intima-media thickness[42] do not predict T deficiency (see **Box 1**). Again, no significant association has been found between serum T levels and drugs used in combination within HAART schemes or parameters of HIV infection (like viral load or CD4 count) (see **Box 1**).[22,24,27]

Box 1
Factors involved in the pathogenesis of male hypogonadism in HIV-infected men and main pathophysiologic mechanisms

Risk factors and predictors of T deficiency

Classical

Age, BMI, weight, waist circumference, visceral adiposity, ethnicity, alcohol, cigarette smoking, sedentary lifestyle, metabolic syndrome, hypertension, diabetes

HIV related

HAART duration, HIV infection duration, lipodystrophy

HIV-related comorbidities

HBV or HCV coinfection, NAFLD, opiates, poor health status, testicular opportunistic infections

Abbreviations: BMI, body mass index; HBV, hepatitis virus B; HCV, hepatitis virus C; NAFLD, nonalcoholic fatty liver disease.

Ethnicity, longer duration of HIV infection, use of injection drugs, and hepatitis C and/or B coinfection seem to be only slightly associated with lower serum T levels in several studies (see **Box 1**).[21,23,26,27,33,35]

That classical risk factors for hypogonadism are not associated with decreased serum T levels does not mean that these factors do not contribute to hypogonadism but simply implies that multiple elements involved in the genesis of hypogonadism coexist in the setting of HIV,[24] which means that each component masks, at least in part, the effects of the others, thus weakening their weight on a statistical point of view, thus suggesting that the pathogenesis of hypogonadism in HIV-infected men is multifactorial.

Pathophysiology of Male Hypogonadism in HIV Infection

Both secondary hypogonadism, due to hypothalamic-pituitary dysfunction, and primary hypogonadism, due to testicular failure, have been described in men with HIV. Secondary (hypogonadotropic) hypogonadism is characterized by reduced or normal levels of circulating gonadotropins, whereas primary (hypergonadotropic) hypogonadism is characterized by increased levels of gonadotropins (**Fig. 1**).

Secondary hypogonadism in men with HIV

Since the first observation of male hypogonadism in patients with HIV/AIDS, researchers pointed their attention to possible causes of T deficiency. In the pre-HAART era, secondary hypogonadism due to hypothalamic-pituitary dysfunction was more frequent than primary hypogonadism due to testicular failure in HIV-infected men.[2,9,11,13,14]

The same results have been obtained from the few studies carried out during HAART treatment in which gonadotropin measurement is available (see **Table 2**).[23–25,32–34] The study involving the greatest number of HIV-infected patients found secondary hypogonadism in 183 of the 212 hypogonadal patients with total serum T levels less than 300 ng/dL (86%).[24] The other studies investigating gonadotropins led to similar results, confirming that hypogonadotropic hypogonadism is more frequent than primary hypogonadism in men with T deficiency.[23,32–34,43,44] Other hypothalamic-pituitary axes, such as the growth hormone–insulin growth factor 1

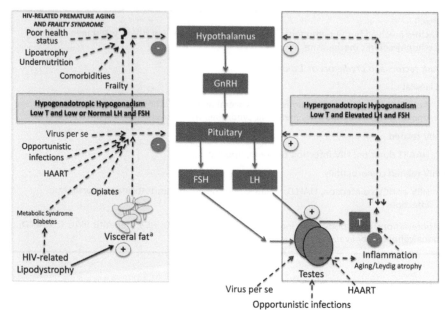

Fig. 1. Pathophysiology of male hypogonadism in HIV-infected men. [a] This mechanism operates through androgen aromatization to estrogen (mainly within adipose tissue), the latter being more potent than androgens in inhibiting gonadotropins secretion at both the hypothalamic and pituitary levels in men. (*Data from* Ashby J, Goldmeier D, Sadeghi-Nejad H. Hypogonadism in human immunodeficiency virus-positive men. Korean J Urol 2014;55(1):9–16.)

axis, are also impaired in HIV-infected patients, suggesting that the function of the hypothalamic-pituitary unit could be more generally altered in HIV infection.[45,46]

How HIV infection leads to the impairment of the hypothalamic-pituitary unit remains a matter of debate.[45,47] Probably, this is the result of multiple associated factors (see **Fig. 1**). Among them, the following might contribute to the development of hypogonadotropic hypogonadism: infections, antiretroviral drugs, increased adiposity, opiates, and poor health status (see **Box 1, Fig. 1**).

The virus per se might influence pituitary function because HIV has been found in pituitary cells in a small percentage of cases (12%) and might account for hypothalamus and pituitary damage.[48,49] In the pre-HAART era, postmortem studies often found signs of infection by opportunistic microorganisms (eg, *Pneumocystis carinii*, *Toxoplasma gondi*), also involving cerebral tissue (see **Fig. 1**).[3,40,44,48,49]

Antiretroviral drugs may directly interfere with several biochemical pathways involved in the control of pituitary hormonal secretion.[47] HIV infection and antiretroviral drugs are indirectly responsible for body composition changes occurring in the context of HIV-related lipodystrophy. Adiposity, mainly visceral fat, can inhibit gonadotropin secretion through increased aromatization of androgens and ultimately through the inhibitory effect of estrogens at both the hypothalamic and pituitary levels (see **Fig. 1**).[50] Visceral fat seems to operate in HIV-infected men because secondary hypogonadism is associated with increased visceral and high estrogen to T ratio (see **Fig. 1**).[24] The increased production of estrogen leads to inhibition of gonadotropins because estradiol is more potent than T in suppressing LH and follicle-stimulating hormone secretion in men, both at the hypothalamic and pituitary levels.[51]

Other factors such as the use of opiates may also contribute to hypogonadotropic hypogonadism. Opiates can suppress the hypothalamic-pituitary axis, and this mechanism might operate in HIV-infected men with a history of use of injection drugs or methadone therapy (see **Fig. 1**).[35]

A possible explanation for the hypogonadotropic hypogonadism in these patients is that a poor health status may induce the hypogonadal state (see **Fig. 1**). Critical illness leads to hypogonadotropic hypogonadism,[52] and T deficiency is common in men suffering from systemic disorders.[53] Low serum T levels were found to be closely associated with poor health status, comorbidities, and frailty in older men[54,55] and in men with high cardiovascular risk.[56] This mechanism could reflect an adaptive response to illness in unhealthy patients similar to hypothalamic hypogonadism observed in anorexia nervosa[57] or similar to low T3 syndrome.[58,59] Thus, low T levels could be considered a biomarker of frailty because it is the consequence of a beneficial adaptation to illness that is reached for avoiding physiologic states that might constitute a risk for the sick patient, such as reproductive behavior, vigorous physical activity, increased energy expenditure, and high cardiovascular rate.[56] This condition might confer an advantage for both the patient (in terms of sparing energy) and the species (preventing fatherhood).[56] HIV-infected men are prone to develop multiple comorbidities, and they resemble older men as a consequence of an accelerated process of aging starting in the 40s. This condition of premature aging[60] leads to the development of a frailty syndrome[61] in these patients, in the context of which hypothalamic hypogonadism might be a valuable mechanism of sparing as in older men,[56,59] as also previously hypothesized.[44]

Primary hypogonadism in men with HIV

In the pre-HAART era, postmortem studies in hypogonadal men with AIDS showed a pattern of inflammation within the testes together with a reduction of Leydig cell number consistent with testicular atrophy.[44,49,62,63] HIV is able to disseminate within the human testis, and in this site could represent a possible source of infection after virus replication and dissemination through sperm, just after having passed the altered blood-testis barrier.[3,49,63] This observation justifies the recovery of HIV virus in the sperm.

In HIV-infected patients treated with HAART (86%), primary hypogonadism was found in 29 of the 212 patients (14%) with total serum T levels less than 300 ng/dL.[24] This small proportion of men with primary hypogonadism is in line with the results of other studies.[25,34,44] However, when preclinical compensated hypogonadism, that is, normal serum T levels despite elevated serum LH levels, was also considered ($n = 396$), men with primary hypogonadism were 8% ($n = 29$), those with secondary hypogonadism 46% ($n = 183$), and those with compensated hypogonadism 46% ($n = 184$).[24] Data from the pre-HAART and HAART periods confirm that a more severe disease is associated with elevated serum LH levels and primary testicular failure.[63] Less evidence of testicular damage, however, is available from studies on men undergoing HAART with good control of the HIV infection.[63,64]

DIAGNOSIS

The diagnostic approach to male hypogonadism in HIV-infected patients should be based on a medical interview to obtain information on both patient's health status and symptoms and on clinical examination, as in the general population.[50] All these information should be thereafter integrated with and substantiated by biochemical testing.[18,50,65]

Signs and Symptoms

Signs and symptoms of male hypogonadism do not differ between HIV-uninfected and HIV-infected men. The main symptoms related to androgen deficiency are hot flashes and the decrease in the following components of male sexual function: sexual desire, sexual activity, sleep-related erections, and erectile function.[18,50,65,66] The most important sign is the reduction of testicular volume followed by reduced secondary sexual characteristics (pubic hair, shaving frequency), and fat redistribution, especially that characterized by visceral fat accumulation.[18,50,65,67] Another important clue is the onset of signs due to osteoporosis (reduced height or occurrence of pathologic fractures), but the signs related to osteoporosis generally appear after a long history of hypogonadism.[18,50,65] Conversely, reduced bone mineral density (BMD) might be a good radiological sign that could be clinically searched for.

Several other symptoms such as mood changes (depression, loss of vitality and motivation, and fatigue) and variation of physical performance are less specific.[18,50,65] The presence and the entity of the symptoms and signs mainly depend on the severity of hypogonadism and individual susceptibility.[68]

In clinical practice, the main problem is that signs and symptoms of hypogonadism are common in several chronic diseases and HIV infection.

Overlap of signs and symptoms of male hypogonadism in HIV infection

The main symptoms of hypogonadism and their occurrence in HIV infection or in other HIV-related diseases are summarized in **Table 3**.

Most of the symptoms of male hypogonadism occur frequently in men with HIV independent of their gonadal status.[44] In 1325 consecutive HIV-infected men, BMD did not differ between hypogonadal men with serum total T levels less than 300 ng/dL and eugonadal men. Accordingly, the same percentages of men with osteoporosis or osteopenia were recorded in the 2 groups.[24] In a subset of 247 HIV-infected men, even parameters of erectile dysfunction did not correlate with hypogonadism,[24] in line with other studies.[22,27] Again, the prevalence of erectile dysfunction did not differ between hypogonadal and eugonadal men.[24] In clinical practice, most of the signs and symptoms of hypogonadism overlap with those of HIV infection (see **Table 3**)[24]; this is because (1) osteoporosis is common among men with HIV[69]; (2) body image changes and the stigma of the disease affect negatively on self-esteem, sexuality, and mood[70,71]; (3) the fear of HIV transmission compromises sexuality[70]; and (4) the coexistence of several comorbidities together with the related poor health status influences negatively both mood and sexuality.[61,71] With this in view, sleep-related erections,[72,73] testes volume, sperm volume, and hot flashes or sweats[68] all remain good indicators of T status because they do not depend on psychological correlates (see **Table 3**).[73] However, these indicators are always present when T deficiency is severe (<100 ng/dL), whereas they are inconstantly present in case of mild to moderate hypogonadism[68,72] or are difficult to objectify and monitor (ie, decreased body hair and beard).

Several symptoms of male hypogonadism are also shared by several other chronic illnesses (see **Table 3**).[44,74]

Several researchers investigated the value of diagnostic tools, such as the aging males' symptoms (AMS) scale, and they concluded that the AMS scale is less sensitive and less specific when used in HIV-infected men,[23,27,75] thus suggesting not using it for the diagnosis of hypogonadism in this specific clinical condition.

All these aspects imply that signs and symptoms of hypogonadism lose their specificity in HIV-infected men and are not reliable for the diagnosis in this setting. Similarly, validated questionnaires for the diagnosis of hypogonadism are less valuable in men

Table 3
Signs and symptoms of hypogonadism in HIV-infected men that overlap with those of HIV infection and other clinical conditions associated with HIV

Not Overlapped	Overlap with HIV Infection Symptoms	Overlap with HIV-Related Comorbidities/Chronic Illness Symptoms
Loss/impaired sleep-related erections	Reduced sexual interest and desire	Obesity, metabolic syndrome, Diabetes type 2
Decrease in testes size	Reduced frequency of sexual activity	Erectile dysfunction
Decreased volume of ejaculate	Erectile dysfunction	Visceral adiposity
Hot flushes, sweats	Mood and behavioral symptoms	Increased waist
Reduction of body hair and beard	Depression	Reduced lean mass
	Decreased vitality	Chronic renal insufficiency
	Reduced motivation	Decreased vitality
	Fatigue	Fatigue
	Varied physical performance	Varied physical performance
	Lipodystrophic symptoms	Osteoporosis
	Visceral adiposity	Reduced BMD
	Increased waist	Height reduction
	HIV-associated weight loss	Bone pain/fractures
	Decreased vitality	Hepatitis (HBV and/or HCV coinfection)
	Fatigue	Reduced sexual interest and desire
	Varied physical performance	Depression
	Reduced lean mass	Decreased vitality
		Reduced motivation
		Fatigue
		Varied physical performance
		CV diseases
		Erectile dysfunction
		Depression
		Decreased vitality
		Reduced motivation
		Fatigue
		Varied physical performance
		Reduced lean mass

Abbreviations: CV, cardiovascular; HBV, hepatitis virus B; HCV, hepatitis virus C.

with HIV. In clinical practice, signs and symptoms should lead the clinician in the workup aiming to exclude the diagnosis of hypogonadism, but it should also be considered that, when present, they might be due to other HIV-related diseases.

Biochemical Diagnosis of Hypogonadism in HIV-Infected Men

The clinical suspicion of hypogonadism should be confirmed by biochemical testing. Several guidelines are available for the diagnosis of hypogonadism in adult men, but most of them are based on the results of studies involving older men.[18,50,63,76] In addition, only the Endocrine Society guidelines provide advice on hypogonadism in men with HIV.[18] If one considers that there is no consensus on (1) what is the best serum T threshold for the diagnosis of hypogonadism, (2) what is the serum T that should be measured (total, free, bioavailable), and (3) what is the best method of assay useful in the clinic,[18,50,65] it becomes clear that one is far from having valuable cutoffs for a correct diagnosis of hypogonadism, especially in men with HIV.

Box 2
Biochemical diagnosis of hypogonadism according to different definitions

Endocrine Society Guidelines, 2010 (XX)

Total serum T<300 ng/dL

Evidence of 2 altered measurements

Serum free T less than the laboratory normal range or less than 50 pg/mL

AACE Guidelines, 2002 (XX)

Total serum T<319 ng/dL (−2.5 standard deviations less than mean T values)

Measurement of serum LH needed

ISA, ISSAM, EAU, EAA, and ASA Recommendations, 2009 (XX)

Total serum T<230 ng/dL

Gray area: 230<total serum T<350, in this range further data on free serum T needed

Consider free serum T in some conditions (obesity)

Threshold for free T: 65 pg/mL

EACS Guidelines version 7.0, 2013 (XX)

If signs of hypogonadism are present, refer to endocrinologist

HIV Medicine Association of the Infectious Diseases Society of America Guidelines, 2013 (XX)

Morning free T preferred

Clinical advice for proper clinical investigations in the diagnosis of hypogonadism

Obtain morning serum sample for T measurement (7–10 AM)

Be aware of the method used for T assay (accuracy reference range)

Obtain 2 different T measurements (the second as confirmatory of T deficiency)

Consider total serum T less than 100 ng/dL as a certain threshold for T deficiency

Consider total serum T less than 200 ng/dL as a reliable threshold for T deficiency

Measure SHBG (for calculated free T) or free serum T (with an accurate method) if total serum T is doubtful, or is in a gray area, or if abnormal T protein binding is suspected (see **Fig. 2**)

Obtain LH and FSH serum levels for a better characterization of hypogonadism

Abbreviations: AACE, American Association of Clinical Endocrinologists; ASA, American Society of Andrology; EAA, European Academy of Andrology; EACS, European AIDS Clinical Society; EAU, European Association of Urology; ISA, International Society of Andrology; ISSAM, International Society for the Study of Aging Male.

The authors summarize the main advice of different guidelines provided by endocrinologists, urologists, and andrologists compared with that provided by experts in HIV medicine (**Box 2**). In general, differently from the past, current guidelines on HIV infection recommend referring to an endocrinologist when hypogonadism is suspected,[76–78] but there is no consensus on how to diagnose hypogonadism in HIV-infected men. Furthermore, several clues useful for limiting misclassification of patients with hypogonadism to appropriately assess clinical investigations are provided (see **Box 2**). Some of them could be obvious for endocrinologists or andrologists, but they could be of great interest for infectious disease physicians managing HIV-infected men in their daily practice.

Table 4
Usefulness of methods for serum T measurement in clinical practice

	Total Serum T	Free Serum T
Gold standard	LC/MS/MS Advantages: most accurate Disadvantages: costly, currently not available for clinical use, locally settled reference range needed Current use: clinical research, clinical purposes	Equilibrium dialysis Advantages: most accurate Disadvantages: costly, currently not available for clinical use Current use: research
Accurate methods	Commercially available kits (RIA, chemiluminescence) Advantages: not expensive, available for clinical use Disadvantages: less accurate Current use: clinical purposes	Calculated free T (from total T and SHBG) Advantages: correlates with the gold standard, not expensive Disadvantages: depends on accuracy of total T and SHBG assays, SHBG not currently available for clinical use Current use: clinical purposes and research
Inaccurate methods	RIA performed after protein extraction or chromatography Advantages: avoid protein interferences and cross-reaction with other steroids Disadvantages: costly, time consuming, not so accurate, currently not available for clinical use Current use: not determined	Bioavailable T Advantages: none Disadvantages: costly, time consuming, frequent bias Current use: research Direct methods (analog free T or others) Advantages: direct measurement of free T Disadvantages: frequent bias, erroneous results Current use: not advisable

Abbreviations: LC/MS/MS, liquid chromatography-tandem mass spectrometry; RIA, radioimmunoassay.

Methods for T measurement

According to the method used for T measurement, the same patient might be classified as hypogonadic or not, depending on the type of the cutoff used (see **Box 2**), the serum T measured (free or total), and the type of assay used (**Table 4**).[17,18,65] In particular, misclassification is more common when serum T level is slightly reduced, whereas it is uncommon when the patient's serum T level is very low (total T<100 ng/dL; free T<50 pg/mL).[50] Several researchers consider a total T level less than 200 ng/dL as a good marker of clinical hypogonadism because such a T value is almost constantly associated with symptoms of hypogonadism in HIV-uninfected men.[50,66–68] All these considerations apply also to HIV-infected men.[30,79]

A further source of misclassification in these patients is consistent with the alteration of SHBG, which is frequent in men with HIV (**Fig. 2**). Obesity, especially visceral adiposity, might increase SHBG synthesis, thus reducing the unbound rate of circulating T (see **Fig. 2**).[80] SHBG levels are often increased in patients with HIV because of the high prevalence of visceral obesity related to lipodystrophic fat redistribution,[11,13,14,20,23,25,27,81] especially in patients with severe liver dysfunction.[82] Thus, several researchers recommend serum free T measurement as a first step in the

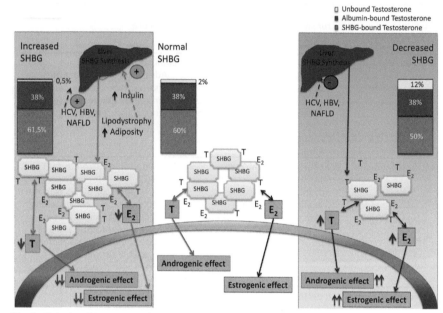

Fig. 2. Relationships among free serum T, total T, and SHBG in HIV-infected men. Hepatitis coinfection could lead to increased or decreased SHBG levels, depending on the degree of liver dysfunction. E₂, estradiol; HBV, hepatitis virus B; HCV, hepatitis virus C; NAFLD, non-alcoholic fatty liver disease.

diagnosis of hypogonadism in HIV-infected men, to avoid false-negative results (about 32%) due to normal serum total T but already impaired free T (see **Fig. 2**).[23,30,79] SHBG levels, however, have also been found normal[31] or reduced[83] in HIV-infected men, the latter especially in patients with severe liver dysfunction (see **Fig. 2**). Hence, liver diseases, which are common in men with HIV and hepatitis virus coinfections, could lead to a decrease[84] or an increase[85] in SHBG levels, adding a further confounding element for the diagnosis of hypogonadism in this setting.

The diagnosis of hypogonadism becomes challenging if all these possible biases related to T measurement methods are considered. **Table 4** summarizes the advantages and disadvantages of several of them.

Data on serum free T should be obtained when possible in HIV-infected men, but it should be borne in mind that direct measurement of free T with commercially available kits are unreliable (see **Table 4**) and that the calculation of serum free T using SHBG and total T should be preferred.[17] However, even this parameter remains of limited value in clinical practice because of the possible sum of errors of each assay, especially when total T is measured with inaccurate tools (see **Table 4**).[59] In addition, in daily practice, SHBG is no longer available in all clinical laboratories (see **Table 4**).

Fig. 3 provides a valuable algorithm for the biochemical diagnosis of male hypogonadism in HIV-infected patients obtained by integrating information available in the literature. Having 2 repeated measurements of morning serum total or free T is the approach most widely used by clinicians to definitely rule out T deficiency in men.[18,50,59] Finally, in the presence of documented secondary hypogonadism, a workup on pituitary function and morphology might be useful in some patients, especially those with very low serum T or with other signs or symptoms of pituitary diseases.[18,50]

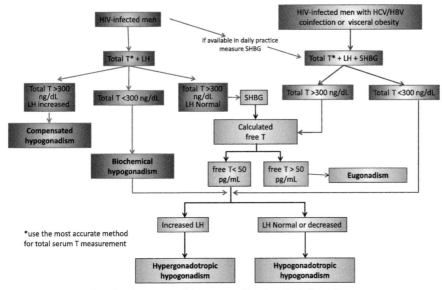

Fig. 3. Algorithm for the diagnosis of hypogonadism in HIV-infected men.

TREATMENT

Decision making concerning the selection of candidate for T replacement is difficult because the interpretation of signs, symptoms, and serum T levels is complex in HIV-infected men. Treatment should be started in all patients with severe T deficiency (total T<100 ng/dL or free T<30 ng/dL). Patients with slightly decreased serum T levels could be monitored and a wait-and-see approach might lead T prescription, especially if a progressive further decrease in T level occurs. Borderline low serum T level should be integrated with the clinical condition of the patient, and decision on T treatment should be individualized. If the patient with a low T level is losing weight and lean mass, treatment is recommended. In case of secondary hypogonadism, fatherhood desire should be investigated to properly plan gonadotropin treatment.[50]

Several preparations are available for T treatment, the choice of which depends on clinician experience, patients' preferences, and the degree of T deficiency (long-acting preparations indicated for severe hypogonadism, oral and transdermal preparations indicated for moderate to mild forms of hypogonadism) (**Table 5**). When a treatment that improves or restores sexual function and activity (such as T) is prescribed to HIV-infected men, it is mandatory to provide them and reinforce counseling on safe sexual practice.[70]

The efficacy of T treatment in HIV-infected men has been demonstrated for some parameters such as weight, lean mass, and sexual function.[18,86,87] As T treatment has been used also in eugonadal HIV-infected men to counteract lost muscle mass in wasting syndrome by providing supraphysiologic doses of androgens,[4,88] the results in terms of benefits and risks of this treatment in HIV-infected men with proven hypogonadism remain to be defined in detail.

Hematocrit, prostatic specific antigen, and prostate digital rectal examination are mandatory for monitoring T treatment and have to be performed even at baseline to

Table 5
Preparations and formulations of exogenous T

Route of Administration (Dosage, Interval)	Advantages	Disadvantages
Oral		
T undecanoate (40 mg, daily)	Not discomfortable	Most of the absorbed T is lost during first passage through the liver
Buccal T tablets (30 mg, twice daily)		
Intramuscular injection		
T enanthate (200–250 mg, 2–3 wk)	Long interval between administration	Injection discomfort
T cypionate (200 mg, 2 wk) T undecanoate (1000 mg, 10–14 wk)	Not physiologic peak and nadir of serum T (T undecanoate only)	Not physiologic peak and nadir of serum T (except for T undecanoate)
Skin disposal		
Transdermal T patches (50 mg, twice daily)	Comfortable application	Possible skin irritation, itch
T gel 1%–25% (40–625 mg/d, daily)		Dishomogeneous, not constant absorption

detect changes and avoid side effects (erythrocytosis, prostate diseases).[50,65,86] Prostate and breast cancers are absolute contraindications to T treatment.[50,63,86]

CURRENT CONTROVERSIES

The best way for the diagnosis of male hypogonadism in men with HIV remains to be precisely defined (see previous paragraph for details).

Screening of male hypogonadism is not recommended in the general population. Due to the elevated prevalence of hypogonadism among HIV-infected men, screening for T deficiency might be useful to identify patients who need replacement treatment. However, if the difficulties in making the diagnosis, the risk of overtreating patients who do not need T replacement, and the risks of cardiovascular disease due to T treatment of men in a poor health status are all considered, it becomes clear that a real estimation of the risks and benefits of a universal screening of HIV-infected patients is still lacking. At present, only men with signs or symptoms of hypogonadism should be screened. Future research may help clarify whether universal screening is beneficial for men with HIV infection.

Whether or not T treatment should be administered to all HIV-infected men with low T levels remains a matter of debate. The possibility that hypogonadism occurs in HIV-infected men as an adaptive mechanism recruited to counteract a condition of poor health status[56] should be considered before starting T treatment in hypogonadal men with HIV. HIV-infected men, in fact, are frail and often have a history of previous minor and/or major cardiovascular events.[61] With this in view, T treatment might result detrimental rather than beneficial in these patients because it has been proved to increase mortality and the number of cardiovascular events in older, frail men,[89] as well as in other cohorts of unhealthy hypogonadal patients.[90] All these considerations suggest caution in considering T treatment of all HIV-infected men with documented biochemical and clinical hypogonadism.

SUMMARY

The management of male hypogonadism needs a multidisciplinary approach involving both the specialist in HIV medicine and the endocrinologist (or andrologist). Based on extensive clinical experience in the management of endocrine disease in patients with HIV infection, the authors organized this multidisciplinary evaluation by providing endocrinological outpatients service directly within the clinic of infectious disease where patients are referred to. This or other similar kind of organizational aspects might be of help in correctly diagnosing and managing the HIV-infected patient with hypogonadism.

Future research probably will clarify the exact mechanism leading to impaired serum T levels in men with HIV.

ACKNOWLEDGMENTS

The authors are indebted to Giulia Brigante, MD, PhD, and Chiara Diazzi, MD, PhD, for their help in searching the literature for useful resources and for their continuous support in the clinical management of HIV-infected patients. They thank Chiara Diazzi, MD, PhD, for technical support in painting digital pictures.

REFERENCES

1. Lefrere JJ, Laplanche JL, Vittecoq D, et al. Hypogonadism in AIDS. AIDS 1988; 2(2):135–6.
2. Dobs AS, Dempsey MA, Ladenson PW, et al. Endocrine disorders in men infected with human immunodeficiency virus. Am J Med 1988;84(3):611–6.
3. Sellmeyer DE, Grunfeld C. Endocrine and metabolic disturbances in human immunodeficiency virus infection and the acquired immune deficiency syndrome. Endocr Rev 1996;17(5):518–32.
4. Grinspoon S, Corcoran C, Askari H, et al. Effects of androgen administration in men with the AIDS wasting syndrome. A randomized, double-blind, placebo-controlled trial. Ann Intern Med 1998;129(1):18–26.
5. Palella FJ Jr, Delaney KM, Moorman AC, et al. Declining morbidity and mortality among patients with advanced human immunodeficiency virus infection. HIV Outpatient Study Investigators. N Engl J Med 1998;338(13):853–60.
6. Available at: http://www.unaids.org/en/media/unaids/contentassets/documents/epidemiology/2013/gr2013/UNAIDS_Global_Report_2013_en.pdf. Accessed May 5, 2013.
7. Croxson TS, Chapman WE, Miller LK, et al. Changes in the hypothalamic-pituitary-gonadal axis in human immunodeficiency virus-infected homosexual men. J Clin Endocrinol Metab 1989;68(2):317–21.
8. Villette JM, Bourin P, Doinel C, et al. Circadian variations in plasma levels of hypophyseal, adrenocortical and testicular hormones in men infected with human immunodeficiency virus. J Clin Endocrinol Metab 1990;70(3):572–7.
9. Raffi F, Brisseau JM, Planchon B, et al. Endocrine function in 98 HIV-infected patients: a prospective study. AIDS 1991;5(6):729–33.
10. Wagner G, Rabkin JG, Rabkin R. Illness stage, concurrent medications, and other correlates of low testosterone in men with HIV illness. J Acquir Immune Defic Syndr Hum Retrovirol 1995;8(2):204–7.
11. Grinspoon S, Corcoran C, Lee K, et al. Loss of lean body and muscle mass correlates with androgen levels in hypogonadal men with acquired immunodeficiency syndrome and wasting. J Clin Endocrinol Metab 1996;81(11):4051–8.

12. Salehian B, Jacobson D, Swerdloff RS, et al. Testicular pathologic changes and the pituitary-testicular axis during human immunodeficiency virus infection. Endocr Pract 1999;5(1):1–9.

13. Arver S, Sinha-Hikim I, Beall G, et al. Serum dihydrotestosterone and testosterone concentrations in human immunodeficiency virus-infected men with and without weight loss. J Androl 1999;20(5):611–8.

14. Laudat A, Blum L, Guéchot J, et al. Changes in systemic gonadal and adrenal steroids in asymptomatic human immunodeficiency virus-infected men: relationship with the CD4 cell counts. Eur J Endocrinol 1995;133(4):418–24.

15. Merenich JA, McDermott MT, Asp AA, et al. Evidence of endocrine involvement early in the course of human immunodeficiency virus infection. J Clin Endocrinol Metab 1990;70(3):566–71.

16. Dobs AS, Few WL 3rd, Blackman MR, et al. Serum hormones in men with human immunodeficiency virus-associated wasting. J Clin Endocrinol Metab 1996; 81(11):4108–12.

17. Rosner W, Auchus RJ, Azziz R, et al. Position statement: utility, limitations, and pitfalls in measuring testosterone: an Endocrine Society position statement. J Clin Endocrinol Metab 2007;92(2):405–13.

18. Bhasin S, Cunningham GR, Hayes FJ, et al. Testosterone therapy in men with androgen deficiency syndromes: an Endocrine Society clinical practice guideline. J Clin Endocrinol Metab 2010;95(6):2536–59.

19. Berger D, Muurahainen N, Wittert H, et al. Hypogonadism and wasting in the era of HAART in HIV-infected patients. Proceedings of 12th International AIDS Conference. [abstract: 32174]. Geneva (Switzerland), June 28 – July 3, 1998.

20. Rietschel P, Corcoran C, Stanley T, et al. Prevalence of hypogonadism among men with weight loss related to human immunodeficiency virus infection who were receiving highly active antiretroviral therapy. Clin Infect Dis 2000;31(5): 1240–4.

21. Fisher A, Desyatnik M, Baaj A. The prevalence of hypogonadism in HIV infected patients receiving HAART. XIII International AIDS Conference. [abstract: Tu-PeB3180]. Durban (South Africa), July 9–14, 2000.

22. Crum-Cianflone NF, Bavaro M, Hale B, et al. Erectile dysfunction and hypogonadism among men with HIV. AIDS Patient Care STDS 2007;21(1):9–19.

23. Moreno-Pérez O, Escoin C, Serna-Candel C, et al. The determination of total testosterone and free testosterone (RIA) are not applicable to the evaluation of gonadal function in HIV-infected males. J Sex Med 2010;7(8):2873–83.

24. Rochira V, Zirilli L, Orlando G, et al. Premature decline of serum total testosterone in HIV-infected men in the HAART-era. PLoS One 2011;6(12):e28512.

25. Pepe J, Isidori AM, Falciano M, et al. The combination of FRAX and Ageing Male Symptoms scale better identifies treated HIV males at risk for major fracture. Clin Endocrinol (Oxf) 2012;77(5):672–8.

26. Monroe AK, Dobs AS, Cofrancesco J Jr, et al. Testosterone and Abnormal Glucose Metabolism in an Inner-City Cohort. J Mens Health 2012;9(3).

27. Sunchatawirul K, Tantiwongse K, Chathaisong P, et al. Hypogonadism among HIV-infected men in Thailand. Int J STD AIDS 2012;23(12):876–81.

28. De Ryck I, Van Laeken D, Apers L, et al. Erectile dysfunction, testosterone deficiency, and risk of coronary heart disease in a cohort of men living with HIV in Belgium. J Sex Med 2013;10(7):1816–22.

29. Blick G. Optimal diagnostic measures and thresholds for hypogonadism in men with HIV/AIDS: comparison between 2 transdermal testosterone replacement therapy gels. Postgrad Med 2013;125(2):30–9.

30. Monroe AK, Dobs AS, Palella FJ, et al. Morning free and total testosterone in HIV-infected men: implications for the assessment of hypogonadism. AIDS Res Ther 2014;11(1):6.

31. Dubé MP, Parker RA, Mulligan K, et al. Effects of potent antiretroviral therapy on free testosterone levels and fat-free mass in men in a prospective, randomized trial: A5005s, a substudy of AIDS Clinical Trials Group Study 384. Clin Infect Dis 2007;45(1):120–6.

32. Collazos J, Esteban M. Has prolactin a role in the hypogonadal status of HIV-infected patients? J Int Assoc Physicians AIDS Care 2009;8(1):43–6.

33. Klein RS, Lo Y, Santoro N, et al. Androgen levels in older men who have or who are at risk of acquiring HIV infection. Clin Infect Dis 2005;41(12):1794–803.

34. Wunder DM, Fux CA, Bersinger NA, et al. Androgen and gonadotropin patterns differ in HIV-1-infected men who develop lipoatrophy during antiretroviral therapy: a case-control study. HIV Med 2008;9(6):427–32.

35. Amini Lari M, Parsa N, Marzban M, et al. Depression, testosterone concentration, sexual dysfunction and methadone use among men with hypogonadism and HIV infection. AIDS Behav 2012;16(8):2236–43.

36. Araujo AB, O'Donnell AB, Brambilla DJ, et al. Prevalence and incidence of androgen deficiency in middle-aged and older men: estimates from the Massachusetts Male Aging Study. J Clin Endocrinol Metab 2004;89(12):5920–6.

37. Schneider HJ, Sievers C, Klotsche J, et al. Prevalence of low male testosterone levels in primary care in Germany: cross-sectional results from the DETECT study. Clin Endocrinol 2009;70(3):446–54.

38. Tajar A, Forti G, O'Neill TW, et al. Characteristics of secondary, primary, and compensated hypogonadism in aging men: evidence from the European Male Ageing Study. J Clin Endocrinol Metab 2010;95(4):1810–8.

39. Kaufman JM, Vermeulen A. Declining gonadal function in elderly men. Baillieres Clin Endocrinol Metab 1997;11(2):289–309.

40. Lo JC, Schambelan M. Reproductive function in human immunodeficiency virus infection. J Clin Endocrinol Metab 2001;86(6):2338–43.

41. Monroe AK, Dobs AS, Xu X, et al. Sex hormones, insulin resistance, and diabetes mellitus among men with or at risk for HIV infection. J Acquir Immune Defic Syndr 2011;58(2):173–80.

42. Monroe AK, Dobs AS, Xu X, et al. Low free testosterone in HIV-infected men is not associated with subclinical cardiovascular disease. HIV Med 2012;13(6):358–66.

43. Ashby J, Goldmeier D, Sadeghi-Nejad H. Hypogonadism in human immunodeficiency virus-positive men. Korean J Urol 2014;55(1):9–16.

44. Mylonakis E, Koutkia P, Grinspoon S. Diagnosis and treatment of androgen deficiency in human immunodeficiency virus-infected men and women. Clin Infect Dis 2001;33(6):857–64.

45. Zirilli L, Orlando G, Carli F, et al. GH response to GHRH plus arginine is impaired in lipoatrophic women with human immunodeficiency virus compared with controls. Eur J Endocrinol 2012;166(3):415–24.

46. Brigante G, Diazzi C, Ansaloni A, et al. Gender differences in GH response to GHRH+ARG in lipodystrophic patients with HIV: a key role for body fat distribution. Eur J Endocrinol 2014;170(5):685–96.

47. Zirilli L, Orlando G, Diazzi C, et al. Hypopituitarism and HIV-infection: a new co-morbidity in the HAART era? J Endocrinol Invest 2008;31(Suppl 9):33–8.

48. Sano T, Kovacs K, Scheithauer BW, et al. Pituitary pathology in acquired immunodeficiency syndrome. Arch Pathol Lab Med 1989;113(9):1066–70.

49. Poretsky L, Can S, Zumoff B. Testicular dysfunction in human immunodeficiency virus-infected men. Metabolism 1995;44(7):946–53.
50. Buvat J, Maggi M, Guay A, et al. Testosterone deficiency in men: systematic review and standard operating procedures for diagnosis and treatment. J Sex Med 2013;10(1):245–84.
51. Rochira V, Zirilli L, Genazzani AD, et al. Hypothalamic-pituitary-gonadal axis in two men with aromatase deficiency: evidence that circulating estrogens are required at the hypothalamic level for the integrity of gonadotropin negative feedback. Eur J Endocrinol 2006;155(4):513–22.
52. Woolf PD, Hamill RW, McDonald JV, et al. Transient hypogonadotropic hypogonadism caused by critical illness. J Clin Endocrinol Metab 1985;60(3):444–50.
53. Morley JE, Melmed S. Gonadal dysfunction in systemic disorders. Metabolism 1979;28(10):1051–73.
54. Travison TG, Araujo AB, Kupelian V, et al. The relative contributions of aging, health, and lifestyle factors to serum testosterone decline in men. J Clin Endocrinol Metab 2007;92(2):549–55.
55. Wu FC, Tajar A, Beynon JM, et al. Identification of late-onset hypogonadism in middle-aged and elderly men. N Engl J Med 2010;363(2):123–35.
56. Corona G, Rastrelli G, Maseroli E, et-al. Low testosterone syndrome protects subjects with high cardiovascular risk burden from major adverse cardiovascular events. Andrology, in press. http://dx.doi.org/10.1111/j.2047-2927.2014.00241.x.
57. Miller KK. Endocrine effects of anorexia nervosa. Endocrinol Metab Clin North Am 2013;42(3):515–28.
58. Warner MH, Beckett GJ. Mechanisms behind the non-thyroidal illness syndrome: an update. J Endocrinol 2010;205(1):1–13.
59. Handelsman DJ. An old emperor finds new clothing: rejuvenation in our time. Asian J Androl 2011;13(1):125–9.
60. Deeks SG, Phillips AN. HIV infection, antiretroviral treatment, ageing, and non-AIDS related morbidity. BMJ 2009;338:a3172.
61. Guaraldi G, Prakash M, Moecklinghoff C, et al. Morbidity in older HIV-infected patients: impact of long-term antiretroviral use. AIDS Rev 2014;16(2):75–89. http://dx.doi.org/10.1093/infdis/jiu258.
62. De Paepe ME, Vuletin JC, Lee MH, et al. Testicular atrophy in homosexual AIDS patients: an immune-mediated phenomenon? Hum Pathol 1989;20(6):572–8.
63. Azu OO. Highly active antiretroviral therapy (HAART) and testicular morphology: current status and a case for a stereologic approach. J Androl 2012;33(6):1130–42.
64. Roulet V, Satie AP, Ruffault A, et al. Susceptibility of human testis to human immunodeficiency virus-1 infection in situ and in vitro. Am J Pathol 2006;169(6):2094–103.
65. Wang C, Nieschlag E, Swerdloff R, et al. Investigation, treatment, and monitoring of late-onset hypogonadism in males: ISA, ISSAM, EAU, EAA, and ASA recommendations. J Androl 2009;30(1):1–9.
66. Travison TG, Morley JE, Araujo AB, et al. The relationship between libido and testosterone levels in aging men. J Clin Endocrinol Metab 2006;91(7):2509–13.
67. Hall SA, Esche GR, Araujo AB, et al. Correlates of low testosterone and symptomatic androgen deficiency in a population-based sample. J Clin Endocrinol Metab 2008;93(10):3870–7.
68. Zitzmann M, Faber S, Nieschlag E. Association of specific symptoms and metabolic risks with serum testosterone in older men. J Clin Endocrinol Metab 2006;91(11):4335–43.

69. Powderly WG. Osteoporosis and bone health in HIV. Curr HIV/AIDS Rep 2012; 9(3):218–22.
70. Santi D, Brigante G, Zona S, et al. Male sexual dysfunction and HIV–a clinical perspective. Nat Rev Urol 2014;11(2):99–109.
71. Guaraldi G, Luzi K, Murri R, et al. Sexual dysfunction in HIV-infected men: role of antiretroviral therapy, hypogonadism and lipodystrophy. Antivir Ther 2007;12(7): 1059–65.
72. Granata AR, Rochira V, Lerchl A, et al. Relationship between sleep-related erections and testosterone levels in men. J Androl 1997;18(5):522–7.
73. Rochira V, Zirilli L, Madeo B, et al. Sex steroids and sexual desire mechanism. J Endocrinol Invest 2003;26(Suppl 3):29–36.
74. Sartorius GA, Handelsman DJ. Testicular dysfunction in systemic diseases. In: Nieschlag E, Behre HM, Nieschlag S, editors. Andrology male reproductive health and dysfunction. 3rd edition. Berlin (Germany): Springer-Verlag; 2010. p. 339–64.
75. Claramonte M, García-Cruz E, Luque P, et al. Prevalence and risk factors of erectile dysfunction and testosterone deficiency symptoms in a rural population in Uganda. Arch Esp Urol 2012;65(7):689–97.
76. Petak SM, Nankin HR, Spark RF, et al, American Association of Clinical Endocrinologists. American Association of Clinical Endocrinologists Medical Guidelines for clinical practice for the evaluation and treatment of hypogonadism in adult male patients–2002 update. Endocr Pract 2002;8(6):440–56.
77. EACS guidelines version 7.0. 2013. Available at: http://www.eacsociety.org/Portals/0/Guidelines_Online_131014.pdf. Accessed May 5, 2014.
78. Aberg JA, Gallant JE, Ghanem KG, et al. Primary care guidelines for the management of persons infected with HIV: 2013 update by the HIV Medicine Association of the Infectious Diseases Society of America. Clin Infect Dis 2014;58(1): 1–10.
79. Monroe AK, Brown TT. Free testosterone for hypogonadism assessment in HIV-infected men. Clin Infect Dis 2014;58(11):1640.
80. Giagulli VA, Kaufman JM, Vermeulen A. Pathogenesis of the decreased androgen levels in obese men. J Clin Endocrinol Metab 1994;79(4):997–1000.
81. Martin ME, Benassayag C, Amiel C, et al. Alterations in the concentrations and binding properties of sex steroid binding protein and corticosteroid-binding globulin in HIV+ patients. J Endocrinol Invest 1992;15(8):597–603.
82. Phongtankuel V, Schrank G, Campbell EN, et al. Elevated testosterone levels in HIV-infected men: case report and a retrospective chart review. J Int Assoc Provid AIDS Care 2013;12(5):315–8.
83. Wasserman P, Segal-Maurer S, Rubin D. Low sex hormone-binding globulin and testosterone levels in association with erectile dysfunction among human immunodeficiency virus-infected men receiving testosterone and oxandrolone. J Sex Med 2008;5(1):241–7.
84. Hua X, Sun Y, Zhong Y, et al. Low serum sex hormone-binding globulin is associated with nonalcoholic fatty liver disease in type 2 diabetic patients. Clin Endocrinol (Oxf) 2014;80(6):877–83.
85. Nguyen HV, Mollison LC, Taylor TW, et al. Chronic hepatitis C infection and sex hormone levels: effect of disease severity and recombinant interferon-alpha therapy. Intern Med J 2006;36(6):362–6.
86. Bhasin S, Storer TW, Javanbakht M, et al. Testosterone replacement and resistance exercise in HIV-infected men with weight loss and low testosterone levels. JAMA 2000;283(6):763–70.

87. Corona G, Rastrelli G, Maggi M. Diagnosis and treatment of late-onset hypogo-nadism: systematic review and meta-analysis of TRT outcomes. Best Pract Res Clin Endocrinol Metab 2013;27(4):557–79.

88. Knapp PE, Storer TW, Herbst KL, et al. Effects of a supraphysiological dose of testosterone on physical function, muscle performance, mood, and fatigue in men with HIV-associated weight loss. Am J Physiol Endocrinol Metab 2008; 294(6):E1135–43.

89. Basaria S, Coviello AD, Travison TG, et al. Adverse events associated with testosterone administration. N Engl J Med 2010;363(2):109–22.

90. Vigen R, O'Donnell CI, Barón AE, et al. Association of testosterone therapy with mortality, myocardial infarction, and stroke in men with low testosterone levels. JAMA 2013;310(17):1829–36.

Gonadal Function and Reproductive Health in Women with Human Immunodeficiency Virus Infection

 CrossMark

Swaytha Yalamanchi, MD[a], Adrian Dobs, MD[a],
Ruth M. Greenblatt, MD[b,c,d,*]

KEYWORDS

• HIV infection • Women • Sex steroids • Reproductive biology

KEY POINTS

• Reproductive health in human immunodeficiency virus (HIV) infection is associated with extent of HIV morbidity; women who receive antiretroviral treatment, suppress viremia, and have normal CD4 lymphocyte counts generally have normal reproductive function.

• Hormonal contraceptives are generally safe, but some debate persists regarding the effects of certain progestins in increasing susceptibility to HIV infection, although the effect size, if this interaction exists, is small.

• There is little evidence that HIV infection causes early menopause, but protracted amenorrhea can be common, particularly among women with advanced HIV disease.

• Complications of pregnancy, such as preeclampsia and gestational diabetes may be more common among women infected with HIV, although more research is needed to evaluate this.

• Puberty occurs normally in girls infected with HIV, and although height attainment may be lessened, later puberty can occur in girls with HIV viremia and CD4 lymphocyte depletion.

Conflicts of interest: None (A. Dobs, R.M. Greenblatt).
[a] Department of Endocrinology, Diabetes and Metabolism, Johns Hopkins University School of Medicine, 1830 Monument Street, Baltimore, MD 21287, USA; [b] Department of Clinical Pharmacy, University of California, San Francisco Schools of Pharmacy and Medicine, 405 Irving Street, Second Floor, San Francisco, CA 94122, USA; [c] Department of Medicine, University of California, San Francisco Schools of Pharmacy and Medicine, 405 Irving Street, Second Floor, San Francisco, CA 94122, USA; [d] Department of Epidemiology and Biostatistics, University of California, San Francisco Schools of Pharmacy and Medicine, 405 Irving Street, Second Floor, San Francisco, CA 94122, USA
* Corresponding author. 405 Irving Street, Second Floor, San Francisco, CA 94122.
E-mail address: ruth.greenblatt@ucsf.edu

Endocrinol Metab Clin N Am 43 (2014) 731–741
http://dx.doi.org/10.1016/j.ecl.2014.05.002
endo.theclinics.com

INTRODUCTION

On a global basis, women account for more than 50% of persons living with human immunodeficiency virus (HIV) infection. In 2011 in the United States, 21% of the estimated 10,257 new HIV diagnoses were made in women, and 84% of these were from heterosexual contact.[1] Most HIV infections occur early in women's reproductive lives, and thus it is important to consider the impact of HIV on reproductive health and reproductive aging. This article addresses the unique implications of HIV infection on reproductive health throughout women's lifetimes, from the time they enter menarche to menopause, with specific impact on the ovulatory cycle, sex steroid hormone production, contraception, fertility, and pregnancy, and the implications of gonadal function for the course and outcomes of HIV infection.

PUBERTY

Information on puberty in girls infected with HIV is based on several US studies that focused on individuals who acquired HIV infection at birth. The most significant differences between girls who are and are not infected with HIV occur among individuals who had not received antiretroviral therapy, or what is now considered adequate therapy. In these studies, HIV infection was associated with reduced height attainment, the severity of which was associated with extent of CD4 lymphocyte depletion.[2] No differences in timing of puberty based on HIV status were found in 1 small US study.[2] The largest analysis of puberty in children with perinatal HIV infection was generated by data combined from large US cohorts, the Adolescent Master Protocol, and the Pediatric AIDS (acquired immunodeficiency syndrome) Clinical Trials Group, which included findings from 2086 children who were infected with HIV and compared these with 453 children who were exposed to HIV but not infected.[3] In this larger study, age at puberty (based on Tanner staging) was significantly later in girls and boys in the group infected with HIV (10.5 vs 10 years for girls, and 11.5 vs 10.7 years for boys, P values<.0001 for both). Extent of pubertal delay was greatest in children with very high HIV RNA levels and very low CD4+ leukocytes. Antiretroviral treatment was associated with age at puberty that was comparable with uninfected girls.

Any delays in puberty related to HIV infection are likely ameliorated by receipt of effective combined antiretroviral therapies (cART).

SEX STEROID LEVELS

Because sex steroids are important immune modulators, the effects of sex steroids on HIV and immune function among women infected with HIV are of great interest. Several in vitro studies have indicated that estrogen and the estrogen receptor (ER) system can interact with HIV components. For example, Szotek and colleagues[4] found that physiologic concentrations of 17beta-estradiol inhibit HIV replication in peripheral blood mononuclear cells via a mechanism involving beta-catenin, transcription factor 4 (TCF-4), and ERα. The Wira group reported that pretreatment of CD4 lymphocytes and macrophages with 17ss-estradiol protected these cells from infection with either C-C chemokine receptor type 5 (CCR-5) –tropic or C-X-C chemokine receptor type 4 (CXCR4)–tropic HIV strains via blockage of cell entry; maximal effect occurred at 5×10^{-8}M, a concentration that saturates cellular ERs.[5] Estradiol treatment after HIV exposure had no effect and ethinyl estradiol did not show the same protective action. These findings have potential implications for the selection of steroid components of hormonal contraceptives. However, caution must be applied if estrogen or androgen treatments are to be considered for use in women infected with HIV because HIV produces a prothrombotic state, which predisposes HIV patients to thrombotic complications.[6]

Multiple studies indicate that sex steroids can interact with HIV components or host responses, but this research is currently of unclear clinical application.

OVULATORY CYCLE AND FUNCTION

After menarche the ovarian follicle is the major source of sex steroids in nonpregnant, premenopausal women. Steroid synthesis occurs in the single follicle that produces a mature oocyte (the preovulatory and ovulatory follicle) during each ovulatory cycle. Sex steroid production varies by ovulatory cycle phase; a steady state is never achieved. The ovulatory cycle is regulated by neuroendocrine actions that respond to feedback elements produced by the follicle. Sex steroid synthesis is greatly reduced if follicle development and ovulation do not occur. Besides the physiologic anovulatory states before menarche and following menopause, anovulation can occur with perturbations of ovarian, hypothalamic, or pituitary functions. Chronic illness and disruptions of energy balance can result in anovulation, which is commonly reported in relationship to wasting illnesses, low body fat, and receipt of a variety of medications and drugs including cancer chemotherapies,[7,8] immune modulators,[9] antiepileptics,[10,11] antipsychotics,[10,12] and opioids.[13,14] Several of these factors, such as wasting,[15] and use of a variety of medications are common among women infected with HIV. In addition, tobacco use, which is also common among women infected with HIV, also can influence levels of neuroendocrine regulators, such as follicle-stimulating hormone (FSH).[16,17]

Studies of the effects of HIV infection on ovulation and sex steroid production are challenging to conduct because the measurement of most sex steroids and gonadotropins must be interpreted by ovulatory cycle phase; few studies of the effects of HIV infection on ovulatory functions have used methods that enable cycle phase interpretation of steroid and gonadotropin levels. Data from women with irregular menstrual cycles may be particularly difficult to interpret. Furthermore, effects of HIV must be differentiated from those of conditions and treatments that are common among women infected with HIV, such as use of opioids and loss of fat mass.

Women infected with HIV are at increased risk for secondary amenorrhea caused by:

- Loss of body fat
- Use of drugs associated with amenorrhea, such as psychiatric and seizure medications, cancer chemotherapies, immune modulators, and long-term opioids.

The Women's Interagency HIV Study (WIHS), a large observational cohort study of US women with, or at high risk for, HIV infection, conducted evaluations of sex steroid levels among women with regular menstrual cycles, who did not receive exogenous sex steroids, and who underwent sample collection during the early follicular ovulatory phase.[18] The women infected with HIV varied widely in their CD4 lymphocyte counts and plasma HIV RNA levels. Estradiol levels were 37.0 pg/mL (95% confidence interval, 27.0, 51.0) in the women infected with HIV versus 43.5 pg/mL (31.0, 58.0) in the uninfected women, a difference that was statistically significant at the $P = .001$ level. There was no statistically significant difference in inhibin-b and FSH levels between the two groups. The study measured dehydroepiandrosterone sulfate (DHEAS), testosterone, and sex hormone binding globulin (SHBG) levels at times not determined by ovulatory phase and found that HIV infection was associated with statistically significant differences in all three measures. Mean DHEAS in women infected with HIV was 73.3 μg/dL (34.0, 123) versus 106.0 μg/dL in uninfected women (65.0, 165; $P<.0001$), mean testosterone in women infected with HIV was 22.7 ng/dL (10.0, 36.9) versus 37.3 ng/dL in uninfected women (22.7, 53.1; $P<.0001$), and mean SHBG in women infected with HIV was significantly higher at 58.5 nmol/L (41.0, 88.0) versus 47.0 nmol/L in uninfected women (32.0, 70.0; $P<.0001$). Use or nonuse of combination antiretroviral regimens and controlling for age, smoking, body mass, and drug use did not influence the hormonal measures in this study, indicating that HIV infection may be associated with reduced sex steroid levels. By contrast, Weinberg and colleagues[19] studied sex steroid levels at 3 time points following menses in 20 HIV infected, and 20 HIV uninfected women who were not pregnant, not receiving exogenous sex steroids, and who had a regular pattern of menstrual bleeding. The group infected with HIV had CD4 lymphocyte counts greater than or equal to 300 cells/μL and plasma HIV RNA levels less than 10,000 copies/mL. No significant differences in estradiol and progesterone levels were found between the HIV infected and uninfected groups. The discordant results may be caused by differences in sample size, but are more likely to result from higher CD4 cell counts and lower HIV RNA levels in the Weinberg versus the WIHS studies, indicating that HIV disease status may influence sex steroid levels.

Clark and colleagues examined FSH and self-reported menstrual pattern among 24 women infected with HIV aged 20 to 42 years who had participated in AIDS Clinical Trials Group studies before 2000 and who had advanced HIV disease. They found that most women had normal FSH levels, but that 48% of the group had not experienced menses in 90 days, which indicated a high occurrence of anovulation. Another study examined 14 WIHS participants who were infected with HIV, aged 19 to 44 years, who reported regular menstrual cycles and who provided weekly blood samples. Twenty-eight percent of the women experienced anovulation as determined by endocrine criteria including early follicular phase estradiol and FSH, periovulatory luteinizing hormone, and midluteal progesterone levels.[20] These studies may indicate that anovulation is associated with extent of HIV morbidity, but the small sample size is a significant limitation.

MENOPAUSE

Menopause is defined by the final menstrual period experienced by a woman, and is preceded by variability in cycle length and eventually periods of amenorrhea lasting greater than or equal to 60 days.[21] The World Health Organization defines menopause as 12 consecutive months without menstruation, with the date of menopause occurring at the end of the year of amenorrhea.[22] Interpretation of published findings on the impact of HIV infection on the age of menopause depends on the how menopause is defined, and whether self-reported amenorrhea is considered to be a reliable indicator of menopause in a chronically ill population. Studies that use self-reported amenorrhea of 12 months' duration as a criterion for menopause tend to find that HIV infection is associated with menopause at an earlier age than occurs among uninfected women.[23,24] Earlier age at menopause is associated with low[25] or higher[26] CD4 lymphocyte counts and recreational drug use.[25–27]

In middle age, women who experience prolonged amenorrhea may report menopause regardless of whether physiologic tests of ovarian reserve (primary and secondary follicles that are capable of forming an ovulatory follicle) have been done to confirm menopause. Cejtin and colleagues[28] published from the WIHS that more than 50% of women infected with HIV who reported greater than or equal to 12 months of amenorrhea did not have FSH levels of more than 25 mIU/mL, indicating that protracted amenorrhea was common in the absence of menopause in this large study. Thus, given the frequency of amenorrhea in association with HIV infection, determination of the relationship between HIV infection and age at menopause supports the use of biological measures of menopause. Seifer and colleagues[29,30] completed 2 analyses of infected and uninfected WIHS participants who had regular menstrual cycles and who were sampled during the early follicular phase, and found no statistically significant difference by HIV status in age at which biological measures indicated diminished ovarian reserve, which is an essential feature of menopause. Overall there is little indication that HIV infection is associated with an earlier age at menopause, but it seems that HIV, and HIV morbidity, is associated with amenorrhea. Prolonged anovulation and amenorrhea both share some medical outcomes with menopause (for example, risk of bone demineralization), so ovulatory dysfunction in HIV infection may have significant health implications.

FERTILITY

Some studies indicate that women infected with HIV who are not receiving antiretroviral treatment may have decreased fertility compared with their uninfected counterparts.[31,32] As a sexually transmitted infection, HIV is also epidemiologically associated with the occurrence of other sexually transmitted infections, some of which cause pelvic inflammatory disease, which in turn may cause tubal factor infertility. In addition, some AIDS-defining conditions, such as tuberculosis or lymphoma, or their treatment, may adversely affect fertility.[33] The odds of pregnancy are greatest in women with less severe HIV morbidity as indicated by disease stage,[34] higher CD4 cell count,[35] and lower number of copies of HIV RNA in plasma (viral load).[36,37] Receipt of potent antiretroviral therapy regimens is associated with increased fertility, an effect that is likely related to the woman's choice in view of a good prognosis,[38] and the increased CD4 cell counts and decreased viral load that results from therapy.[35]

CONCEPTION

Significant concerns are often expressed regarding the risk of HIV transmission in couples with 1 partner infected with HIV. Greater HIV disease infirmity, lower CD4 lymphocyte counts, and increased HIV RNA in plasma or genital fluids are associated with increased likelihood of HIV transmission. The efficacy of potent antiretroviral regimens in suppressing HIV replication and resultant viremia and shedding of virus in genital secretions has changed the approach to prevention of transmission of HIV in couples who are discordant for infection. A large number of studies have shown that treatment with potent antiretroviral regimens (cART) of the partner infected with HIV and suppression of detectable viremia results in a high degree of protection from sexual HIV transmission.[39,40] Computational models indicate that reduction in plasma HIV RNA levels to less than 100 copies decreases heterosexual transmission by 91% (79%–96%).[41] The risk of transmission approaches zero when analysis is limited to cART recipients who succeed in reducing HIV RNA to less than the level of assay detection (less than 50 copies per milliliter of plasma).[42] Additional protection can be provided by preexposure treatment of the uninfected partner (so-called pre-exposure prophy-laxis) in which an uninfected individual who is at risk for the sexual acquisition of HIV consistently takes a regimen of 2 antiretroviral nucleosides to prevent transmis-sion.[43–45] Other options for reduction of transmission risk include the use of insemina-tion with processing of semen to wash sperm and eliminate leukocytes,[46–48] and general care for reproductive health issues, such as any sexual transmitted infections.[43,49]

PREGNANCY

Before the introduction of effective antiretroviral therapy, approximately one-quarter of pregnancies among women infected with HIV resulted in transmission to their new-borns.[50] The first great success in the prevention of HIV transmission was reported in 1994, with demonstration that azidothymidine, a single nucleoside, was effective in reducing transmission to 8.3% of births. Since that time, use of cART has been shown to be virtually 100% effective in prevention of transmission from mother to infant when maternal treatment is initiated during pregnancy and plasma HIV RNA is less than the assay detection level.[51] It is now common for women infected with HIV to contemplate pregnancy with the expectation of a healthy infant, and the outcomes of pregnancy among women infected with HIV are generally good. Elective cesarean section is rec-ommended for women with HIV RNA levels greater than 50 copies/mL before onset of labor.[51] Several concerns regarding pregnancy complications in women infected with HIV have arisen, including some evidence of increased occurrence of preeclampsia, gestational diabetes, and low infant birth weight. Although initial concerns were focused on the possible role of antiretroviral drugs in preeclampsia, more recent data from Botswana indicate that preeclampsia in women infected with HIV is inde-pendently associated with high pretreatment plasma HIV RNA levels and low levels of placental growth factor.[52] The Frankfort HIV Cohort group reported that, in the cART era, preterm birth among women infected with HIV declined compared with earlier times, but preeclampsia and gestational diabetes did not change with the advent of cART, and remained more common than was reported for the general pop-ulation.[53] These findings are not definitive, but they support the current recommenda-tions that pregnant women infected with HIV should receive careful prenatal care including provision of cART.

CONTRACEPTION

Research on contraception and HIV infection has largely focused on 2 topics: the po-tential effects of hormonal contraceptives on susceptibility to HIV infection, and the impact of antiretroviral drugs on hormonal contraceptive effectiveness.

HIV Susceptibility

Because hormonal contraceptives are among the most commonly used medications globally and users tend to be young, sexually active women, the impact of hormonal contraceptive exposure on risk of HIV infection has been the focus of multiple research studies. Overall, the research findings are not conclusive and even in studies that indi-cate that exposure to contraceptive steroids may confer risk, the effect size is modest. The greatest concern regards depot injectable medroxyprogesterone acetate (DMPA) or Depo-Provera, which is a widely used, inexpensive, and effective contraceptive. The consensus is that combination oral contraceptives likely have no effect on HIV susceptibility. With regard to DMPA, no consensus has been reached, and study find-ings are mixed.[54] DMPA has significant glucocorticoid mimetic effects that could influence HIV susceptibility.[55] Several alternative contraceptive progestins do not influence HIV viral effects that are mediated via the glucocorticoid receptor; DMPA does.[56] However, studies of human vaginal histology do not indicate that DMPA produces epithelial thinning,[57] which was postulated as a basis for increased risk with this contraceptive. Overall, careful review of current research provides no clear answer,[58] and a switch from DMPA to oral contraceptives has significant monetary and social disadvantages.[59]

The contradictory evidence related to hormonal contraceptives and increased susceptibility to HIV infection most often implicates DMPA, but the effect size is small. The high efficacy and low cost of this contraceptive must be taken into consideration as well.

Contraceptive Effectiveness

Because many antiretroviral drugs, particularly protease inhibitors and non-nucleoside reverse transcriptase inhibitors, can influence the activity of key drug metabolism pathways, drug-drug interactions between hormonal contraceptives and antiretroviral treatment (ART) are possible. Of greatest concern is the potential for ART to decrease levels of contraceptive estrogens and progestins, resulting in contraceptive failure, although most studies focus on pharmacologic end points and not contraceptive efficacy.[60] El-Ibiary and Cocohoba[61] reviewed studies dated to 2006 and identified many potential interactions that are specific to both the antiretroviral drug and to the steroid component of the contraceptive. In general, the greatest concern occurred in the setting of regimens that contain ritonavir, a protease inhibitor that is a potent inducer and inhibitor of several metabolic enzymes, but the investigators noted that more research is greatly needed. Robinson and colleagues[62] did a similar analysis up to 2012 but did not focus on the effects of concurrent ritonavir. They noted that DMPA and the levonorgestrel intrauterine system both were almost free of interactions with ART. Nanda and colleagues[63] studied 402 premenopausal South African women and found no significant effect of nevirapine on the efficacy of low-dose combination oral contraceptives. Landolt and colleagues[64] similarly found that nevirapine did not adversely influence levels of contraceptive progestins, but efavirenz did in a small study of Thai women, but DMPA levels and breakthrough ovulation were not influenced by efavirenz in another study.[65] Limited data indicate that hormonal contraceptives do not adversely influence ARV levels, although the range of such studies is limited.[60]

SUMMARY

The availability of potent combination antiretroviral therapies has greatly improved the overall health and survival of women infected with HIV. Access to and use of cART is the major predictor of outcome of HIV infection among women. Many questions remain to be answered related to the impact of menopause on the course of HIV infection, and whether contraceptive steroids influence risk of HIV transmission or alter concentrations of antiretroviral drugs. In addition, although conception can be achieved without transmission of HIV to an uninfected partner and to the newborn, further research is needed to determine whether complications of pregnancy such as preeclampsia and gestational diabetes are more common among women infected with HIV, and, if so, how HIV infection or its treatment contributes to these pathogenic conditions.

REFERENCES

1. Centers for Disease Control and Prevention. HIV surveillance report 2011. vol. 23. February, 2013.
2. Kessler M, Kaul A, Santos-Malave C, et al. Growth patterns in pubertal HIV-infected adolescents and their correlation with cytokines, IGF-1, IGFBP-1, and IGFBP-3. J Pediatr Endocrinol Metab 2013;26(7–8):639–44.
3. Williams PL, Abzug MJ, Jacobson DL, et al. Pubertal onset in children with perinatal HIV infection in the era of combination antiretroviral treatment. AIDS 2013; 27(12):1959–70.
4. Szotek EL, Narasipura SD, Al-Harthi L. 17beta-Estradiol inhibits HIV-1 by inducing a complex formation between beta-catenin and estrogen receptor alpha on the HIV promoter to suppress HIV transcription. Virology 2013;443(2):375–83.
5. Rodriguez-Garcia M, Biswas N, Patel MV, et al. Estradiol reduces susceptibility of CD4+ T cells and macrophages to HIV-infection. PLoS One 2013;8(4):e62069.
6. Auerbach E, Aboulafia DM. Venous and arterial thromboembolic complications associated with HIV infection and highly active antiretroviral therapy. Semin Thromb Hemost 2012;38(8):830–8.
7. Torino F, Barnabei A, De Vecchis L, et al. Recognizing menopause in women with amenorrhea induced by cytotoxic chemotherapy for endocrine-responsive early breast cancer. Endocr Relat Cancer 2012;19(2):R21–33.
8. Dieudonne AS, Vandenberghe J, Geerts I, et al. Undetectable antimullerian hormone levels and recovery of chemotherapy-induced ovarian failure in women with breast cancer on an oral aromatase inhibitor. Menopause 2011;18(7):821–4.
9. Harward LE, Mitchell K, Pieper C, et al. The impact of cyclophosphamide on menstruation and pregnancy in women with rheumatologic disease. Lupus 2013;22(1):81–6.
10. Joffe H, Hayes FJ. Menstrual cycle dysfunction associated with neurologic and psychiatric disorders: their treatment in adolescents. Ann N Y Acad Sci 2008; 1135:219–29.
11. Verrotti A, D'Egidio C, Coppola G, et al. Epilepsy, sex hormones and antiepileptic drugs in female patients. Expert Rev Neurother 2009;9(12):1803–14.
12. Thangavelu K, Geetanjali S. Menstrual disturbance and galactorrhea in people taking conventional antipsychotic medications. Exp Clin Psychopharmacol 2006;14(4):459–60.
13. Vuong C, Van Uum SH, O'Dell LE, et al. The effects of opioids and opioid analogs on animal and human endocrine systems. Endocr Rev 2010;31(1):98–132.
14. Daniell HW. Opioid endocrinopathy in women consuming prescribed sustained-action opioids for control of nonmalignant pain. J Pain 2008;9(1):28–36.
15. Diamanti A, Ubertini GM, Basso MS, et al. Amenorrhea and weight loss: not only anorexia nervosa. Eur J Obstet Gynecol Reprod Biol 2012;161(1):111–2.
16. Freour T, Masson D, Dessolle L, et al. Ovarian reserve and in vitro fertilization cycles outcome according to women smoking status and stimulation regimen. Arch Gynecol Obstet 2012;285(4):1177–82.
17. Schuh-Huerta SM, Johnson NA, Rosen MP, et al. Genetic variants and environmental factors associated with hormonal markers of ovarian reserve in Caucasian and African American women. Hum Reprod 2012;27(2):594–608.
18. Karim R, Mack WJ, Kono N, et al. Gonadotropin and sex steroid levels in HIV-infected premenopausal women and their association with subclinical atherosclerosis in HIV-infected and -uninfected women in the women's interagency HIV study (WIHS). J Clin Endocrinol Metab 2013;98(4):E610–8.

19. Weinberg A, Enomoto L, Marcus R, et al. Effect of menstrual cycle variation in female sex hormones on cellular immunity and regulation. J Reprod Immunol 2011;89(1):70–7.

20. Greenblatt R, Ameli N, Grant R, et al. Impact of the ovulatory cycle on virologic and immunologic markers in HIV-infected women. J Infect Dis 2000;181:181–90.

21. Harlow SD, Gass M, Hall JE, et al. Executive summary of the stages of reproductive aging workshop + 10: addressing the unfinished agenda of staging reproductive aging. J Clin Endocrinol Metab 2012;97(4):1159–68.

22. Utian WH. Menopause-related definitions. In: Daya S, Harrison RF, Kempers RD, editors. Advances in Fertility and Reproductive Medicine: Proceedings of the 18th World Congress on Fertility and Sterility. Montreal, 2004. p. 133–8.

23. Ferreira CE, Pinto-Neto AM, Conde DM, et al. Menopause symptoms in women infected with HIV: prevalence and associated factors. Gynecol Endocrinol 2007; 23(4):198–205.

24. Conde DM, Silva ET, Amaral WN, et al. HIV, reproductive aging, and health implications in women: a literature review. Menopause 2009;16(1):199–213.

25. de Pommerol M, Hessamfar M, Lawson-Ayayi S, et al. Menopause and HIV infection: age at onset and associated factors, ANRS CO3 Aquitaine cohort. Int J STD AIDS 2011;22(2):67–72.

26. Schoenbaum EE, Hartel D, Lo Y, et al. HIV infection, drug use and onset of natural menopause. Clin Infect Dis 2005;41:1517–24.

27. Fantry L, Zhan M, Taylor G, et al. Age of menopause and menopausal symptoms in HIV-infected women. AIDS Patient Care STDS 2005;19:703–11.

28. Cejtin HE, Kalinowski A, Bacchetti P, et al. Effects of human immunodeficiency virus on protracted amenorrhea and ovarian dysfunction. Obstet Gynecol 2006; 108(6):1423–31.

29. Seifer DB, Golub ET, Lambert-Messerlian G, et al. Biologic markers of ovarian reserve and reproductive aging: application in a cohort study of HIV infection in women. Fertil Steril 2007;88(6):1645–52.

30. Seifer DB, Golub ET, Lambert-Messerlian G, et al. Variations in serum mullerian inhibiting substance between white, black, and Hispanic women. Fertil Steril 2009;92(5):1674–8.

31. Zaba B, Gregson S. Measuring the impact of HIV on fertility in Africa. AIDS 1998; 12(Suppl 1):S41–50.

32. Gray RH, Wawer MJ, Serwadda D, et al. Population-based study of fertility in women with HIV-1 infection in Uganda. Lancet 1998;351(9096):98–103.

33. Kushnir VA, Lewis W. Human immunodeficiency virus/acquired immunodeficiency syndrome and infertility: emerging problems in the era of highly active antiretrovirals. Fertil Steril 2011;96(3):546–53.

34. Ross A, Van der Paal L, Lubega R, et al. HIV-1 disease progression and fertility: the incidence of recognized pregnancy and pregnancy outcome in Uganda. AIDS 2004;18(5):799–804.

35. Makumbi FE, Nakigozi G, Reynolds SJ, et al. Associations between HIV antiretroviral therapy and the prevalence and incidence of pregnancy in Rakai, Uganda. AIDS Res Treat 2011;2011:519492.

36. Massad LS, Springer G, Jacobson L, et al. Pregnancy rates and predictors of conception, miscarriage and abortion in US women with HIV. AIDS 2004; 18(2):281–6.

37. Nguyen RH, Gange SJ, Wabwire-Mangen F, et al. Reduced fertility among HIV-infected women associated with viral load in Rakai district, Uganda. Int J STD AIDS 2006;17(12):842–6.

38. Kaida A, Laher F, Strathdee SA, et al. Childbearing intentions of HIV-positive women of reproductive age in Soweto, South Africa: the influence of expanding access to HAART in an HIV hyperendemic setting. Am J Public Health 2011; 101(2):350–8.

39. Cohen MS, Chen YQ, McCauley M, et al. Prevention of HIV-1 infection with early antiretroviral therapy. N Engl J Med 2011;365(6):493–505.

40. Nosyk B, Audoin B, Beyrer C, et al. Examining the evidence on the causal effect of HAART on transmission of HIV using the Bradford Hill criteria. AIDS 2013; 27(7):1159–65.

41. Baggaley RF, White RG, Hollingsworth TD, et al. Heterosexual HIV-1 infectiousness and antiretroviral use: systematic review of prospective studies of discordant couples. Epidemiology 2013;24(1):110–21.

42. Loutfy MR, Wu W, Letchumanan M, et al. Systematic review of HIV transmission between heterosexual serodiscordant couples where the HIV-positive partner is fully suppressed on antiretroviral therapy. PLoS One 2013;8(2):e55747.

43. Matthews LT, Smit JA, Cu-Uvin S, et al. Antiretrovirals and safer conception for HIV-serodiscordant couples. Curr Opin HIV AIDS 2012;7(6):569–78.

44. Aaron E, Cohan D. Preexposure prophylaxis for the prevention of HIV transmission to women. AIDS 2013;27(1):F1–5.

45. Baeten JM, Celum C. Antiretroviral preexposure prophylaxis for HIV prevention. N Engl J Med 2013;368(1):83–4.

46. Garrido N, Meseguer M, Remohi J, et al. Semen characteristics in human immunodeficiency virus (HIV)- and hepatitis C (HCV)-seropositive males: predictors of the success of viral removal after sperm washing. Hum Reprod 2005;20(4): 1028–34.

47. Eke AC, Oragwu C. Sperm washing to prevent HIV transmission from HIV-infected men but allowing conception in sero-discordant couples. Cochrane Database Syst Rev 2011;(1):CD008498.

48. Bujan L, Hollander L, Coudert M, et al. Safety and efficacy of sperm washing in HIV-1-serodiscordant couples where the male is infected: results from the European CREAThE network. AIDS 2007;21(14):1909–14.

49. Fidler S, Anderson J, Azad Y, et al. Position statement on the use of antiretroviral therapy to reduce HIV transmission, January 2013: the British HIV Association (BHIVA) and the Expert Advisory Group on AIDS (EAGA). HIV Med 2013; 14(5):259–62.

50. Connor EM, Sperling RS, Gelber R, et al. Reduction of maternal-infant transmission of human immunodeficiency virus type 1 with zidovudine treatment. Pediatric AIDS Clinical Trials Group Protocol 076 Study Group. N Engl J Med 1994; 331(18):1173–80.

51. Senise J, Bonafe S, Castelo A. The management of HIV-infected pregnant women. Curr Opin Obstet Gynecol 2012;24(6):395–401.

52. Powis KM, McElrath TF, Hughes MD, et al. High viral load and elevated angiogenic markers associated with increased risk of preeclampsia among women initiating highly active antiretroviral therapy in pregnancy in the Mma Bana study, Botswana. J Acquir Immune Defic Syndr 2013;62(5):517–24.

53. Reitter A, Stucker A, Linde R, et al. Pregnancy complications in HIV-positive women: 11-year data from the Frankfurt HIV Cohort. HIV Med 2014. [Epub ahead of print].

54. Lutalo T, Musoke R, Kong X, et al. Effects of hormonal contraceptive use on HIV acquisition and transmission among HIV-discordant couples. AIDS 2013; 27(Suppl 1):S27–34.

55. Hapgood JP, Ray RM, Govender Y, et al. Differential glucocorticoid receptor-mediated effects on immunomodulatory gene expression by progestin contraceptives: implications for HIV-1 pathogenesis. Am J Reprod Immunol 2014; 71(6):505–12.

56. Tomasicchio M, Avenant C, Du Toit A, et al. The progestin-only contraceptive medroxyprogesterone acetate, but not norethisterone acetate, enhances HIV-1 Vpr-mediated apoptosis in human CD4+ T cells through the glucocorticoid receptor. PLoS One 2013;8(5):e62895.

57. Bahamondes MV, Castro S, Marchi NM, et al. Human vaginal histology in long-term users of the injectable contraceptive depot-medroxyprogesterone acetate. Contraception 2014. [Epub ahead of print].

58. Murphy K, Irvin SC, Herold BC. Research gaps in defining the biological link between HIV risk and hormonal contraception. Am J Reprod Immunol 2014. [Epub ahead of print].

59. Jain AK. Hormonal contraception and HIV acquisition risk: implications for individual users and public policies. Contraception 2012;86(6):645–52.

60. Thurman AR, Anderson S, Doncel GF. Effects of hormonal contraception on antiretroviral drug metabolism, pharmacokinetics and pharmacodynamics. Am J Reprod Immunol 2014;71(6):523–30.

61. El-Ibiary SY, Cocohoba JM. Effects of HIV antiretrovirals on the pharmacokinetics of hormonal contraceptives. Eur J Contracept Reprod Health Care 2008;13(2):123–32.

62. Robinson JA, Jamshidi R, Burke AE. Contraception for the HIV-positive woman: a review of interactions between hormonal contraception and antiretroviral therapy. Infect Dis Obstet Gynecol 2012;2012:890160.

63. Nanda K, Delany-Moretlwe S, Dube K, et al. Nevirapine-based antiretroviral therapy does not reduce oral contraceptive effectiveness. AIDS 2013;27(Suppl 1): S17–25.

64. Landolt NK, Phanuphak N, Ubolyam S, et al. Efavirenz, in contrast to nevirapine, is associated with unfavorable progesterone and antiretroviral levels when co-administered with combined oral contraceptives. J Acquir Immune Defic Syndr 2013;62(5):534–9.

65. Nanda K, Amaral E, Hays M, et al. Pharmacokinetic interactions between depot medroxyprogesterone acetate and combination antiretroviral therapy. Fertil Steril 2008;90(4):965–71.

Vitamin D and Calcium Abnormalities in the HIV-Infected Population

Gerome V. Escota, MD[a], Sara Cross, MD[b],
William G. Powderly, MD[a],*

KEYWORDS

- Vitamin D • Vitamin D deficiency/insufficiency • Vitamin D supplementation
- Calcium • HIV • AIDS

KEY POINTS

- Vitamin D is involved in several extraskeletal functions.
- Vitamin D deficiency is highly prevalent in the HIV-infected population.
- The adverse outcomes associated with vitamin D deficiency mirror several comorbidities that frequently occur among HIV-infected persons, including osteopenia and osteoporosis, cardiovascular disease, diabetes and the metabolic syndrome, and cancer. ·
- Studies investigating the effectiveness of vitamin D supplementation in the HIV-infected population are conflicting.
- Standard recommendation regarding screening and treatment of vitamin D deficiency in the HIV-infected population is lacking.

INTRODUCTION

Vitamin D, an essential hormone that maintains normal serum calcium,[1] was shown in the early 1900s to cure and prevent rickets.[2,3] Osteomalacia has long been recognized as a bone disorder, but it was not until 1967 that vitamin D deficiency was implicated in its cause. More recently, vitamin D has been suggested as a key factor in several extraskeletal functions and disease processes. It has been associated with cardiovascular disease,[4] diabetes,[5] muscle weakness and falls,[6,7] autoimmune disorders,[8] and certain malignancies including colon, prostate, and breast cancer.[9–11]

The use of combination antiretroviral therapy (cART) has dramatically reduced HIV-associated morbidity and mortality.[12] Non-AIDS defining illnesses (NADIs; eg, cardiovascular disease, diabetes, osteoporosis, cancer) become more prevalent as HIV-infected individuals grow older.[13] Modification and prevention of risk factors

[a] Division of Infectious Diseases, Washington University School of Medicine, 660 South Euclid, St Louis, MO 63110, USA; [b] Division of Infectious Diseases, University of Tennessee Health Sciences Center, 956 Court Avenue, E336 Coleman Building, Memphis, TN 38163, USA
* Corresponding author.
E-mail address: wpowderl@wustl.edu

Endocrinol Metab Clin N Am 43 (2014) 743–767
http://dx.doi.org/10.1016/j.ecl.2014.05.005
0889-8529/14/$ – see front matter © 2014 Elsevier Inc. All rights reserved.

associated with these comorbidities are currently active areas of research. Given the suggested role of vitamin D deficiency in many of these chronic illnesses, the impact of vitamin D deficiency in the HIV-infected population is an important topic that is reviewed here.

VITAMIN D METABOLISM

Vitamin D sources include exposure to sunlight, "oily fish," cod liver oil, shiitake mushrooms, egg yolks, fortified foods, and supplements.[14–16] Vitamin D from the skin and diet is transported to the liver and metabolized to 25-hydroxyvitamin D (25-OHD), its major circulating form. 25-OHD is then further metabolized in the kidney to form its biologically active metabolite, 1,25-dihydroxyvitamin D (1,25-OHD). 1,25-OHD maintains calcium in the normal range by facilitating absorption of renal calcium and intestinal calcium and phosphorus.[15] Most experts define vitamin D deficiency as serum 25-OHD less than 20 ng/mL, and vitamin D insufficiency as 25-OHD between 21 and 29 ng/mL. Based on the findings that intestinal calcium absorption is maximized at 25-OHD greater than 32 ng/mL, that nadir parathyroid hormone (PTH) is reached at 25-OHD between 30 and 40 ng/mL, and that secondary hyperparathyroidism is seen at 25-OHD less than 32 ng/mL, a 25-OHD level of at least 30 ng/mL is generally accepted as sufficient.[17]

EPIDEMIOLOGY OF VITAMIN D DEFICIENCY/INSUFFICIENCY

Vitamin D deficiency is common worldwide, with an estimated 1 billion people with either vitamin D deficiency or insufficiency. In the United States, data from the 2003 to 2006 National Health and Nutrition Examination Survey (NHANES) estimate the prevalence of vitamin D deficiency at 38%, whereas that of either vitamin D insufficiency or deficiency at 79% among adults.[17]

Vitamin D deficiency is also highly prevalent in the HIV-infected population. Among 253 cART-naïve subjects in London, 58% were found to be vitamin D–deficient, whereas 13% were severely deficient (25-OHD <10 ng/mL).[18] Using a more stringent definition of vitamin D deficiency (25-ODH <12 ng/mL), Mueller and colleagues[19] demonstrated a 42% prevalence of vitamin D deficiency among 211 cART-naïve participants in the Swiss HIV Cohort Study. Approximately one-fourth of participants on stable cART have 25-OHD less than 10 to 14 ng/mL, as shown by 2 separate observational studies in New York and the Netherlands.[20,21] Similar to the general population, the prevalence of vitamin D deficiency in these studies was influenced by the season when 25-OHD measurements were obtained.[18,19]

Despite these high estimates, the prevalence rates of vitamin D deficiency in the HIV-infected and uninfected populations are comparable. The Study to Understand the Natural History of HIV and AIDS in the Era of Effective Therapy (SUN Study) investigators evaluated the vitamin D status of 672 participants compared with age-matched, race-matched, and sex-matched adult subjects from the NHANES. They found modestly lower vitamin D deficiency prevalence among HIV-infected persons (29.7%) compared with controls (38.8%). The same trend was also observed for vitamin D deficiency/insufficiency.[22]

FACTORS ASSOCIATED WITH VITAMIN D DEFICIENCY/INSUFFICIENCY

Several HIV-related and non-HIV-related risk factors are associated with vitamin D deficiency (**Box 1**).[19,22–27] All non-HIV-related factors are similar to those found among HIV-uninfected cohorts with the exception of intravenous drug use (IDU), which has

Box 1
Non-HIV-related factors associated with vitamin D deficiency
Dark skin pigmentation
Obesity
Winter season
Low sun exposure
Low alimentary vitamin D intake
Intravenous drug use
Physical inactivity
Tobacco use
Renal disease
Liver disease
Malabsorption

not been extensively studied in the general population.[6,28–33] Few HIV-related factors have been elucidated.

The role of antiretroviral medications in vitamin D deficiency has been extensively studied, and the nonnucleoside reverse transcriptase inhibitor (NNRTI) efavirenz has consistently been associated with vitamin D deficiency.[19,22,25,26,34] Efavirenz affects vitamin D metabolism by inducing the enzyme 24-hydroxylase, which hydrolyzes active vitamin D into its inactive form (calcitroic acid). A recent study of 1077 patients (33% with severe vitamin D deficiency) found that efavirenz was associated with 2-fold increased odds of having vitamin D deficiency.[34] Brown and McComsey[35] evaluated 87 participants who were initiated on cART and found a 1.8 times higher risk of vitamin D deficiency in those started on efavirenz-based cART compared with non-efavirenz-based treatment regimen. More recently, Wohl and colleagues[36] showed that initiation of efavirenz resulted in a significant decrease in vitamin D levels, whereas initiation of rilpivirine had little effect on vitamin D. The MONET trial included 256 subjects who switched cART from either NNRTI-based or protease inhibitor (PI)-based therapy to boosted darunavir. At baseline, those on efavirenz had lower vitamin D levels. Switching participants from efavirenz to boosted darunavir led to a significant increase in vitamin D levels.[37] Of note, vitamin D deficiency does not represent an NNRTI class effect. The NNRTIs nevirapine and rilpivirine have not been found to be associated with vitamin D deficiency.[36,38]

PIs inhibit 25-α-hydroxylase and 1-α-hydroxylase enzymes and consequently decrease production of the active form of vitamin D.[39] Lower bone mineral density (BMD) has been shown in several studies of subjects receiving PIs[22,40,41]; however, a causal relationship with vitamin D deficiency has not been established.

Active IDU and acquisition of HIV through nonhomosexual exposure have been associated with vitamin D deficiency. Mueller and colleagues[19] found that active IDU was associated with lower vitamin D levels in their study of 211 participants. The EuroSIDA study group found that HIV infection through nonhomosexual exposure was associated with vitamin D deficiency in their large study of 2000 participants. Limited sunlight exposure and malnutrition likely contributed to vitamin D deficiency in these populations.[42]

Studies evaluating history of AIDS diagnosis as a factor contributing to vitamin D deficiency have shown inconsistent results. A large study of 810 subjects showed that a history of AIDS was independently associated with vitamin D deficiency.[24] Theodorou and colleagues[26] also found a positive association between AIDS diagnosis and vitamin D deficiency among 2044 participants. Conversely, 3 large studies that included a total of 3877 subjects found no relationship between vitamin D deficiency and previous AIDS diagnosis.[19,22,25]

Results of studies examining the role of CD4 count in vitamin D deficiency have also been inconclusive.[22,24–26] Subjects with low CD4 counts are immunocompromised and possibly malnourished. Their lack of sunlight exposure because of generally poor health status may also be contributory.

Other possible HIV-associated factors such as duration of HIV diagnosis and viral suppression have been studied with conflicting results. The SUN investigators found no relationship between duration since HIV diagnosis and vitamin D deficiency.[22] Allavena and colleagues[25] also reached the same conclusion among 2994 participants. Conversely, in a smaller study, Mueller and colleagues[19] found that vitamin D levels were higher in those with longer HIV diagnosis. They suggested that the general health status of participants recently diagnosed with HIV infection might be poorer, leading to lower levels of vitamin D. Recently, Cervero and colleagues[23] showed that lack of viral suppression was associated with a 3.5 times higher risk of vitamin D deficiency. On the contrary, Welz and colleagues[34] found no association between HIV viral load and vitamin D deficiency.

OUTCOMES ASSOCIATED WITH VITAMIN D DEFICIENCY/INSUFFICIENCY

Among HIV-uninfected individuals, several adverse outcomes are associated with vitamin D deficiency. These outcomes considerably overlap with NADIs that have recently become more prevalent in the HIV-infected population (**Fig. 1**).

Musculoskeletal Disease

Osteopenia and osteoporosis

Low BMD is 4 to 6 times more prevalent among HIV-infected persons compared with the general population.[43] It is also more commonly seen among vitamin D–deficient

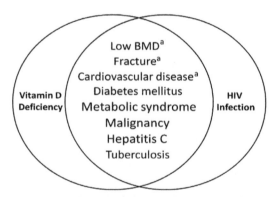

Fig. 1. Adverse outcomes shared by HIV infection and vitamin D deficiency. These outcomes, which are highly prevalent in both the HIV-infected and the HIV-uninfected vitamin D–deficient populations, overlap with some of the deleterious sequelae associated with persistent chronic inflammation. The latter is also characteristic of HIV infection and associated with vitamin D deficiency in the general population. [a] Independently associated with vitamin D deficiency in the general population and with HIV infection.

HIV-uninfected individuals.[44–46] Prolonged vitamin D deficiency is known to cause hypocalcemia, which leads to secondary hyperparathyroidism and subsequent bone demineralization.[47] Despite this mechanistic basis of bone loss, it is important to note that there are studies in the general population that fail to show a link between vitamin D deficiency and low BMD.[48–50]

In the HIV-infected population, most studies show no association between vitamin D and BMD. Among 672 participants in the SUN Study, the proportion of subjects with dual X-ray absorptiometry (DXA) T score less than or equal to -1 was not statistically different between the vitamin D sufficient and insufficient groups.[22] Sherwood and colleagues[51] found no association between vitamin D deficiency and low BMD and observed no correlation between 25-OHD and DXA T scores among 271 subjects. Similarly, Casado and colleagues[52] demonstrated that secondary factors such as hepatitis C co-infection and chronic kidney disease were significantly associated with low BMD, but no association was found with 25-OHD less than 20 ng/mL. Likewise, Amiel and colleagues[53] showed that the significantly lower BMD among their HIV-infected male subjects compared with HIV-uninfected controls was not attributable to differences in vitamin D levels between the 2 groups. In other studies, median vitamin D levels were not significantly different among HIV-infected persons with normal BMD and those with either osteopenia or osteoporosis.[54–56] The level of PTH was also not associated with low BMD in most of these studies.[51,53,55,56]

An association between vitamin D and BMD has only been shown by a few investigators. Among 100 HIV-infected women, Dolan and colleagues[57] showed that baseline 25-OHD was positively correlated with higher baseline hip BMD. However, when these participants were followed for a median of 24 months, baseline vitamin D level failed to predict significant reduction in BMD. In another study, baseline 25-OHD less than 20 ng/mL was predictive of greater than 3% femoral neck BMD decline among 100 premenopausal women enrolled in the Women's Interagency HIV Study (WIHS) after a median follow-up of 2.5 years.[58] Other investigators have also observed a correlation between vitamin D levels and BMD but only in the lumbar spine and among Hispanic subjects but not in other sites or among African American participants.[59]

Fracture, muscle strength, and fall risk

Low BMD comprises only a part of the composite risk for fragility fracture. Risk of fall comprises the other component.[60,61] Several[62–64] but not all[65,66] observational studies in the general population show that vitamin D deficiency is associated with risk of fragility fracture. Similarly, several studies suggest an association between vitamin D deficiency and increased fall risk,[67,68] muscle weakness, and poor performance on physical function testing.[69] These associations may, in part, be explained by the effect of vitamin D on skeletal muscles, which also contain vitamin D receptors.[70] Atrophy, fibrosis, and fat infiltration are often seen in muscle biopsy of vitamin D–deficient individuals.[70] Although the optimum serum concentration of vitamin D that prevents fracture remains controversial in the general population, hip and nonvertebral fractures were prevented in several studies when 25-OHD increased to 40 ng/mL after vitamin D supplementation.[71]

The impact of vitamin D deficiency on fracture risk has not been investigated in the HIV-infected population. However, in a recent study, Ansemant and colleagues[72] showed that 25-OHD less than 10 ng/mL was significantly associated with increased fall risk in a cohort of 263 HIV-infected persons in France after adjustment for age, sex, hepatitis B or C co-infection, and tobacco use. HIV-infected persons often have several risk factors for falling, such as having several concurrent comorbidities (ie, cardiovascular disease, hypertension), polypharmacy, cognitive impairment, peripheral neuropathy, psychiatric illness, and frailty.[73] The latter, for instance, is a geriatric syndrome characterized by low endurance, poor strength, and low physical activity that occurs at an earlier age among HIV-infected persons compared with the general population.[74] However, 25-OHD level has not been found to be correlated with the occurrence of frailty among HIV-infected persons.[75,76]

Cardiovascular Disease

Either because of an excess of traditional risk factors (eg, 2 to 3 times higher prevalence of smoking)[77] in the HIV-infected population or because of HIV infection itself,[78–81] the risk of cardiovascular disease is significantly greater among HIV-infected persons compared with the general population. An independent association between vitamin D deficiency and cardiovascular disease has also been demonstrated in several large observational studies among HIV-uninfected individuals.[4,82] Suppression of the renin-angiotensin system and stimulation of cellular proliferation and differentiation induced by binding of 1,25 OHD to vitamin D receptors in the heart, the endothelium, and the vascular smooth muscle are some of the proposed mechanisms of how vitamin D influences cardiovascular health.[32,83]

In the HIV-infected population, only a handful of studies investigating the association of vitamin D deficiency and cardiovascular disease is available. Among participants with mostly suppressed viremia in the Hawaii Aging with HIV-Cardiovascular Cohort Study, an increased likelihood of having coronary artery calcium (CAC) was demonstrated among vitamin D–deficient subjects.[84] In addition, higher levels of vitamin D were also shown in this study to be positively correlated with higher brachial artery flow-mediated dilatation (FMD). Possibly because of a small sample size, no association was seen with carotid artery intima-media thickness (cIMT). In another cross-sectional study, an independent, graded, stepwise increase in cIMT with decreasing vitamin D levels was demonstrated among 139 HIV-infected participants even after adjusting for age, sex, hypertension, elevated cholesterol, and tobacco use.[85] Similarly, Ross and colleagues,[86] in a study among 149 HIV-infected individuals, demonstrated that for each standard deviation decrease in vitamin D level, there is a 10-fold increased risk of having a cIMT above the median range. Using computed tomographic coronary angiography in a cohort of 674 HIV-infected African Americans (48% cocaine users), Lai and colleagues[87] identified 64 (10%) participants with significant asymptomatic coronary artery stenosis (ie, ≥50% obstruction). On multivariate analysis, participants with 25-OHD less than 10 ng/mL were found to have a 2-fold risk of having prevalent coronary artery stenosis independent of sex, cocaine use, hypertension, elevated cholesterol, diabetes, body mass index (BMI), and tobacco use. In a follow-up study wherein cocaine users with low Framingham risk score (ie, score <10%) and who did not have significant carotid artery stenosis at enrollment were followed over time, the same authors found that incident coronary artery stenosis was significantly greater in participants with vitamin D deficiency compared with subjects who had higher vitamin D levels (11/100 person-years vs 2/100 person-years). The time interval for the development of significant coronary artery stenosis among vitamin D–deficient participants was also significantly shorter compared with vitamin D–sufficient subjects. On multivariate analysis, after adjustment for traditional risk factors, vitamin D deficiency was shown to be the only risk factor independently associated with incident carotid artery stenosis.[88]

Asymptomatic cardiovascular disease, as demonstrated by cIMT, CAC, and brachial artery FMD, has been strongly linked with cardiovascular event occurrence in the general population.[89–91] These markers of silent coronary artery disease have also been independently associated with vitamin D deficiency among HIV-uninfected individuals.[92–94] However, studies showing association of vitamin D deficiency with cardiovascular events (eg, myocardial infarction, unstable angina) are lacking in the HIV-infected population, and there is no evidence that repletion of vitamin D affects cardiovascular outcomes.

Diabetes, Insulin Resistance, and the Metabolic Syndrome

In animal models, vitamin D deficiency is associated with impaired pancreatic β-cell function and insulin resistance.[95] Studies in the general population have demonstrated independent association of vitamin D deficiency with diabetes[5] and with the metabolic syndrome.[96] On the other hand, in the HIV-infected population, independent association with vitamin D deficiency has only been demonstrated with diabetes and not with the metabolic syndrome. In a cross-sectional study of 1811 HIV-infected persons in Italy, vitamin D deficiency was shown to be the strongest independent risk factor for diabetes after adjustment for sex, age, BMI, and hepatitis C coinfection (odds ratio: 1.85; 95% confidence interval: 1.03–3.32).[97] No association between vitamin D deficiency and the metabolic syndrome was seen after adjustment for confounders in this study. Furthermore, among 754 HIV-infected women enrolled in WIHS, vitamin D deficiency was not shown to be independently associated with insulin resistance as measured by the homeostasis model assessment after adjustment for multiple covariables.[98] Even though the prevalence of the metabolic syndrome and the incidence of diabetes among HIV-infected persons are comparable to the general population,[99,100] the high prevalence of the metabolic syndrome in the HIV-infected population (11%–45%)[101] remains concerning because of the significant risk of cardiovascular disease in this population.

Tuberculosis, Hepatitis C, HIV Disease Progression

Tuberculosis

The discovery that vitamin D plays a role in monocyte/macrophage differentiation and activation led to research on the immunomodulatory and antimicrobial function of vitamin D.[102,103] Monocyte activation upregulates vitamin D receptors and triggers 1,25-OHD synthesis, which then initiates a cascade of mechanisms that have been shown to inhibit growth of *Mycobacterium tuberculosis*, including synthesis of cathelicidin and induction of phagolysosomal fusion and autophagy.[104–106] In the general population, persons with 25-OHD less than 4 ng/mL were shown to have 3-fold odds of having active tuberculosis.[107] Vitamin D has also been historically used to treat pulmonary tuberculosis during the preantibiotic era with mixed results.[108]

A cross-sectional study among 174 HIV-infected and 196 HIV-uninfected individuals in Cape Town, South Africa showed that vitamin D deficiency is independently associated with active tuberculosis and that this association is greater among HIV-infected persons.[109] In a cohort study of participants with smear-positive tuberculosis initiating antimicrobial treatment in Tanzania, of whom 344 (51%) were HIV-infected, Mehta and colleagues[110] showed that serum 25-OHD less than 30 ng/mL was independently associated with disease relapse 1 month after tuberculosis treatment initiation. Surprisingly, vitamin D level less than 20 ng/mL was not associated with this outcome. In another prospective cohort study done in Tanzania that enrolled 1103 HIV-infected persons initiating highly active antiretroviral therapy (HAART) and enrolled in a randomized controlled trial (RCT) of a vitamin D–free multivitamin supplementation, baseline 25-OHD less than 20 ng/mL was associated with higher incident smear-positive tuberculosis after a median follow-up of 20.6 months.[111] Reverse causality (ie, that vitamin D deficiency occurred as a result of tuberculosis) was ruled out in this study by the exclusion of patients who developed tuberculosis within 1 month of enrollment.

Hepatitis C

Hepatitis C virus (HCV) infection occurs at a significantly higher rate among HIV-infected persons compared with the general population.[112] HIV/HCV coinfected individuals also have a considerably lower response rate to traditional HCV treatment and higher progression to advanced liver disease compared with HCV mono-infected persons.[113,114] Vitamin D has been shown to act in synergy with interferon and ribavirin in inducing sustained virologic response.[115–117] Studies conducted among Hepatitis C monoinfected patients have shown independent association of vitamin D deficiency with treatment failure and severe liver fibrosis.[118–120] The exact mechanism of its antiviral effect is unknown, although it was recently shown to amplify the innate antiviral immune response by upregulating the expression of interferon-β and the MxA gene and dampening IP-10 expression.[115,121] Furthermore, vitamin D has been shown to directly inhibit the proliferation and the profibrotic effect of hepatic stellate cells.[122]

Studies conducted among HIV-HCV coinfected persons also show association between vitamin D and liver fibrosis. Among 189 subjects, Terrier and colleagues[123] demonstrated that low 25-OHD was independently associated with severe liver fibrosis on biopsy and also correlated with serum markers of fibrosis. A similar finding was also observed by Milazzo and colleagues[124] in a more recent study. On the other hand, studies investigating the association between sustained virologic response and vitamin D level have shown varying results with some studies demonstrating an association,[125,126] whereas other studies do not.[123,127]

HIV disease progression

Preclinical experiments have demonstrated that treatment of peripheral blood mononuclear cells with 1,25-OHD decreased the cells' susceptibility to HIV infection by inhibiting viral entry, modulating expression of CD4+ cell surface antigen, damping viral p24 production, and limiting monocyte proliferation.[128,129] Thereafter, several observational studies have shown significant association between higher levels of vitamin D and rates of immune recovery.[130–132]

Studies have also been conducted to investigate the association of vitamin D and clinical outcomes. Among 884 HIV-infected pregnant women in Tanzania who were followed for a median of 70 months, baseline 25-OHD less than 32 ng/mL was shown to be independently associated with progression to more advanced HIV stage and that women with 25-OHD in the highest quintile had a 42% lower risk of all-cause mortality than women with levels in the lowest quintile.[133] The same observations were also demonstrated in a large European study involving almost 2000 participants.[42] In this study, subjects with baseline 25-OHD greater than 12 ng/mL had statistically significant lower 5-year all-cause mortality risk and clinical progression to AIDS compared with those with lower 25-OHD level. Vitamin D deficiency has also been associated with incident severe anemia, low BMI, acute upper respiratory infections, and oral thrush.[134] It should be noted that other studies have failed to demonstrate an association between vitamin D level and clinical outcomes. Sherwood and colleagues,[51] in a study involving 271 US participants followed for at least 8 years, failed to show significant association between baseline 25-OHD less than 20 ng/mL and all-cause mortality, clinical progression to AIDS, respiratory disease, hospitalizations, and malignancies. However, this study was limited because of its small sample size and modest number of observed clinical outcomes.

Malignancy and Chronic Inflammation

Malignancy

The association of vitamin D deficiency with risk of cancer in the HIV-infected population remains to be determined. However, vitamin D deficiency in the general population has been linked with higher cancer risk including colon cancer (2-fold risk),[135] breast cancer (4-fold risk),[136] prostate cancer (3-fold risk),[137] and ovarian cancer (4-fold risk).[138] In experimental studies, vitamin D has been demonstrated to exert antitumor effects by suppressing tumor angiogenesis, restricting cancer proliferation by contact inhibition, and stimulating cellular differentiation and apoptosis.[135,139] It is important to note that regardless of vitamin D status, HIV-infected persons have a high cancer risk. HIV infection may slightly increase the risk of some non-AIDS malignancies, independent of known risk factors.[140] However, vitamin D deficiency has not been implicated in any study of HIV and cancer.

Chronic inflammation

HIV infection is associated with chronic inflammation (ie, elevated tumor necrosis factor [TNF], interleukin-6 [IL-6], C-reactive protein [CRP]) and immune system activation (ie, increased soluble CD14, CXCL10) that persist even after achieving full virologic suppression and immune recovery with the use of HAART.[141,142] Elevated markers of inflammation have been shown in the HIV-infected population to be independent predictors of cardiovascular events,[143,144] diabetes and the metabolic syndrome,[145,146] low BMD,[147] malignancies,[148] neurocognitive impairment,[149] frailty,[150] and all-cause mortality.[151–153] Chronic inflammation has also been associated with these outcomes, including all-cause mortality, in the general population.[154–156] Thus, there is a considerable overlap in the outcomes associated with vitamin D deficiency and chronic inflammation in both the HIV-infected and HIV-uninfected populations.

Because most cells in the immune system bear vitamin D receptors, vitamin D serves as a powerful immune modulator. It inhibits T-cell proliferation and activation[157–159] and suppresses the development of Th1[160] and Th17 cells.[161] The shift of the cytokine balance toward a proinflammatory Th1/Th17 response may be one of the mechanisms behind the association of vitamin D deficiency with several autoimmune diseases including multiple sclerosis,[162] rheumatoid arthritis,[163] systemic lupus erythematosus,[164] and type 1 diabetes mellitus.[165]

The role of vitamin D deficiency in HIV-associated chronic inflammation is an area of active research. In one study involving 316 participants in Nepal, the risk of having high-sensitivity C-reactive protein (hsCRP) greater than 3 mg/L, a level considered by the American Heart Association as high risk for cardiovascular events,[166] was 3-fold greater among subjects with 25-OHD less than 20 ng/mL compared with those with higher vitamin D levels.[167] In other studies, levels of 25-OHD were shown to correlate positively with levels of interleukin-6 (IL-6) ($r = 0.14$, $P = .02$),[72] tumor necrosis factor-α (TNF-α) ($r = -0.21$, $P = .03$),[168] and T-cell activation markers ($r = -0.3$, $P = .01$).[168]

BENEFITS OF VITAMIN D SUPPLEMENTATION

Recommendations regarding vitamin D supplementation in the general population are mostly derived from studies on bone health. Several large RCTs demonstrate beneficial effects of vitamin D plus calcium on BMD[169] and fracture risk.[170] Meta-analyses show that supplementing vitamin D with calcium is superior to using vitamin D alone for preventing fracture.[170] On the other hand, the evidence for vitamin D use on clinical outcomes beyond skeletal health, on diabetes, the metabolic syndrome, cardiovascular disease, cancer, immune response, falls, are inconsistent and insufficient to base general recommendations (**Table 1**).

Table 1
Summary of vitamin D supplementation studies in the HIV-infected population compared to the general population

Outcome	Intervention	Change in 25-OHD	Results	Studies in the General Population
Musculoskeletal disease				
Etiminani-Esfahani et al,[171] 2012	Vitamin D 300,000 IU once	Modest increase	Net bone formation was observed based on longitudinal changes in BTM	Significant improvement in BMD[169,172]
Bang et al,[173] 2013	Calcitriol 0.5–1 μg + cholecalciferol 1,200 IU + calcium 800 g vs cholecalciferol 1,200 IU + calcium 800 g for 16 weeks	Modest increase	Net bone formation was observed based on longitudinal changes in BTM	Variable effects on fracture prevention[174,175]
Piso et al,[176] 2013	Cholecalciferol 300,000 IU once		No effect on BTM, but PTH declined in subjects receiving tenofovir	
Havens, et al,[177] 2012	Cholecalciferol 50,000 IU at 0, 4, 8 weeks	95% had 25-OHD >20 ng/mL at 12 weeks compared with 48% at baseline in the vitamin D group		
van den Bout-van den Beukel et al,[178] 2008	Cholecalciferol 2,000 IU daily for 14 weeks, then 1,000 IU daily until 48 weeks	Significantly increased from baseline	No statistically significant BMD change was observed	
Mondy et al,[179] 2005	Vitamin D 400 IU + calcium 1 g daily for 48 weeks	No measurement performed	No statistically significant BMD change was observed	
McComsey et al,[180] 2007	Vitamin D 400 IU + calcium 1 g daily for 48 weeks	Not measured before and after treatment	BMD increased by 1.3% at the total hip but not at other sites	
Arpadi et al,[181] 2012	Cholecalciferol 100,000 IU every 2 months + calcium 1 g daily for 2 years	Significantly increased	Increased BMD not statistically significant compared with placebo	
Overton et al,[182] 2014	Cholecalciferol 4,000 IU daily + calcium 1 g daily for 48 weeks	Significantly increased enough to reach sufficient level	Lesser BMD decline at the total hip compared with placebo; lower bone resorption marker increase compared with placebo	
Yin et al,[183] 2010	Self-reported vitamin D and calcium intake	Not provided	No association with incident fracture	

Study	Intervention	Vitamin D level	Outcome	Conclusion
Cardiovascular disease				
Longenecker et al,[184] 2012	Cholecalciferol 4,000 IU daily for 12 weeks	Significantly increased but not enough to reach sufficient level	No change in brachial artery FMD	Role remains to be established[185]
Insulin resistance				
Longenecker et al,[184] 2012	Cholecalciferol 4,000 IU daily for 12 weeks	Significantly increased but not enough to reach sufficient level	Significant increased HOMA-IR in the vitamin D group but not statistically different from placebo	No improvement in fasting glucose, HgbA(1c), or insulin resistance[186]
van den Bout-van den Beukel et al,[178] 2008	Cholecalciferol 2,000 IU daily for 14 weeks, then 1,000 IU daily until 48 weeks	Significantly increased from baseline	Increased insulin resistance	
Chronic inflammation				
Longenecker et al,[184] 2012	Cholecalciferol 4,000 IU daily for 12 weeks	Significantly increased but not enough to reach sufficient level	Not associated with change in markers of inflammation	Role remains to be established[187]
van den Bout-van den Beukel et al,[178] 2008	Cholecalciferol 2,000 IU daily for 14 weeks, then 1000 IU daily until 48 weeks	Significantly increased from baseline	Not associated with change in markers of inflammation	
Giacomet et al,[188] 2013	Cholecalciferol 100,000 IU every 3 months for 4 doses	20% remained vitamin D deficient in the vitamin D group compared with 60% in the placebo	Resulted in a shift to an anti-inflammatory T-cell phenotype	
HIV disease progression				
Giacomet et al,[188] 2013	Cholecalciferol 100,000 IU every 3 months for 4 doses	20% remained vitamin D deficient in the vitamin D group compared with 60% in the placebo	No change in CD4+ cell count	N/A
Kakalia et al,[189] 2011	Vitamin D 5,600 IU/week vs 11,200 IU/week	Significantly increased but only 67% reached sufficiency level	No change in CD4+ cell count	

Abbreviations: 25-OHD, 25-hyroxyvitamin D; BMD, bone mineral density; BTM, bone turnover markers; HgbA(1c), hemoglobin A(1c); HOMA-IR, homeostasis model assessment-insulin resistance; IU, international units; PTH, parathyroid hormone.

Data from Refs.[171,173,176–184]

Bone Turnover Markers, Bone Mineral Density, and Fracture

In the HIV-infected population, several prospective studies show that vitamin D supplementation results in net bone formation by assessing changes in bone turnover markers (BTM) over time. Among 107 subjects taking efavirenz in Iran, one-time intramuscular dose of vitamin D 300,000 IU led to a significant increase in serum osteocalcin (a bone formation marker) and collagen type 1 C-telopeptide (CTx; a bone resorption marker) after 3 months. Because the increase in osteocalcin (208%) was greater in magnitude compared with CTx (60%), the investigators concluded that vitamin D supplementation led to net bone formation.[171] Other studies confirmed this finding even with only modest increases in 25-OHD with the use of high-dose cholecalciferol alone or a combination of calcitriol and cholecalciferol.[173,176] On the other hand, a study conducted in a US cohort of 203 youths between 18 and 25 years of age failed to demonstrate significant change in BTM at 12 weeks among subjects randomized to receive cholecalciferol 50,000 IU at 0, 4, and 8 weeks, compared with placebo.[177]

The effect of vitamin D supplementation on longitudinal changes in BMD is underwhelming. In a small nonrandomized study among 20 participants with 25-OHD less than 10 to 14 ng/mL in the Netherlands, supplementation with cholecalciferol 2,000 IU/day for 14 weeks followed by 1,000 IU/day until 48 weeks did not result in a significant change in BMD at week 48 even with significant increases in 25-OHD. The authors attributed this finding to the low prevalence of osteopenia and osteoporosis at baseline among their participants.[178] Similarly, Mondy and colleagues,[179] in a cohort of 31 participants originally enrolled in an RCT powered to detect lumbar spine BMD change with the use of alendronate, showed that among subjects randomized to receive only calcium 1 g/day plus vitamin D 400 IU daily, lumbar spine BMD increased by 1.3% at 48 weeks compared with baseline (vs 5.2% in the alendronate group). This change, however, was not statistically significant. In another RCT comparing alendronate with fixed dose calcium and vitamin D, a significant but mild increase in BMD was observed at the total hip (1.3%, $P = .03$), but not at other sites among participants receiving only calcium and vitamin D.[180]

Two RCTs compared vitamin D with placebo. The first study was conducted among 59 children aged 6 to 16 years in the United States who were randomized to receive either cholecalciferol 100,000 IU every 2 months plus calcium 1 g/day or calcium 1 g/day alone for 2 years. Total body and spine BMD significantly increased in both arms after 2 years but no between-group difference was observed.[181] The second study was more recent and conducted among 165 adult participants initiating efavirenz-based cART. Participants were randomized to receive cholecalciferol 4,000 IU daily plus calcium 1 g/day or placebo for 48 weeks. BMDs before and after 48 weeks of cART initiation were compared. Participants who received cholecalciferol plus calcium had statistically significant lower total hip BMD decline (1.46%) compared with those who received placebo (3.19%) and also had lower CTx increase compared with the placebo group.[182] The results of this study suggest that vitamin D plus calcium supplementation during cART initiation could potentially prevent bone loss that is consistently seen with cART initiation.[190]

There are few studies on fracture risk and vitamin D supplementation. Among 2391 women (1728 HIV-infected, 663 HIV-uninfected) followed over a median time of 5.4 years, fracture incidence did not differ according to HIV status. There were more HIV-infected than HIV-uninfected women taking vitamin D supplements at baseline (42% vs 28%, $P \leq .001$). However, self-reported vitamin D or calcium intake was not associated with lower incidence of fracture in either group.[183]

Other Effects

The authors could only find one study investigating the effect of vitamin D supplementation on cardiovascular outcomes in the HIV-infected population. In an RCT involving 45 subjects with 25-OHD less than 20 ng/mL, 12-week supplementation with daily oral cholecalciferol 4,000 IU did not result in a statistically significant change in brachial artery FMD compared with placebo.[184] In the same study, insulin resistance increased from baseline with vitamin D supplementation but was not statistically different from the placebo arm. Baseline inflammatory markers (ie, CRP, IL-6, sTNFR1) also did not change significantly with vitamin D supplementation compared with placebo. These results could partly be attributed to the modest increase in 25-OHD (5 ng/mL) among subjects receiving vitamin D supplementation. A smaller prospective study in the Netherlands also failed to demonstrate benefit of vitamin D supplementation on insulin resistance and inflammatory markers (ie, IL-6, TNF-α) after 48 weeks.[178]

In an RCT involving 52 mostly virologically suppressed vertically infected youths aged 8 to 26 years with 25-OHD less than 30 ng/mL, Giacomet and colleagues[188] showed that 12-month supplementation with cholecalciferol 100,000 IU every 3 months for 4 doses resulted in an anti-inflammatory T-cell phenotype (ie, decrease in Th17:Treg ratio) at 3 months. This effect was no longer seen at 12 months. There was also no significant change in baseline CD4+ cell count observed between the treatment and placebo arms despite that only 20% of the participants in the treatment group remained vitamin D–deficient compared with 60% in the placebo group ($P = .007$). The lack of effect of vitamin D supplementation on gain in CD4+ cell count over time despite increases in 25-OHD was also demonstrated among 53 children (85% with 25-OHD <20 ng/mL) with preserved immune function.[189]

Screening and Treatment Recommendations

The Endocrine Society published guidelines for the general population on screening and treatment of vitamin D deficiency in 2011. For screening, they recommend that only patients at risk for vitamin D deficiency be screened by checking serum 25-OHD. In adults with vitamin D deficiency, they recommend treatment with 50,000 IU weekly of ergocalciferol or cholecalciferol, or 6,000 IU daily until 25-OHD serum levels reach 30 ng/mL.[16]

In the HIV-infected population, the European AIDS Clinical Society's most recent guidelines suggest checking vitamin D status in patients with a history of low BMD or fracture, those with high risk of fracture, or those with other factors associated with vitamin D deficiency. For persons with 25-OHD less than 10 ng/mL, they advocate for vitamin D replacement. For those with 25-OHD between 10 and 20 ng/mL, supplementation is recommended only for patients with osteoporosis, osteomalacia, or increased PTH.[191]

McComsey and colleagues[192] developed recommendations for bone disease in HIV infection, addressing vitamin D deficiency as well. They recommend 50,000 IU of vitamin D weekly for 8 to 12 weeks and then monthly thereafter, or 2,000 IU daily for 12 weeks and then 1,000 to 2,000 IU daily thereafter. Vitamin D levels after replacement should be measured. They recommend supplementation to achieve 25-OHD greater than 32 ng/mL.

Several small studies have evaluated vitamin D supplementation in the HIV-infected population. Childs and colleagues[193] reported on dose response data in HIV-infected patients on vitamin D supplementation. A total of 74 subjects were supplemented, with higher doses given to those with lower baseline 25-OHD (2,800 IU for <10 ng/mL; 1,800 for 10–20 ng/mL; and 800 IU for 20–30 ng/mL). At 16 weeks, in those patients reporting

100% adherence, 25-OHD increased by 15 ng/mL, with the greatest increase in those with the lowest baseline 25-OHD. Recently, Falasca and colleagues[194] enrolled 153 participants in a vitamin D supplementation study and provided 67 subjects with 25,000 IU cholecalciferol monthly for 10 months. They achieved an increase in 25-OHD from 15.7 to 27.4 ng/mL. Several other vitamin D dosing regimens have been tried with varying effects on baseline 25-OHD (see **Table 1**).

Vitamin D toxicity, characterized by hypercalcemia, is rarely seen. Hathcock and colleagues[195] evaluated numerous dosing studies and did not find any cases of intoxication in individuals taking up to 10,000 IU daily of cholecalciferol. They suggested this dose for cholecalciferol as the tolerable upper intake level. Rare cases of vitamin D intoxication have been seen in some patients taking long-term nonprescription dietary supplements who were not monitored, in those patients with other comorbidities such as renal insufficiency, and in those who were also on confounding medications such as hydrochlorothiazide and prednisone.[195]

SUMMARY

The prevalence of vitamin D deficiency among HIV-infected persons is substantial and comparable with the general population. The factors associated with vitamin D deficiency are similar for both populations, but additional factors (ie, use of certain antiretroviral agents) also contribute to vitamin D deficiency among HIV-infected persons. The adverse outcomes associated with vitamin D deficiency considerably overlap with NADIs that are increasingly becoming widespread in the aging HIV-infected population. However, there is scant evidence to support any causal inference. Firm recommendations regarding vitamin D deficiency screening and treatment are lacking in the HIV-infected population reflecting the lack of studies that show unequivocal benefit of vitamin D supplementation in this group of individuals. Further studies are evidently warranted as efforts to identify and address modifiable risk factors contributing to NADIs continue.

REFERENCES

1. Heaney RP. Vitamin D and calcium interactions: functional outcomes. Am J Clin Nutr 2008;88(suppl):541S–4S.
2. Hess AF, Lewis JM, Rivkin H. Newer aspects of the therapeutics of viosterol (irradiated ergosterol). JAMA 1930;94:1885.
3. Hess AF, Unger LF. The cure of infantile rickets by sunlight. JAMA 1921;77:39.
4. Kendrick J, Targher G, Smits G, et al. 25-Hydroxyvitamin D deficiency is independently associated with cardiovascular disease in the Third National Health and Nutrition Examination Survey. Atherosclerosis 2009;205(1):255–60.
5. Mattila C, Knekt P, Mannisto S, et al. Serum 25-hydroxyvitamin D concentration and subsequent risk of type 2 diabetes. Diabetes Care 2007;30(10):2569–70.
6. Wicherts IS, van Schoor NM, Boeke AJ, et al. Vitamin D status predicts physical performance and its decline in older persons. J Clin Endocrinol Metab 2007;92(6):2958–65.
7. Snijder MB, van Schoor NM, Pluijm SM, et al. Vitamin D status in relation to one-year risk of recurrent falling in older men and women. J Clin Endocrinol Metab 2006;91(8):2980–5.
8. Cooper JD, Smyth DJ, Walker NM, et al. Inherited variation in vitamin D genes is associated with predisposition to autoimmune disease type 1 diabetes. Diabetes 2011;60(5):1624–31.

9. Tangpricha V, Flanagan JN, Whitlach LW, et al. 25-hydroxyvitamin D-1alpha-hydroxylase in normal and malignant colon tissue. Lancet 2001;357(9269): 1673–4.

10. Kovalenko PL, Zhang Z, Yu JG, et al. Dietary vitamin D and vitamin D receptor level modulate epithelial cell proliferation and apoptosis in the prostate. Cancer Prev Res (Phila) 2011;4(10):1617–25.

11. Rose AA, Elser C, Ennis M, et al. Blood levels of vitamin D and early stage breast cancer prognosis: a systematic review and meta-analysis. Breast Cancer Res Treat 2013;141(3):331–9.

12. Palella FJ Jr, Delaney KM, Moorman AC, et al. Declining morbidity and mortality among patients with advanced human immunodeficiency virus infection. HIV Outpatient Study Investigators. N Engl J Med 1998;338(13):853–60.

13. Effros RB, Fletcher CV, Gebo K, et al. Workshop on HIV infection and aging: what is known and future research directions. Clin Infect Dis 2008;47(4):542–53.

14. Hollick MF. McCollum Award Lecture. Vitamin D: new horizons for the 21st century. Am J Clin Nutr 1994;60:619–30.

15. DeLuca HF. Overview of general physiologic features and functions of vitamin D. Am J Clin Nutr 2004;80(6 Suppl):1689S–96S.

16. Holick MF, Binkley NC, Bischoff-Ferrari HA, et al. Evaluation, treatment, and prevention of vitamin D deficiency: an Endocrine Society clinical practice guideline. J Clin Endocrinol Metab 2011;96(7):1911–30.

17. National Center for Health Statistics, Centers for Disease Control and Prevention, National health and nutrition examination survey. Available at: http://www.cdc.gov/nchs/nhanes/about_nhanes.htm. Accessed March 10, 2014.

18. Gedela K, Edwards SG, Benn P, et al. Prevalence of vitamin D deficiency in HIV-positive, antiretroviral treatment-naïve patients in a single centre study. Int J STD AIDS 2013;25(7):488–92.

19. Mueller NJ, Fux CA, Ledergerber B, et al. High prevalence of severe vitamin D deficiency in combined antiretroviral therapy-naive and successfully treated Swiss HIV patients. AIDS 2010;24(8):1127–34.

20. Kim JH, Gandhi V, Psevdos G Jr, et al. Evaluation of vitamin D levels among HIV-infected patients in New York City. AIDS Res Hum Retroviruses 2012;28(3): 235–41.

21. Van Den Bout-Van Den Beukel CJ, Fievez L, Michels M, et al. Vitamin D deficiency among HIV type 1-infected individuals in the Netherlands: effects of antiretroviral therapy. AIDS Res Hum Retroviruses 2008;24(11):1375–82.

22. Dao CN, Patel P, Overton ET, et al. Low vitamin D among HIV-infected adults: prevalence of and risk factors for low vitamin D levels in a cohort of HIV-infected adults and comparison to prevalence among adults in the US general population. Clin Infect Dis 2011;52:396–405.

23. Cervero M, Agud JL, Garcia-Lacalle C, et al. Prevalence of vitamin D deficiency and its related risk factor in a Spanish cohort of adult HIV-infected patients: effects of antiretroviral therapy. AIDS Res Hum Retroviruses 2012;28(9): 963–71.

24. Vescini F, Cozzi-Lepri A, Borderi M, et al. Prevalence of hypovitaminosis D and factors associated with vitamin D deficiency and morbidity among HIV-infected patients enrolled in a large Italian cohort. J Acquir Immune Defic Syndr 2011; 58(2):163–72.

25. Allavena C, Delpierre C, Cuzin L, et al. High frequency of vitamin D deficiency in HIV-infected patients: effects of HIV-related factors and antiretroviral drugs. J Antimicrob Chemother 2012;67:2222–30.

26. Theodorou M, Serté T, Van Gossum M, et al. Factors associated with vitamin D deficiency in a population of 2044 HIV-infected patients. Clin Nutr 2014;2:274–9.
27. Crutchley RD, Gathe J, Mayberry C, et al. Risk factors for vitamin D deficiency in HIV-infected patients in the south central United States. AIDS Res Hum Retroviruses 2012;28(5):454–9.
28. Holick MF. Vitamin D and bone health. J Nutr 1996;126(4 Suppl):1159S–64S.
29. Holick MF, Chen TC. Vitamin D deficiency: a worldwide problem with health consequences. Am J Clin Nutr 2008;87(Suppl):1080S–6S.
30. Adeyemi OM, Agniel D, French AL. Vitamin D deficiency in HIV-infected and HIV-uninfected women in the United States. J Acquir Immune Defic Syndr 2011;57(3):197–204.
31. Hermann AP, Brot C, Gram J, et al. Premenopausal smoking and bone density in 2015 perimenopausal women. J Bone Miner Res 2000;15(4):780–7.
32. Holick MF. Vitamin D deficiency. N Engl J Med 2007;357(3):266–81.
33. Dusso AS, Brown AJ, Slatopolsky E. Vitamin D. Am J Physiol Renal Physiol 2005; 289:F8–28.
34. Welz T, Childs K, Ibrahim F, et al. Efavirenz is associated with severe vitamin D deficiency and increased alkaline phosphatase. AIDS 2010;24:1923–8.
35. Brown TT, McComsey GA. Association between initiation of antiretroviral therapy with efavirenz and decreases in 25-hydroxyvitamin D. Antivir Ther 2010;15(3): 425–9.
36. Wohl DA, Orkin C, Doroana M. Change in vitamin D levels and risk of severe vitamin D deficiency over 48 weeks among HIV-1 infected, treatment-naïve adults receiving rilpivirine or efavirenz in a Phase III trial (ECHO). Antivir Ther 2014;19(2):191–200.
37. Fox J, Peters B, Prakash M, et al. Improvement in vitamin D deficiency following antiretroviral regime change: results from the MONET trial. AIDS Res Hum Retroviruses 2011;27(1):29–34.
38. Lattuada E, Lanzafame M, Zoppini G, et al. No influence of nevirapine on vitamin D deficiency in HIV-infected patients. AIDS Res Hum Retroviruses 2009;25(8): 849–50.
39. Cozzolino M, Vidal M, Vittoria Arcidiacono M, et al. HIV-protease inhibitors impair vitamin D bioactivation to 1,25-dihydroxyvitamin D. AIDS 2003;17: 513–20.
40. Briot K, Kolta S, Flandre P, et al. Prospective one-year bone loss in treatment-naïve HIV+ men and women on single or multiple drug HIV therapies. Bone 2011;48(5):1133–9.
41. Mallizia AP, Cotter E, Chew N. HIV protease inhibitors selectively induce gene expression alterations associated with reduced calcium deposition in primary human osteoblasts. AIDS Res Hum Retroviruses 2007;23(2):243–50.
42. Viard JP, Souberbielle JC, Kirk O, et al. Vitamin D and clinical disease progression in HIV infection: results from the EuroSIDA study. AIDS 2011;25(10): 1305–15.
43. Brown TT, Qaqish RB. Antiretroviral therapy and the prevalence of osteopenia and osteoporosis: a meta-analytic review. AIDS 2006;20:2165–74.
44. Ooms ME, Lips P, Van Lingen A, et al. Determinants of bone mineral density and risk factors for osteoporosis in healthy elderly women. J Bone Miner Res 1993; 8(6):669–75.
45. Bischoff-Ferrari HA, Dietrich T, Orav EJ, et al. Positive association between 25-hydroxyvitamin D levels and bone mineral density: a population-based study of younger and older adults. Am J Med 2004;116(9):634–9.

46. Kuchuk NO, Pluijm SM, van Schoor NM, et al. Relationships of serum 25-hydroxy-vitamin D to bone mineral density and serum parathyroid hormone and markers of bone turnover in older persons. J Clin Endocrinol Metab 2009;94(4):1244–50.
47. Lips P. Vitamin D deficiency and secondary hyperparathyroidism in the elderly: consequences for bone loss and fractures and therapeutic implications. Endocr Rev 2001;22(4):477–501.
48. Hosseinpanah F, Rambod M, Hossein-Nejad A, et al. Association between vitamin D and bone mineral density in Iranian postmenopausal women. J Bone Miner Metab 2008;26(1):86–92.
49. Sigurdsson G, Franzson L, Steingrimsdottir L, et al. The association between parathyroid hormone, vitamin D and bone mineral density in 70-year-old Icelandic women. Osteoporos Int 2000;11(12):1031–5.
50. Tsai KS, Hsu SH, Cheng JP, et al. Vitamin D stores of urban women in Taipei: effect on bone density and bone turnover, and seasonal variation. Bone 1997; 20(4):371–4.
51. Sherwood JE, Mesner OC, Weintrob AC, et al. Vitamin D deficiency and its association with low bone mineral density, HIV-related factors, hospitalization, and death in a predominantly black HIV-infected cohort. Clin Infect Dis 2012;55(12): 1727–36.
52. Casado JL, Bañon S, Andrés R, et al. Prevalence of causes of secondary osteoporosis and contribution to lower bone mineral density in HIV-infected patients. Osteoporos Int 2014;25(3):1071–9.
53. Amiel C, Ostertag A, Slama L, et al. BMD is reduced in HIV-infected men irrespective of treatment. J Bone Miner Res 2004;19:402–9.
54. Rachid T, Devitt E, Meryron I, et al. No association of vitamin D levels with individual antiretroviral agents, duration of HIV infection, alkaline phosphatase levels nor bone mineral density findings. Abstracts presented at: 18th International AIDS Conference. Vienna, Austria, July 21, 2010.
55. Ramayo E, González-Moreno MP, Macías J, et al. Relationship between osteopenia, free testosterone, and vitamin D metabolite levels in HIV-infected patients with and without highly active antiretroviral therapy. AIDS Res Hum Retroviruses 2005;21(11):915–21.
56. Mondy K, Yarasheski K, Powderly WG, et al. Longitudinal evolution of bone mineral density and bone markers in human immunodeficiency virus-infected individuals. Clin Infect Dis 2003;36:482–90.
57. Dolan SE, Kanter JR, Grinspoon S. Longitudinal analysis of bone density in human immunodeficiency virus-infected women. J Clin Endocrinol Metab 2006; 91(8):2938–45.
58. Yin MT, Lu D, Cremers S, et al. Short-term bone loss in HIV-infected premenopausal women. J Acquir Immune Defic Syndr 2010;53(2):202–8.
59. Stein EM, Yin MT, McMahon DJ, et al. Vitamin D deficiency in HIV-infected postmenopausal Hispanic and African-American women. Osteoporos Int 2011; 22(2):477–87.
60. Dontas IA, Yiannakopoulos CK. Risk factors and prevention of osteoporosis-related fractures. J Musculoskelet Neuronal Interact 2007;7(3):268–72.
61. McClung MR. The relationship between bone mineral density and fracture risk. Curr Osteoporos Rep 2005;3(2):57–63.
62. Cauley JA, Lacroix AZ, Wu L, et al. Serum 25-hydroxyvitamin D concentrations and risk for hip fractures. Ann Intern Med 2008;149(4):242–50.
63. Looker AC. Serum 25-hydroxyvitamin D and risk of major osteoporotic fractures in older U.S. adults. J Bone Miner Res 2013;28(5):997–1006.

64. Edwards BJ, Langman CB, Bunta AD, et al. Secondary contributors to bone loss in osteoporosis related hip fractures. Osteoporos Int 2008;19(7):991–9.

65. Garnero P, Munoz F, Sornay-Rendu E, et al. Associations of vitamin D status with bone mineral density, bone turnover, bone loss and fracture risk in healthy post-menopausal women. The OFELY study. Bone 2007;40(3):716–22.

66. Rothenbacher D, Klenk J, Denkinger MD, et al. Prospective evaluation of renal function, serum vitamin D level, and risk of fall and fracture in community-dwelling elderly subjects. Osteoporos Int 2014;25(3):923–32.

67. Roddam AW, Neale R, Appleby P, et al. Association between plasma 25-hydroxyvitamin D levels and fracture risk: the EPIC-Oxford study. Am J Epidemiol 2007; 166(11):1327–36.

68. Murad MH, Elamin KB, Abu Elnour NO, et al. The effect of vitamin D on falls: a systematic review and meta-analysis. J Clin Endocrinol Metab 2011;96(10): 2997–3006.

69. Dam TT, von Muhlen D, Barrett-Connor EL. Sex-specific association of serum vitamin D levels with physical function in older adults. Osteoporos Int 2009; 20(5):751–60.

70. Boland R. Role of vitamin D in skeletal muscle function. Endocr Rev 1986;7(4): 434–48.

71. Bischoff-Ferrari HA, Giovannucci E, Willett WC, et al. Estimation of optimal serum concentrations of 25-hydroxyvitamin D for multiple health outcomes. Am J Clin Nutr 2006;84(1):18–28.

72. Ansemant T, Mahy S, Piroth C, et al. Severe hypovitaminosis D correlates with increased inflammatory markers in HIV infected patients. BMC Infect Dis 2013;13:7.

73. Erlandson KM, Allshouse AA, Jankowski CM, et al. Risk factors for falls in HIV-infected persons. J Acquir Immune Defic Syndr 2012;61(4):484–9.

74. Desquilbet L, Jacobson LP, Fried LP, et al. HIV-1 infection is associated with an earlier occurrence of a phenotype related to frailty. J Gerontol A Biol Sci Med Sci 2007;62(11):1279–86.

75. Onen N, Patel P, Baker J, et al. Frailty and pre-frailty in a contemporary cohort of HIV-infected adults in the SUN Study. Presented at the 19th Conference on Retroviruses and Opportunistic Infections. Seattle, WA, March 5–8, 2012 [abstract: 858].

76. Erlandson KM, Allshouse AA, Jankowski CM, et al. Functional impairment is associated with low bone and muscle mass among persons aging with HIV infection. J Acquir Immune Defic Syndr 2013;63(2):209–15.

77. Niaura R, Shadel WG, Morrow K, et al. Human immunodeficiency virus infection, AIDS, and smoking cessation: the time is now. Clin Infect Dis 2000;31(3):808–12.

78. Currier JS, Taylor A, Boyd F, et al. Coronary heart disease in HIV-infected individuals. J Acquir Immune Defic Syndr 2003;33(4):506–12.

79. Triant VA, Lee H, Hadigan C, et al. Increased acute myocardial infarction rates and cardiovascular risk factors among patients with human immunodeficiency virus disease. J Clin Endocrinol Metab 2007;92(7):2506–12.

80. Lo J, Abbara S, Shturman L, et al. Increased prevalence of subclinical coronary atherosclerosis detected by coronary computed tomography angiography in HIV-infected men. AIDS 2010;24(2):243–53.

81. Chow FC, Regan S, Feske S, et al. Comparison of ischemic stroke incidence in HIV-infected and non-HIV-infected patients in a US health care system. J Acquir Immune Defic Syndr 2012;60(4):351–8.

82. Wang TJ, Pencina MJ, Booth SL, et al. Vitamin D deficiency and risk of cardiovascular disease. Circulation 2008;117(4):503–11.

83. Yc Li, Kong J, Wei M, et al. 1,25-Dihydroxyvitamin D(3) is a negative endocrine regulator of the renin-angiotensin system. J Clin Invest 2002;110(2): 229–38.

84. Shikuma CM, Seto T, Liang CY, et al. Vitamin D levels and markers of arterial dysfunction in HIV. AIDS Res Hum Retroviruses 2012;28(8):793–7.

85. Choi A, Lo JC, Mulligan K, et al. Association of vitamin D insufficiency with carotid intima-media thickness in HIV-infected persons. Clin Infect Dis 2011;52(7): 941–4.

86. Ross AC, Judd S, Kumari M, et al. Vitamin D is linked to carotid intima-media thickness and immune reconstitution in HIV-positive individuals. Antivir Ther 2011;16(4):555–63.

87. Lai H, Gerstenblith G, Fishman EK, et al. Vitamin D deficiency is associated with silent coronary artery disease in cardiovascularly asymptomatic African Americans with HIV infection. Clin Infect Dis 2012;54(12):1747–55.

88. Lai H, Fishman EK, Gerstenblith G, et al. Vitamin D deficiency is associated with development of subclinical coronary artery disease in HIV-infected African American cocaine users with low Framingham-defined cardiovascular risk. Vasc Health Risk Manag 2013;9:729–37.

89. Polak JF, Pencina MJ, Pencina KM, et al. Carotid intima-media thickness and cardiovascular events. N Engl J Med 2011;365(3):213–21.

90. Kondros GT, Hoff JA, Sevrukov A, et al. Electron-beam tomography coronary artery calcium and cardiac events: a 37-month follow-up of 5635 initially asymptomatic low- to intermediate-risk adults. Circulation 2003;107(20):2571–6.

91. Schechter M, Shechter A, Koren-Moraq N, et al. Usefulness of brachial artery flow-mediated dilation to predict long-term cardiovascular events in subjects without heart disease. Am J Cardiol 2014;113(1):162–7.

92. Targher G, Bertolini L, Padovani R, et al. Serum 25-hydroxyvitamin D3 concentrations and carotid intima-media thickness among type 2 diabetic patients. Clin Endocrinol (Oxf) 2006;65(5):593–7.

93. De Boer IH, Kestenbaum B, Shoben AB, et al. 25-hydroxyvitamin D levels inversely associate with risk for developing coronary artery calcification. J Am Soc Nephrol 2009;20(8):1805–12.

94. Tarcin O, Yavuz DG, Ozben B, et al. Effect of vitamin D deficiency and replacement on endothelial function in asymptomatic subjects. J Clin Endocrinol Metab 2009;94(10):4023–30.

95. Chertow BS, Sivitz WI, Baranetsky NG, et al. Cellular mechanisms of insulin release: the effects of vitamin D deficiency and repletion on rat insulin secretion. Endocrinology 1983;113(4):1511–8.

96. Ford ES, Ajani UA, McGuire LC, et al. Concentrations of serum vitamin D and the metabolic syndrome among U.S. adults. Diabetes Care 2005;28(5):1228–30.

97. Szep Z, Guaraldi G, Shah SS, et al. Vitamin D deficiency is associated with type 2 diabetes mellitus in HIV infection. AIDS 2001;25(4):525–9.

98. Adeyemi OM, Livak B, Orsi J, et al. Vitamin D and insulin resistance in non-diabetic women's interagency HIV study participants. AIDS Patient Care STDS 2013;27(6):320–5.

99. Mondy K, Overton ET, Grubb J, et al. Metabolic syndrome in HIV-infected patients from an urban, Midwestern US outpatient population. Clin Infect Dis 2007;44(5):726–34.

100. Tien PC, Schneider MF, Cole SR, et al. Antiretroviral therapy exposure and incidence of diabetes mellitus in the Women's Interagency HIV Study. AIDS 2007; 21(13):1739–45.

101. Paula AA, Falcao MC, Pacheco AG. Metabolic syndrome in HIV-infected individuals: underlying mechanism and epidemiological aspects. AIDS Res Ther 2013; 10(1):32. http://dx.doi.org/10.1186/1742-6405-10-32.

102. Rook GA, Steele J, Fraher L, et al. Vitamin D3, gamma interferon, and control of proliferation of Mycobacterium tuberculosis by human monocytes. Immunology 1986;57(1):159–63.

103. Crowle AJ, Ross EJ, May MH. Inhibition by 1,25(OH)2-vitamin D3 of the multiplication of virulent tubercle bacilli in cultured human macrophages. Infect Immun 1987;55(12):2945–50.

104. Realgegeno S, Modlin RL. Shedding light on the vitamin D-tuberculosis-HIV connection. Proc Natl Acad Sci U S A 2011;109(47):18861–2.

105. Martineau AR, Wilkinson KA, Newton SM, et al. IFN-gamma- and TNF-independent vitamin D-inducible human suppression of mycobacteria: the role of cathelicidin LL-37. J Immunol 2007;178(11):7190–8.

106. Yuk JM, Shin DM, Lee HM, et al. Vitamin D3 induces autophagy in human monocytes/macrophages via cathelicidin. Cell Host Microbe 2009;6(3):231–43.

107. Wilkinson RJ, Llewelyn M, Toossi Z, et al. Influence of vitamin D deficiency and vitamin D receptor polymorphisms on tuberculosis among Gujarati Asians in west London: a case-control study. Lancet 2000;355(9204):618–21.

108. Martineau AR, Honecker FU, Wilkinson RJ, et al. Vitamin D in the treatment of pulmonary tuberculosis. J Steroid Biochem Mol Biol 2007;103(3–5):793–8.

109. Martineau AR, Timms PM, Bothamley GH, et al. High-dose vitamin D(3) during intensive-phase antimicrobial treatment of pulmonary tuberculosis: a double-blind randomised controlled trial. Lancet 2011;377(9761):242–50.

110. Mehta S, Mugusi FM, Bosch RJ, et al. Vitamin D status and TB treatment outcomes in adult patients in Tanzania: a cohort study. BMJ Open 2013;3(11): e003703.

111. Sudfeld CR, Giovannucci EL, Isanaka S, et al. Vitamin D status and incidence of pulmonary tuberculosis, opportunistic infections, and wasting among HIV-infected Tanzanian adults initiating antiretroviral therapy. J Infect Dis 2013; 207(3):378–85.

112. Armstrong GL, Wasley A, Simard EP, et al. The prevalence of hepatitis C virus infection in the United States, 1999 through 2002. Ann Intern Med 2006; 144(10):705–14.

113. Torriani FJ, Rodriguez-Torres M, Rockstroh JK, et al. Peginterferon Alfa-2a plus ribavirin for chronic hepatitis C virus infection in HIV-infected patients. N Engl J Med 2004;351(5):438.

114. McGovern BH. Hepatitis C in the HIV-infected patient. J Acquir Immune Defic Syndr 2007;45(Suppl 2):S47.

115. Gal-Tanamy M, Bachmetov L, Ravid A, et al. Vitamin D: an innate antiviral agent suppressing hepatitis C virus in human hepatocytes. Hepatology 2011;54(5): 1570–9.

116. Abu-Mouch S, Fireman Z, Jarchovsky J, et al. Vitamin D supplementation improves sustained virologic response in chronic hepatitis C (genotype 1)-naïve patients. World J Gastroenterol 2011;17(47):5184–90.

117. Bitetto D, Fabris C, Fornasiere E, et al. Vitamin D supplementation improves response to antiviral treatment for recurrent hepatitis C. Transpl Int 2011; 24(1):43–50.

118. Villar LM, Del Campo JA, Ranchal I, et al. Association between vitamin D and hepatitis C virus infection: a meta-analysis. World J Gastroenterol 2013;19(35): 5917–24.

119. Petta S, Cammà C, Scazzone C, et al. Low vitamin D serum level is related to severe fibrosis and low responsiveness to interferon-based therapy in genotype 1 chronic hepatitis C. World J Gastroenterol 2011;17(47):5184–90.

120. Lange CM, Bojunga J, Ramos-Lopez E, et al. Vitamin D deficiency and a CYP27B1-1260 promoter polymorphism are associated with chronic hepatitis C and poor response to interferon-alfa based therapy. J Hepatol 2011;54(5): 887–93.

121. Kondo Y, Kato T, Kimura O, et al. 1(OH) vitamin D3 supplementation improves the sensitivity of the immune-response during Peg-IFN/RBV therapy in chronic hepatitis C patients-case controlled trial. PLoS One 2013;8(5):e63672.

122. Abramovitch S, Dahan-Bachar L, Sharvit E, et al. Vitamin D inhibits proliferation and profibrotic marker expression in hepatic stellate cells and decreases thioacetamide-induced liver fibrosis in rats. Gut 2011;60(12):1728–37.

123. Terrier B, Carrat F, Geri G, et al. Low 25-OH vitamin D serum levels correlate with severe fibrosis in HIV-HCV co-infected patients with chronic hepatitis. J Hepatol 2011;55(4):756–61.

124. Milazzo L, Mazzali C, Bestetti G, et al. Liver-related factors associated with low vitamin D levels in HIV and HIV/HCV co-infected patients and comparison to general population. Curr HIV Res 2001;9(3):186–93.

125. Soumekh A, Bichoupan K, Constable C, et al. Two novel finding about interferon/ribavirin treatment: serum calcium falls and 25-hydroxyvitamin D increases. Hepatology 2011;54(Suppl 1):856A.

126. Mandorfer M, Reiberger T, Payer BA, et al. Low vitamin D levels are associated with impaired virologic response to PEGIFN + RBV therapy in HIV-hepatitis C virus coinfected patients. AIDS 2013;27(2):227–32.

127. Branch AD, Kang M, Hollabaugh K, et al. In HIV/hepatitis C virus co-infected patients, higher 25-hydroxyvitamin D concentrations were not related to hepatitis C virus treatment responses but were associated with ritonavir use. Am J Clin Nutr 2013;98(2):423–9.

128. Connor RI, Rigby WF. 1 alpha,25-dihydroxyvitamin D3 inhibits productive infection of human monocytes by HIV-1. Biochem Biophys Res Commun 1991;176(2):852–9.

129. Schuitemaker H, Kootstra NA, Koppelman MH, et al. Proliferation-dependent HIV-1 infection of monocytes occurs during differentiation into macrophages. J Clin Invest 1992;89(4):1154–60.

130. Haug C, Müller F, Aukrust P, et al. Subnormal serum concentration of 1,25-vitamin D in human immunodeficiency virus infection: correlation with degree of immune deficiency and survival. J Infect Dis 1994;169(4):889–93.

131. Teichmann J, Stephan E, Discher T, et al. Changes in calciotropic hormones and biochemical markers of bone metabolism in patients with human immunodeficiency virus infection. Metabolism 2000;49(9):1134–9.

132. Aziz M, Livak B, Burke-Miller J, et al. Vitamin D insufficiency may impair CD4 recovery among Women's Interagency HIV Study participants with advanced disease on HAART. AIDS 2013;27(4):573–8.

133. Mehta S, Giovannucci E, Mugusi FM, et al. Vitamin D status of HIV-infected women and its association with HIV disease progression, anemia, and mortality. PLoS One 2010;5(1):e8770.

134. Mehta S, Mugusi FM, Spiegelman D, et al. Vitamin D status and its association with morbidity including wasting and opportunistic illnesses in HIV-infected women in Tanzania. AIDS Patient Care STDS 2011;25(10):579–85.

135. Garland CF, Garland FC, Gorham ED, et al. The role of vitamin D in cancer prevention. Am J Public Health 2006;96(2):252–61.

136. Colston KW, Lowe LC, Mansi JL, et al. Vitamin D status and breast cancer risk. Anticancer Res 2006;26(4A):2573–80.
137. Ahonen MH, Tenkanen L, Teppo L, et al. Prostate cancer risk and prediagnostic serum 25-hydroxyvitamin D levels (Finland). Cancer Causes Control 2000;11(9): 847–52.
138. Bakhru A, Mallinger JB, Buckanovich RJ, et al. Casting light on 25-hydroxyvitamin D deficiency in ovarian cancer: a study from the NHANES. Gynecol Oncol 2010;119(2):314–8.
139. Holick MF. High prevalence of vitamin D inadequacy and implications for health. Mayo Clin Proc 2006;81(3):353–73.
140. Sigel K, Wisnivesky J, Gordon K, et al. HIV as an independent risk factor for incident lung cancer. AIDS 2012;26(8):1017–25.
141. French MA, King MS, Tschampa JM, et al. Serum immune activation markers are persistently increased in patients with HIV infection after 6 years of antiretroviral therapy despite suppression of viral replication and reconstitution of CD4+ T cells. J Infect Dis 2009;200(8):1212–5.
142. Ostrowski SR, Katzenstein TL, Pedersen BK, et al. Residual viraemia in HIV-1-infected patients with plasma viral load <or=20 copies/ml is associated with increased blood levels of soluble immune activation markers. Scand J Immunol 2008;68(6):652–60.
143. Duprez DA, Neuhaus J, Kuller LH, et al. Inflammation, coagulation and cardiovascular disease in HIV-infected individuals. PLoS One 2012;7(9):e44454.
144. De Luca A, de Gaetano Donati K, Colafigli M, et al. The association of high-sensitivity c-reactive protein and other biomarkers with cardiovascular disease in patients treated for HIV: a nested case-control study. BMC Infect Dis 2013; 13:414.
145. Brown TT, Tassiopoulos K, Bosch RJ, et al. Association between systemic inflammation and incident diabetes in HIV-infected patients after initiation of antiretroviral therapy. Diabetes Care 2010;33(10):2244–9.
146. Biron A, Bobin-Dubigeon C, Volteau C, et al. Metabolic syndrome in French HIV-infected patients: prevalence and predictive factors after 3 years of antiretroviral therapy. AIDS Res Hum Retroviruses 2012;28(12):1672–8.
147. Gazzola L, Bellistri GM, Tincati C, et al. Association between peripheral T-Lymphocyte activation and impaired bone mineral density in HIV-infected patients. J Transl Med 2013;11:51.
148. Borges ÁH, Silverberg MJ, Wentworth D, et al. Predicting risk of cancer during HIV infection: the role of inflammatory and coagulation biomarkers. AIDS 2013; 27(9):1433–41.
149. Ancuta P, Kamat A, Kunstman KJ, et al. Microbial translocation is associated with increased monocyte activation and dementia in AIDS patients. PLoS One 2008;3(6):e2516.
150. Margolick J, Jacobson L, Lopez J. Frailty and circulating concentrations of proinflammatory cytokines and chemokines in HIV-infected and -uninfected men in the Multicenter AIDS Cohort Study (MACS). Abstract presented at: 3rd International Workshop on HIV and Aging. Baltimore, November 5–6, 2012.
151. Tien PC, Choi AI, Zolopa AR, et al. Inflammation and mortality in HIV-infected adults: analysis of the FRAM study cohort. J Acquir Immune Defic Syndr 2010;55(3):316–22.
152. Kuller LH, Tracy R, Belloso W, et al. Inflammatory and coagulation biomarkers and mortality in patients with HIV infection. PLoS Med 2008;5(10):e203.

153. Sandler NG, Wand H, Roque A, et al. Plasma levels of soluble CD14 independently predict mortality in HIV infection. J Infect Dis 2011;203(6):780–90.
154. Currie CJ, Poole CD, Conway P. Evaluation of the association between the first observation and the longitudinal change in C-reactive protein, and all-cause mortality. Heart 2008;94(4):457–62.
155. Cao JJ, Arnold AM, Manolio TA, et al. Association of carotid artery intima-media thickness, plaques, and C-reactive protein with future cardiovascular disease and all-cause mortality: the Cardiovascular Health Study. Circulation 2007; 116(1):32–8.
156. Hearps AC, Martin GE, Rajasuriar R, et al. Inflammatory co-morbidities in HIV+ individuals: learning lessons from healthy ageing. Curr HIV/AIDS Rep 2014; 11(1):20–34.
157. Rigby WF, Stacy T, Fanger MW. Inhibition of T lymphocyte mitogenesis by 1,25-dihydroxyvitamin D3 (calcitriol). J Clin Invest 1984;74(4):1451–5.
158. Penna G, Adorini L. 1 Alpha,25-dihydroxyvitamin D3 inhibits differentiation, maturation, activation, and survival of dendritic cells leading to impaired alloreactive T cell activation. J Immunol 2000;164(5):2405–11.
159. Helming L, Böse J, Ehrchen J, et al. 1alpha,25-Dihydroxyvitamin D3 is a potent suppressor of interferon gamma-mediated macrophage activation. Blood 2005; 106(13):4351–8.
160. Cantorna MT, Zhu Y, Froicu M, et al. Vitamin D status, 1,25-dihydroxyvitamin D3, and the immune system. Am J Clin Nutr 2004;80(6 Suppl):1717S–20S.
161. Chang SH, Chung Y, Dong C. Vitamin D suppresses Th17 cytokine production by inducing C/EBP homologous protein (CHOP) expression. J Biol Chem 2010; 285(50):38751–5.
162. Soilu-Hänninen M, Laaksonen M, Laitinen I, et al. A longitudinal study of serum 25-hydroxyvitamin D and intact parathyroid hormone levels indicate the importance of vitamin D and calcium homeostasis regulation in multiple sclerosis. J Neurol Neurosurg Psychiatry 2008;79(2):152–7.
163. Rossini M, Maddali Bongi S, La Montagna G, et al. Vitamin D deficiency in rheumatoid arthritis: prevalence, determinants and associations with disease activity and disability. Arthritis Res Ther 2010;12(6):R216.
164. Ritterhouse LL, Crowe SR, Niewold TB, et al. Vitamin D deficiency is associated with an increased autoimmune response in healthy individuals and in patients with systemic lupus erythematosus. Ann Rheum Dis 2011;70(9):1569–74.
165. Littorin B, Blom P, Schölin A, et al. Lower levels of plasma 25-hydroxyvitamin D among young adults at diagnosis of autoimmune type 1 diabetes compared with control subjects: results from the nationwide Diabetes Incidence Study in Sweden (DISS). Diabetologia 2006;49(12):2847–52.
166. Myers GL, Rifai N, Tracy RP, et al. Workshop on markers of inflammation and cardiovascular disease: application to clinical and public health practice: report from the laboratory science discussion group. Circulation 2004;110(25):e545–9.
167. Poudel-Tandukar K, Poudel KC, Jimba M, et al. Serum 25-hydroxyvitamin d levels and C-reactive protein in persons with human immunodeficiency virus infection. AIDS Res Hum Retroviruses 2013;29(3):528–34.
168. Hoffman R, Lake J, Tseng CH, et al. Lower 25-hydroxy vitamin D levels are associated with elevated TNF-α and CD8+ T cell activation in HIV-infected patients on suppressive antiretroviral therapy. Abstract presented at: 7th IAS Conference on HIV Pathogenesis and Treatment: Abstract no. PUB002. Kuala Lumpur, Malaysia, 30 June–3 July, 2013.

169. Daly RM, Brown M, Bass S, et al. Calcium- and vitamin D3-fortified milk reduces bone loss at clinically relevant skeletal sites in older men: a 2-year randomized controlled trial. J Bone Miner Res 2006;21(3):397.

170. Chung M, Lee J, Terasawa T, et al. Vitamin D with or without calcium supplementation for prevention of cancer and fractures: an updated meta-analysis for the U.S. Preventive Services Task Force. Ann Intern Med 2011;155(12):827.

171. Etminani-Esfahani M, Khalili H, Jafari S, et al. Effects of vitamin D supplementation on the bone specific biomarkers in HIV infected individuals under treatment with efavirenz. BMC Res Notes 2012;5:204.

172. Jackson RD, LaCroix AZ, Gass M, et al. Calcium plus vitamin D supplementation and the risk of fractures. N Engl J Med 2006;354(7):669.

173. Bang UC, Kolte L, Hitz M, et al. The effect of cholecalciferol and calcitriol on biochemical bone markers in HIV type 1-infected males: results of a clinical trial. AIDS Res Hum Retroviruses 2013;29(4):658–64.

174. Cranney A, Weiler HA, O'Donnell S, et al. Summary of evidence-based review on vitamin D efficacy and safety in relation to bone health. Am J Clin Nutr 2008;88(2):513S.

175. Moyer VA. Vitamin D and calcium supplementation to prevent fractures in adults: U.S. Preventive Services Task Force recommendation statement. Ann Intern Med 2013;158(9):691.

176. Piso RJ, Rothen M, Rothen JP, et al. Per oral substitution with 300000 IU vitamin D (Cholecalciferol) reduces bone turnover markers in HIV-infected patients. BMC Infect Dis 2013;6(13):577.

177. Havens PL, Stephensen CB, Hazra R, et al. Vitamin D3 decreases parathyroid hormone in HIV-infected youth being treated with tenofovir: a randomized, placebo-controlled trial. Clin Infect Dis 2012;54(7):1013–25.

178. van den Bout-van den Beukel CJ, van den Bos M, Oyen WJ, et al. The effect of cholecalciferol supplementation on vitamin D levels and insulin sensitivity is dose related in vitamin D-deficient HIV-1-infected patients. HIV Med 2008; 9(9):771–9.

179. Mondy K, Powderly WG, Claxton SA, et al. Alendronate, vitamin D, and calcium for the treatment of osteopenia/osteoporosis associated with HIV infection. J Acquir Immune Defic Syndr 2005;38(4):426–31.

180. McComsey GA, Kendall MA, Tebas P, et al. Alendronate with calcium and vitamin D supplementation is safe and effective for the treatment of decreased bone mineral density in HIV. AIDS 2007;21(18):2473–82.

181. Arpadi SM, McMahon DJ, Abrams EJ, et al. Effect of supplementation with cholecalciferol and calcium on 2-y bone mass accrual in HIV-infected children and adolescents: a randomized clinical trial. Am J Clin Nutr 2012;95(3): 678–85.

182. Overton ET, Chan ES, Brown TT, et al. High-dose vitamin D and calcium attenuates bone loss with ART initiation: results from ACTG A5280. CROI 2014. Conference on Retroviruses and Opportunistic Infections. Boston, March 3–6, 2014 [abstract: 133].

183. Yin MT, Shi Q, Hoover DR, et al. Fracture incidence in HIV-infected women: results from the Women's Interagency HIV Study. AIDS 2010;24(17):2679–86.

184. Longenecker CT, Hileman CO, Carman TL, et al. Vitamin D supplementation and endothelial function in vitamin D deficient HIV-infected patients: a randomized placebo-controlled trial. Antivir Ther 2012;17(4):613–21.

185. Norman PE, Powell JT. Vitamin D and cardiovascular disease. Circ Res 2014; 114(2):379–93.

186. George PS, Pearson ER, Witham MD. Effect of vitamin D supplementation on glycaemic control and insulin resistance: a systematic review and meta-analysis. Diabet Med 2012;29(8):e142–50.
187. Antico A, Tampoia M, Tozzoli R, et al. Can supplementation with vitamin D reduce the risk or modify the course of autoimmune diseases? A systematic review of the literature. Autoimmun Rev 2012;12(2):127–36.
188. Giacomet V, Vigano A, Manfredini V, et al. Cholecalciferol supplementation in HIV-infected youth with vitamin D insufficiency: effects on vitamin D status and T-cell phenotype: a randomized controlled trial. HIV Clin Trials 2013;14(2): 51–60.
189. Kakalia S, Sochett EB, Stephens D, et al. Vitamin D supplementation and CD4 count in children infected with human immunodeficiency virus. J Pediatr 2011; 159(6):951–7.
190. Bolland MJ, Wang TK, Grey A, et al. Stable bone density in HAART-treated individuals with HIV: a meta-analysis. J Clin Endocrinol Metab 2011;96(9): 2721–31.
191. European AIDS Clinical Society. European AIDS Clinical Society guidelines: prevention and management of non-infectious comorbidities in HIV. October 2013. Available at: http://www.eacsociety.org/Portals/0/Guidelines_Online_131014. pdf. Accessed April 1, 2014.
192. McComsey GA, Tebas P, Shane E, et al. Bone disease in HIV infection: a practical review and recommendations for HIV care providers. Clin Infect Dis 2010; 51(8):937–46.
193. Childs K, Fishman S, Factor S, et al. First report of dose/response data of HIV-infected men treated with vitamin D3 supplements. 16th Conference on Retroviruses and Opportunistic Infections, Montreal, Canada, February 8–11, 2009.
194. Falasca K, Ucciferri C, Di Nicola M, et al. Different strategies of 25OH vitamin D supplementation in HIV+ subjects. Int J STD AIDS 2014. [Epub ahead of print].
195. Hathcock JN, Shao A, Vieth R, et al. Risk assessment for vitamin D. Am J Clin Nutr 2007;85:6–18.

Osteoporosis and Fracture Risk Associated with HIV Infection and Treatment

Juliet Compston, MD, FRCP, FRCPath, FMedSci

KEYWORDS

- Osteoporosis • Fracture • HIV infection • Antiretroviral therapy
- Bone mineral density

KEY POINTS

- Fracture risk is modestly increased in HIV-infected individuals.
- HIV-infected individuals have multiple risk factors for fracture.
- Significant bone loss from the spine and hip occurs during the first 1 to 2 years after initiation of antiretroviral therapy.
- In individuals with a high fracture probability, bisphosphonate therapy may be appropriate.

INTRODUCTION

With the development of effective treatments for HIV-infected individuals and the resulting increase in life expectancy, osteoporosis has emerged as an important co-morbidity. The mechanisms responsible for its evolution are only partially understood, but factors related to both HIV infection and its treatment have been implicated. This review focuses on our current knowledge of the prevalence and incidence of osteoporosis and fracture in HIV-infected individuals and the factors responsible for their development. Management strategies aimed at reducing fracture risk also are discussed.

OSTEOPOROSIS: DEFINITION, DIAGNOSIS, AND FRACTURE RISK ASSESSMENT

Osteoporosis is characterized by reduced bone mass and increased bone fragility, resulting in increased risk of fracture. In the general population, the incidence of fragility fractures increases steeply with age; these fractures cause significant morbidity and mortality in the elderly population and impose huge costs on health care services.[1] In recent years, there have been significant advances in fracture risk

Department of Medicine, Addenbrookes Hospital, Cambridge Biomedical Campus, Box 157, Cambridge CB2 0QQ, UK
E-mail address: jec1001@cam.ac.uk

Endocrinol Metab Clin N Am 43 (2014) 769–780
http://dx.doi.org/10.1016/j.ecl.2014.05.001
0889-8529/14/$ – see front matter © 2014 Elsevier Inc. All rights reserved.

endo.theclinics.com

assessment, enabling more accurate targeting of treatment. Furthermore, a range of therapeutic options with proven antifracture efficacy is now available. However, most of the research leading to these advances has been conducted in postmenopausal women and, to a lesser extent, in older men, and its extrapolation to younger age groups is uncertain.

In 1994, a working group of the World Health Organization (WHO) proposed a classification of osteoporosis based on bone mineral density (BMD) measured by dual energy x-ray absorptiometry (DXA). According to this classification, osteoporosis is defined as a BMD T score of −2.5 or less at the lumbar spine or proximal femur, osteopenia as a BMD T score between −1.0 and −2.5, and severe or established osteoporosis as a T score of −2.5 or less together with 1 or more fragility fractures, the T score being the number of SDs above or below peak bone mass in healthy young adults.[2] This classification is based on the inverse relationship between BMD and fracture risk in postmenopausal women and older men. In premenopausal women and younger men, much less is known about this relationship, and the WHO classification should not be used. In these younger individuals, BMD is expressed as a Z-score (SD score based on age-matched and gender-matched values) and osteoporosis should be diagnosed only in the presence of 1 or more fragility fractures. Z-scores between −2 and +2 are regarded as within the expected range for age and Z-scores below −2 as below the expected range for age.[3]

FRACTURE RISK ASSESSMENT

Although BMD, assessed by DXA, is widely used in clinical practice to predict fracture risk, its sensitivity is relatively low, and most fragility fractures occur in individuals with osteopenia, not osteoporosis.[4] Addition of certain clinical risk factors, the influence of which on fracture risk is partially independent of BMD, improves fracture prediction and forms the basis of fracture risk algorithms, the most widely used of which is the WHO Fracture Risk Assessment Tool (FRAX) (**Box 1**).[5] FRAX can be used with or

---

Box 1
Clinical risk factors used in the World Health Organization Fracture Risk Assessment Tool (FRAX) algorithm

- Age
- Gender
- Body mass index
- Previous fracture
- Parental hip fracture
- Glucocorticoid therapy
- Rheumatoid arthritis
- Tobacco use
- Alcohol abuse
- Secondary osteoporosis*
- Femoral neck bone mineral density (BMD) (optional)

* If both secondary osteoporosis and BMD are entered, only the BMD result will influence the fracture probability estimation, as it is assumed that the effects of secondary osteoporosis are mediated solely through effects on BMD.

without BMD to estimate the 10-year probability of a hip fracture or a major osteoporotic fracture (hip, spine, wrist, or humerus). However, it can be used only in individuals aged 40 years or older because the evidence used to construct the algorithm was confined to people over this age. When use of FRAX is appropriate, country-specific versions, where available, should be used because of geographic variations in the epidemiology of fracture and of mortality, which is incorporated into the fracture probability calculations.

RISK FACTORS FOR OSTEOPOROSIS AND FRACTURE IN HIV-POSITIVE INDIVIDUALS

A number of risk factors for fracture are likely to contribute to the lower BMD and increased fracture risk in the HIV-infected population. These include low body mass index (BMI), smoking, alcohol abuse, glucocorticoid therapy, inflammation, hypogonadism, growth hormone deficiency, and vitamin D insufficiency. Initiation of antiretroviral therapy (ART) is associated with bone loss, and several of the comorbidities associated with HIV infection, including renal disease, hepatitis, and diabetes, may be associated with bone loss and/or increased fracture risk. Increased levels of trauma also increase the risk of fracture, particularly in drug abusers.

BMD IN HIV-INFECTED INDIVIDUALS

Lower spine and hip BMD in HIV-infected than in noninfected individuals has been reported in many cross-sectional studies, both in younger adults and in postmenopausal women and older men.[6–17] A meta-analysis, published in 2006, demonstrated a more than threefold greater prevalence of osteoporosis in HIV-infected individuals compared with noninfected controls; ART-exposed and protease inhibitor–exposed individuals having a higher prevalence than their respective controls.[18] However, most prospective studies of HIV-infected individuals established on ART show stable or increasing BMD,[19–27] although bone loss has been reported in postmenopausal Hispanic and African American women.[28] It has been suggested that the lower BMD in HIV-infected individuals reported in earlier studies may reflect a lower BMI before or shortly after the initiation of ART, and that when BMD is adjusted for body weight, differences between HIV-infected individuals and noninfected controls largely disappear.[29] Thus, earlier diagnosis and prompt initiation of effective ART may reduce adverse effects of HIV infection on bone mass largely through beneficial effects on body weight.

Nonetheless, there is consistent evidence that ART in previously treatment-naïve HIV-infected individuals is associated with bone loss from the spine and hip of up to 6% during the first 12 to 24 months after initiation.[30–37] This bone loss is accompanied by increases in biochemical markers of bone resorption and formation, indicating that bone loss is due to increased bone turnover.[34] Tenofovir-containing regimens are associated with the greatest bone loss,[34–37] and in the A5224s substudy, regimens that included the use of protease inhibitors were associated with greater bone loss at the spine,[35] although this finding has not been consistent. Conversely, recent studies indicate that regimens containing the integrase inhibitor raltegravir may be associated with less bone loss.[38] The causes of bone loss after initiation of ART have not been established; the fact that it is seen with many different treatment regimens suggests that general as well as drug-related factors are involved. It has been suggested that activation of CD4 cells and immune reconstitution following treatment may result in increased levels of proinflammatory, proresorptive cytokines, but further studies are required.[39–41]

Given the stable or increasing BMD reported in HIV-infected individuals established on ART, the clinical significance of transient bone loss after initiation of ART could be questioned. It is possible that during this bone loss, alterations in bone microstructure occur that are irreversible, even though bone mass subsequently increases. Quantitative assessment of cortical and trabecular microstructure have revealed some differences in ART-treated HIV-infected individuals when compared with noninfected individuals. Calmy and colleagues[42] reported significantly lower tibial trabecular density and trabecular number, and significantly decreased radial cortical density, in 22 HIV-infected premenopausal women compared with age-matched controls. In a study of 46 postmenopausal HIV-infected women, lower tibial cortical thickness and cortical area were demonstrated, but there were no significant differences from noninfected controls in the radius in any of the structural parameters assessed.[43] In 30 HIV-infected African American or Hispanic men aged 20 to 25 years, comparison with 15 noninfected controls revealed significantly lower tibial and radial total and trabecular volumetric BMD, and significantly lower cortical and trabecular thickness. A reduction in bone stiffness also was shown by finite element analysis.[44]

Although these studies indicate that differences in trabecular and bone structure may be found in HIV-infected compared with noninfected individuals, the populations investigated have been relatively small and further research is required to establish more definitively alterations in bone microstructure associated with HIV infection and their contribution to increased bone fragility and fracture.

FRACTURE ASSOCIATED WITH HIV INFECTION

Studies of fracture prevalence and incidence in HIV-infected individuals have differed in their design, sample size, ethnicity, age, and gender of the populations studied, the means by which fractures were ascertained (self-reported vs coded via the *International Classification of Diseases*), and type of fracture included (all fractures vs low-energy fractures). Despite this heterogeneity, most have demonstrated a significant increase in fracture risk, although this finding has not been universal.

In a study of 559 men aged 49 years or older, Arnsten and colleagues[16] found a higher fracture incidence in HIV-infected versus noninfected individuals, although this difference was not statistically significant. In a large population-based study from the United States, Triant and colleagues[45] reported a significantly increased prevalence of all fractures in HIV-infected men and women (n = 8525), when compared with noninfected individuals (n = 2,208,792); comparison of ethnic groups revealed a higher prevalence in the HIV-infected cohort among African American and Caucasian women and Caucasian men. However, Yin and colleagues[46] reported no significant difference in fracture incidence rates by HIV status in a cohort of 2391 predominantly premenopausal women, 1928 of whom were HIV-infected. In 119,318 male veterans enrolled in the Veterans Aging Cohort Study Virtual Cohort (VACS-VC), one-third of whom were HIV-positive, the hazard ratio (HR) for incident fracture was significantly higher in HIV-infected men both before and after adjustment for risk factors when compared with noninfected men (HRs 1.32, 95% confidence intervals [CIs] 1.20–1.47 and 1.24, 1.11–1.39, respectively).[47] In the US HIV Outpatient Study (HOPS), Young and colleagues[48] reported that age-adjusted fracture rates in 5826 HIV-infected individuals were significantly higher than those of the general US population. Using Danish health registries, Hansen and colleagues[49] reported a significantly higher incidence of fracture (incidence rate ratio [IRR] 1.5, 1.4–1.7) in HIV-infected men and women (n = 5306) when compared with noninfected case controls (n = 26,230), this increase in risk remaining when only low-energy fractures were included. A more recent study from Danish national health registries of 124,655 fracture cases and 373,962 controls also found a significant increase in fracture risk associated with HIV infection, with an odds ratio of 2.89 (1.99–4.18) after adjustment for age and gender.[50] In a large population-based database from Catalonia, Spain, a significant increase in fracture risk was found in HIV-infected individuals (n = 2489) when compared with noninfected individuals (n = 1,115,667), the age and sex-adjusted HR being 6.2 (3.5–10.9) for hip fracture and 2.7 (2.01–3.5) for major fractures (hip, clinical spine, pelvis, tibia, multiple rib, and proximal humerus), respectively. However, because there were only 12 hip fractures in the HIV cohort, the high fracture risk at this site should be interpreted with caution.[51]

In a systematic review and meta-analysis of incident fractures in HIV-infected individuals, 13 studies were found to be eligible, of which 7 included controls.[52] A significant increase in the risk for all fractures and for fragility fractures was demonstrated (IRR 1.58, 1.25–2.00 and 1.35, 1.10–1.65), respectively. However, the investigators acknowledge that because the test for heterogeneity was significant for the pooled risk estimate for fragility fracture, those results should be treated with some caution. They also documented wide variation in the incidence rates of fracture in HIV-infected individuals across studies, possibly as a result of the different demographics of study populations. It should be noted that the systematic search and meta-analysis did not include the 2 recent large studies of Prieto-Alhambra and colleagues[51] and Güerri-Fernandez and colleagues.[50]

A number of known risk factors for fracture have been identified in HIV-infected individuals. These include older age,[45,46,48] tobacco use,[46,47,49] alcohol or substance abuse,[48] use of glucocorticoids,[53] proton pump inhibitors[47] or anticonvulsants,[53] comorbidities,[47–49] and low BMI.[47]

Non-black or white race has been identified as a significant predictor of fracture in several studies.[16,46,47,49,54] Female gender has not emerged as a significant risk factor and Gedmintas and colleagues[55] recently reported similar rates of fracture in men and women in a cohort of 3161 HIV-infected individuals with a total of 587 fractures.

Factors specific to HIV infection also have been implicated. Low CD4 counts have been associated with increased risk of fragility fracture in some studies.[48,53,56] The potential role of ART is of particular interest, given the well-documented bone loss that occurs during the first 1 to 2 years after initiation. ART exposure was found to be a significant risk factor for fragility fracture in the study of Hansen and colleagues.[49] In an analysis of HIV-infected individuals from 26 randomized trials of ART, fracture rates in the 3398 participants who were ART naïve at baseline were higher within the first 2 years after initiation of ART than in subsequent years.[57] Exposure to tenofovir[54] and to protease inhibitors[47] also has been associated with fragility fracture in some studies, although this association has not been consistently demonstrated.

Coinfection with hepatitis C (HCV) has been demonstrated in a number of studies to be an independent risk factor both for fragility and other fractures in the HIV-infected population, coinfection being associated with a onefold to twofold increase in risk compared with mono-infection with HIV. In a large retrospective cohort study of Medicaid enrollees, HCV/HIV coinfection was associated with a significantly greater risk of hip fracture when compared with HCV mono-infected, HIV mono-infected, or noninfected individuals; the adjusted HR for hip fracture in coinfected versus HCV mono-infected individuals being 1.38 (1.25–1.53).[58] Maalouf and colleagues[59] recently reported similar findings in 55,660 HIV-infected individuals enrolled in the Veterans Affairs' Clinical Case Registry between 1984 and 2009. The risk of osteoporotic fracture (defined as closed wrist, vertebral, or hip fracture) was significantly higher in HCV/HIV coinfected than in HIV mono-infected individuals, the respective fracture rates being

2.57 versus 2.07 per 1000 patient years ($P<.0001$); cirrhosis was a strong predictor of fracture in the coinfected individuals.

Taken together, these studies indicate that HIV infection is associated with increased risk of both fragility and nonfragility fractures. A number of risk factors have been identified, some of which are traditional and apply to the general population and others of which are specific to HIV infection. Important gaps in our knowledge include data on the prevalence and incidence of vertebral fracture and on the contribution of falls to the pathogenesis of fractures.

MECHANISMS OF BONE LOSS IN HIV-INFECTED INDIVIDUALS

The mechanisms underlying reduced bone mass and increased bone fragility associated with HIV infection have not been clearly established. Bone histomorphometric data are restricted to one study, in which iliac crest bone biopsies were obtained from 22 HIV-infected ART-naïve young adults.[60] The results demonstrated significantly lower bone turnover in these individuals in comparison with a control group of healthy kidney donors. In addition, bone formation at the level of individual bone multicellular unit was significantly reduced, indicating reduced osteoblastic activity.

Biochemical markers of bone resorption and formation have been used to assess bone turnover in HIV-infected individuals. It should be noted that these studies have been performed in ART-treated patients, so that effects on bone turnover resulting from the disease per se and its treatment could not be distinguished. Higher levels of bone turnover markers have been reported in Hispanic or African American postmenopausal HIV-infected women when compared with noninfected controls,[28] and in one longitudinal study, higher levels of bone turnover markers were associated with greater bone loss.[61]

From the studies discussed previously, it is difficult to draw conclusions regarding mechanisms of bone loss in HIV-infected individuals. The early study of Serrano and colleagues[60] suggests that in those who are ART-naïve, low bone turnover and reduced bone formation predominate, but extrapolation of these findings to the more common contemporary scenario in which individuals are taking ART is problematic. Although the studies conducted in patients initiating ART suggest that the increase in bone turnover markers may be transient, in the study of Yin and colleagues,[28] baseline levels of bone markers were elevated even though the mean duration of ART exposure was 4.5 years. However, that study was limited to postmenopausal Hispanic or African American women, and further investigations are required to establish whether bone turnover remains increased in individuals receiving long-term ART.

MANAGEMENT OF BONE DISEASE ASSOCIATED WITH HIV INFECTION
Fracture Risk Assessment

Risk factors for fracture have not been fully characterized in the HIV-infected population and recommendations for screening for bone disease therefore have to be largely based on traditional risk factors. The European AIDS Clinical Society recommends that measurement of BMD by DXA should be considered in HIV-infected postmenopausal women and men aged 50 years or older; in addition, a previous history of fracture, glucocorticoid therapy, or clinical hypogonadism may be considered as indications for DXA.[62] FRAX can be used to assess 10-year fracture probability in individuals older than 40 years, but not in younger people. If BMD is low (ie, Z-score lower than -2 in premenopausal women and men younger than 50 years, or T score lower than -2.5 in postmenopausal women and older men), causes of secondary osteoporosis should be excluded. Lateral imaging of the spine also should be considered in those with low spine BMD, height loss, or kyphosis, to establish whether or not vertebral fractures are present. This is important because most vertebral fractures do not come to clinical attention, but all vertebral fractures, whether or not they are symptomatic, are associated with significantly increased risk of future fracture.[63]

General Measures

Risk factors for fracture, where present, should be addressed. This includes advice to stop smoking, reduce alcohol intake, and to maintain reasonable levels of physical activity. Vitamin D deficiency/insufficiency should be corrected and calcium intakes of 750 to 1000 mg per day advised, using dietary measures where possible. The risk of falling should be assessed and, if increased, appropriate measures taken. Nutritional advice should be aimed at maintaining a normal body weight, because low BMI is associated with lower BMD and higher fracture risk.[64] In patients at increased fracture risk, avoidance of tenofovir should be considered.

Pharmacologic Intervention

Several studies have addressed the use of bisphosphonates (alendronate or zoledronic acid) in HIV-infected individuals. These studies have been limited to investigation of changes in BMD and have not been powered for fracture outcomes. Nevertheless, based on their proven effectiveness in reducing fracture in non–HIV-infected postmenopausal women, it seems reasonable to assume that comparable BMD changes in the 2 populations are likely to indicate similar antifracture efficacy. A Cochrane review of 3 randomized controlled trials in osteopenic or osteoporotic HIV-infected patients using oral alendronate, 70 mg once weekly, reported significant gains in lumbar spine and hip BMD after 1 and 2 years, but no decrease in fracture risk (Relative risk 1.28, 0.20–8.21).[65] In 2 of these studies, calcium and vitamin D supplements also were given[66,67]; in the third, dietary counseling was given to achieve adequate calcium intake, but vitamin D supplements were not administered.[68] Subsequently, McComsey and colleagues[69] reported significant increases in spine and hip BMD in a cohort of 82 HIV-infected patients treated with alendronate 70 mg once weekly, calcium, and vitamin D when compared with those treated with calcium and vitamin D alone, and Rozenberg and colleagues[70] recently reported similar benefits in a cohort of 44 HIV-infected adults with osteoporosis in a 96-week study.

Two groups have investigated the use of intravenous zoledronic acid in HIV-infected individuals. In a 2-year randomized controlled trial of intravenous zoledronic acid, 4 mg annually, in 43 HIV-infected men, Bolland and colleagues[71] reported increases in lumbar spine BMD of 8.9% versus 2.6% in the control group, with corresponding changes in the total hip of 3.8% versus −0.8%. An extension study demonstrated persistence of the effect of these 2 annual doses on BMD and bone turnover markers for at least 5 years after the second dose.[72] Huang and colleagues[73] studied the effect of a single intravenous infusion of 5 mg zoledronic acid in 30 HIV-infected men and women with osteopenia or osteoporosis. One year after the infusion, individuals treated with zoledronic acid showed significantly higher BMD in the spine and hip when compared with controls. In both of these studies, calcium and vitamin D supplements were given to both the treatment and placebo groups.

These treatment studies with alendronate and zoledronic acid indicate beneficial effects on BMD similar to those reported in non–HIV-infected postmenopausal women and older men. Defining the indications for pharmacologic intervention in HIV-infected individuals is complex, particularly in the younger population in whom absolute fracture risk is likely to be low, and because of concerns about adverse effects of bisphosphonates, including atypical femoral fractures and osteonecrosis of the jaw,[74–76] treatment should be restricted to those at high fracture risk. In postmenopausal women and older men, fracture probability can be estimated using algorithms such as FRAX and treatment advised according to national intervention thresholds. In younger individuals, bisphosphonate treatment generally should be restricted to those with a history of fragility fracture and referral to a bone specialist may be appropriate. Finally, osteomalacia, which also results in low BMD, should be excluded before starting bisphosphonate therapy.

Because treatment adherence with alendronate is likely to be particularly poor in HIV-infected individuals because of the inconvenience of the dosing regimen, annual zoledronic acid infusions are regarded as the preferable option in most cases. The data of Bolland and colleagues[72] suggest that a dosing frequency of less than once annually may be sufficient, although it should be stressed that no fracture data are available. Calcium and/or vitamin D supplements should be coadministered with bisphosphonate therapy in patients with an inadequate dietary calcium intake and/or vitamin D insufficiency.

SUMMARY

The increase in fracture risk that has been demonstrated in HIV-infected individuals arises from both HIV-specific and nonspecific traditional risk factors, many of which are modifiable. Prediction of fracture risk from BMD values and clinical risk factors has not been well documented in the HIV-infected population but may be valid, particularly in older individuals. In those with a high fracture probability, bisphosphonate therapy should be considered. Better management of nutrition, prompt treatment of HIV infection, and avoidance of known lifestyle risk factors also may help to reduce fractures and their associated morbidity.

REFERENCES

1. Cauley JA. Public health impact of osteoporosis. J Gerontol A Biol Sci Med Sci 2013;68:1243–5.
2. World Health Organization. Assessment of fracture risk and its application to screening for postmenopausal osteoporosis. Technical Report Series. Geneva (Switzerland): WHO; 1994.
3. Schousboe JT, Shepherd JA, Bilezikian JP, et al. Executive summary of the 2013 International Society for Clinical Densitometry Position Development Conference on bone densitometry. J Clin Densitom 2013;16:455–66.
4. Siris ES, Chen YT, Abbott TA, et al. Bone mineral density thresholds for pharmacological intervention to prevent fractures. Arch Intern Med 2004;164:1108–12.
5. Kanis JA, on behalf of the World Health Organization Scientific Group. Assessment of osteoporosis at the primary healthcare level. Technical Report. Sheffield (United Kingdom): WHO Collaborating Centre for Metabolic Bone Disease, University of Sheffield; 2008. Available at: http://www.shef.ac.uk/FRAX.
6. Carr A, Miller J, Eisman JA, et al. Osteopenia in HIV-infected men: association with asymptomatic lactic acidaemia and lower weight pre-antiretroviral therapy. AIDS 2001;15:703–9.
7. Knobel H, Guelar A, Vallecillo G, et al. Osteopenia in HIV-infected patients: is it the disease or is it the treatment? AIDS 2001;15:807–8.
8. Bruera D, Luna N, David DO, et al. Decreased bone mineral density in HIV-infected patients is independent of retroviral therapy. AIDS 2003;17:1917–23.

9. Teichmann J, Stephan E, Lange U, et al. Osteopenia in HIV-infected women prior to highly active antiretroviral therapy. J Infect 2003;46:221–7.
10. Dolan SE, Huang JS, Killilea KM, et al. Reduced bone density in HIV-infected women. AIDS 2004;18:475–83.
11. Amiel C, Ostertag A, Slama L, et al. BMD is reduced in HIV-infected men irrespective of treatment. J Bone Miner Res 2004;19:402–9.
12. Yin M, Dobkin J, Brudney K, et al. Bone mass and mineral metabolism in HIV+ postmenopausal women. Osteoporos Int 2005;16:1345–52.
13. Arnsten JH, Freeman R, Howard AA, et al. HIV and bone mineral density in middle-aged women. Clin Infect Dis 2006;42:1014–20.
14. Brown TT, McComsey GA. Osteopenia and osteoporosis in patients with HIV: a review of current concepts. Curr Infect Dis Rep 2006;8:162–70.
15. Amorosa V, Tebas P. Bone disease and HIV infection. Clin Infect Dis 2006;42:108–14.
16. Arnsten JH, Freeman R, Howard AA, et al. Decreased bone mineral density and increased fracture risk in aging men with or at risk for HIV infection. AIDS 2007;21:617–23.
17. Mulligan K, Harris DR, Emmanuel P, et al. Low bone mass in behaviorally HIV-infected young men on antiretroviral therapy: Adolescent Trials Network Study 021B. Clin Infect Dis 2012;55:461–8.
18. Brown TT, Qaqish RB. Antiretroviral therapy and the prevalence of osteopenia and osteoporosis: a meta-analytic review. AIDS 2006;20:2165–74.
19. Nolan D, Upton R, McKinnon E, et al. Stable or increasing bone mineral density in HIV-infected patients treated with nelfinavir or indinavir. AIDS 2001;15:1275–80.
20. Fernandez-Rivera J, Garcia R, Lozano F, et al. Relationship between low bone mineral density and highly active retroviral therapy including protease inhibitors in HIV-infected patients. HIV Clin Trials 2003;4:337–46.
21. Mondy K, Yarasheski K, Powderly WG, et al. Longitudinal evolution of bone mineral density and bone markers in human immunodeficiency virus-infected individuals. Clin Infect Dis 2003;36:482–90.
22. Bolland MJ, Grey AB, Horne AM, et al. Bone mineral density is not reduced in HIV-infected Caucasian men treated with highly active retroviral therapy. Clin Endocrinol 2006;65:191–7.
23. Dolan SE, Frontera W, Librizzi J, et al. Effects of a supervised home-based aerobic and progressive resistance training regimen in women infected with human immunodeficiency virus: a randomized trial. Arch Intern Med 2006;166:1225–31.
24. Dolan SE, Kanter JR, Grinspoon S. Longitudinal analysis of bone density in human immunodeficiency-infected women. J Clin Endocrinol Metab 2006;91:2938–45.
25. Bolland MJ, Grey AB, Horne AM, et al. Bone mineral density remains stable in HAART-treated HIV-infected men over 2 years. Clin Endocrinol 2007;67:270–5.
26. Yin MT, Lu D, Cremers S, et al. Short-term bone loss in HIV-infected premenopausal women. J Acquir Immune Defic Syndr 2010;53:202–8.
27. Bolland MJ, Wang TK, Grey A, et al. Stable bone density in HAART-treated individuals with HIV: a meta-analysis. J Clin Endocrinol Metab 2001;96:2721–31.
28. Yin MT, Zhang CA, McMahon DJ, et al. Higher rates of bone loss in postmenopausal HIV-infected women: a longitudinal study. J Clin Endocrinol Metab 2012;97:554–62.
29. Bolland MJ, Grey AB, Gamble GD, et al. Low body weight mediates the relationship between HIV infection and low bone mineral density: a meta-analysis. J Clin Endocrinol Metab 2007;92:4522–8.

30. Cassetti I, Madruga JV, Suleiman JM, et al, Study 903E Team*. The safety and efficacy of tenofovir DF in combination with lamivudine and efavirenz through 6 years in antiretroviral-naïve HIV-1-infected patients. HIV Clin Trials 2007;8: 164–72.

31. Brown TT, McComsey GA, King MS, et al. Loss of bone mineral density after antiretroviral therapy initiation, independent of antiretroviral regimen. J Acquir Immune Defic Syndr 2009;51:554–61.

32. Duvivier C, Kolta S, Assoumou L, et al, ANRS 121 Hippocampe study group. Greater decrease in bone mineral density with protease inhibitor regimens compared with nonnucleoside reverse transcriptase inhibitor regimens in HIV-1 infected naive patients. AIDS 2009;23:817–24.

33. Grund B, Peng G, Gibert C, et al. Continuous antiretroviral therapy decreases bone mineral density. AIDS 2009;23:1519–29.

34. Stellbrink HJ, Orkin C, Arribas JR, et al. Comparison of changes in bone density and turnover with abacavir-lamivudine versus tenofovir-emtricitabine in HIV-infected adults: 48-week results from the ASSERT study. Clin Infect Dis 2010; 51:963–72.

35. McComsey GA, Kitch D, Daar ES, et al. Bone mineral density and fractures in antiretroviral-naive persons randomized to receive abacavir-lamivudine or tenofovir disoproxil fumarate-emtricitabine along with efavirenz or atazanavir-ritonavir: AIDS Clinical Trials Group A5224s, a substudy of ACTG A5202. J Infect Dis 2011;203:1791–801.

36. Haskelberg H, Hoy JF, Amin J, et al. Changes in bone turnover and bone loss in HIV-infected patients changing treatment to tenofovir-emtricitabine or abacavir-lamivudine. PLoS One 2012;7:e38377.

37. Assoumou L, Katlama C, Viard JP, et al, ANRS Osteovir study group. Changes in bone mineral density over a 2-year period in HIV-1-infected men under combined antiretroviral therapy with osteopenia. AIDS 2013;27:2425–30.

38. Martin A, Moore C, Mallon PW, et al. Bone mineral density in HIV participants randomized to raltegravir and lopinavir/ritonavir compared with standard second line therapy. AIDS 2013;27:2403–11.

39. Kong YY, Feige U, Sarosi I, et al. Activated T cells regulate bone loss and joint destruction in adjuvant arthritis through osteoprotegerin ligand. Nature 1999; 402:304–9.

40. Won HY, Lee J-A, Park ZS, et al. Prominent bone loss mediated by RANKL and IL-17 produced by CD4+ T cells in TallyHo/JngJ Mice. PLoS One 2011;6: e18168.

41. Barkhordarian A, Ajaj R, Ramchandani MH, et al. Osteoimmunopathology in HIV/AIDS: a translational evidence-based perspective. Patholog Res Int 2011; 2011:359242.

42. Calmy A, Chevalley T, Delhumeau C, et al. Long-term HIV infection and antiretroviral therapy are associated with bone microstructure alterations in premenopausal women. Osteoporos Int 2013;24:1843–52.

43. Yin MT, Shu A, Zhang CA, et al. Trabecular and cortical microarchitecture in postmenopausal HIV-infected women. Calcif Tissue Int 2013;92:557–65.

44. Yin MT, Lund E, Shah J, et al. Lower peak bone mass and abnormal trabecular and cortical microarchitecture in young men infected with HIV early in life. AIDS 2014;28:345–53.

45. Triant VA, Brown TT, Lee H, et al. Fracture prevalence among human immunodeficiency virus (HIV)-infected versus non-HIV-infected patients in a large U.S. healthcare system. J Clin Endocrinol Metab 2008;93:3499–504.

46. Yin MT, Shi Q, Hoover DR, et al. Fracture incidence in HIV-infected women: results from the Women's Interagency HIV Study. AIDS 2010;24:2679–86.
47. Womack JA, Goulet JL, Gibert C, et al. Increased risk of fragility fractures among HIV infected compared to uninfected male veterans. PLoS One 2011; 6:e17217.
48. Young B, Dao CN, Buchacz K, et al, the HIV Outpatient Study (HOPS) Investigators. Increased rates of bone fracture among HIV-infected persons in the HIV Outpatient Study (HOPS) compared with the US general population, 2000–2006. Clin Infect Dis 2011;52:1061–8.
49. Hansen AB, Gerstoft J, Kronborg G, et al. Incidence of low and high-energy fractures in persons with and without HIV infection: a Danish population-based cohort study. AIDS 2012;26:285–93.
50. Güerri-Fernandez R, Vestergaard P, Carbonell C, et al. HIV infection is strongly associated with hip fracture risk, independently of age, gender, and comorbidities: a population-based cohort study. Osteoporos Int 2013;24:1843–52.
51. Prieto-Alhambra D, Güerri-Fernández R, De Vries F, et al. HIV Infection and its association with an excess risk of clinical fractures: a nationwide case-control study. J Bone Miner Res 2013;28:1259–63.
52. Shiau S, Broun EC, Arpadi SM, et al. Incident fractures in HIV-infected individuals: a systematic review and meta-analysis. AIDS 2013;27:1949–57.
53. Yong MK, Elliott JH, Woolley IJ, et al. Low CD4 count is associated with an increased risk of fragility fracture in HIV-infected patients. J Acquir Immune Defic Syndr 2011;57:205–10.
54. Bedimo R, Maalouf NM, Zhang S, et al. Osteoporotic fracture risk associated with cumulative exposure to tenofovir and other antiretroviral agents. AIDS 2012;26:825–31.
55. Gedmintas L, Wright EA, Losina E, et al. Comparative risk of fracture in men and women with HIV. J Clin Endocrinol Metab 2014;99:486–90.
56. Hasse B, Ledergerber B, Furrer H, et al. Morbidity and aging in HIV-infected persons: the Swiss HIV cohort study. Clin Infect Dis 2011;53:1130–9.
57. Yin MT, Kendall MA, Wu X, et al. Fractures after antiretroviral initiation. AIDS 2012;26:2175–84.
58. Lo Re V 3rd, Volk J, Newcomb CW, et al. Risk of hip fracture associated with hepatitis C virus infection and hepatitis C/human immunodeficiency virus coinfection. Hepatology 2012;56:1688–98.
59. Maalouf NM, Zhang S, Drechsler H, et al. Hepatitis C co-infection and severity of liver disease as risk factors for osteoporotic fractures among HIV-infected patients. J Bone Miner Res 2013;28:2577–83.
60. Serrano S, Marinoso ML, Soriano JC, et al. Bone remodeling in human immunodeficiency virus-1-infected patients. A histomorphometric study. Bone 1995;16: 185–91.
61. Brown TT, Fredrick L, Warren D, et al. Decreased total bone mineral density in treatment-naive subjects taking lopinavir/ritonavir combined with raltegravir or tenofovir/emtricitabine. In: 14th European AIDS Conference. Brussels, 2013.
62. European AIDS Clinical Society Guidelines 2013. Available at: http://eacsociety.org/Guidelines.aspx. Accessed May 10, 2014.
63. Harvey N, Dennison E, Cooper C. Osteoporosis: impact on health and economics. Nat Rev Rheumatol 2010;6:99–105.
64. De Laet C, Kanis JA, Oden A, et al. Body mass index as a predictor of fracture risk: a meta-analysis. Osteoporos Int 2005;16:1330–8.

65. Lin D, Rieder MJ. Interventions for the treatment of decreased bone mineral density associated with HIV infection. Cochrane Database Syst Rev 2007;(2): CD005645.
66. Gueraldi G, Orlando G, Madeddu G, et al. Alendronate reduces bone resorption in HIV-associated osteopenia/osteoporosis. HIV Clin Trials 2004;5:269–77.
67. Mondy K, Powderly WG, Claxton SA, et al. Alendronate, vitamin D and calcium for the treatment of osteopenia/osteoporosis associated with HIV infection. J Acquired Immune Defic Syndr 2005;38:426–31.
68. Negredo E, Martinez-Lopez E, Paredes R, et al. Reversal of HIV-1-associated osteoporosis with once weekly alendronate. AIDS 2005;19:343–5.
69. McComsey GA, Kendall MA, Tebas P, et al. Alendronate with calcium and vitamin D supplementation is safe and effective for the treatment of decreased bone mineral density in HIV. AIDS 2007;21:2473–82.
70. Rozenberg S, Lanoy E, Bentata M, et al, ANRS 120 Fosivir Study Group. Effect of alendronate on HIV-associated osteoporosis: a randomized, double-blind, placebo-controlled, 96-week trial (ANRS 120). AIDS Res Hum Retroviruses 2012;28:972–80.
71. Bolland MJ, Grey AB, Horne AM, et al. Annual zoledronate increases bone density in highly active antiretroviral therapy-treated human immunodeficiency virus-infected men: a randomized controlled trial. J Clin Endocrinol Metab 2007;92:1283–8.
72. Bolland MJ, Grey A, Horne AM, et al. Effects of intravenous zoledronate on bone turnover and bone density persist for at least five years in HIV-infected men. J Clin Endocrinol Metab 2012;97:1922–8.
73. Huang J, Meixner L, Fernandez S, et al. A double-blinded, randomized controlled trial of zoledronate therapy for HIV-associated osteopenia and osteoporosis. AIDS 2009;23:51–7.
74. Shane E, Burr D, Abrahamsen B, et al. Atypical subtrochanteric and diaphyseal femoral fractures: second report of a task force of the American Society for Bone and Mineral Research. J Bone Miner Res 2014;29:1–23.
75. Suresh F, Pazianas M, Abrahamsen B. Safety issues with bisphosphonate therapy for osteoporosis. Rheumatology 2014;53:19–31.
76. Compston J. Pathophysiology of atypical femoral fractures and osteonecrosis of the jaw. Osteoporos Int 2011;22:2951–61.

Thyroid Abnormalities

Anthony P. Weetman, MD, DSc*

KEYWORDS

- Thyroid function • Infective thyroiditis • Immune reconstitution
- Inflammatory syndrome • Graves disease • Non-thyroidal illness

KEY POINTS

- Most patients with early human immunodeficiency virus (HIV) infection with no weight loss have normal thyroid function.
- As disease progresses, subtle abnormalities in thyroid function occur in some patients, including subclinical hypothyroidism and isolated low free thyroxine levels.
- Immune reconstitution in the first 3 years after highly active antiretroviral therapy is associated with the development of Graves disease and other autoimmune disorders in a small number of patients.
- In advanced HIV infection, unusual opportunistic infections may cause acute or subacute thyroiditis.

Many endocrine and metabolic abnormalities have been identified after infection with human immunodeficiency virus (HIV), typically comprising endocrine gland involvement by neoplasms or after opportunistic infection, hormone abnormalities resulting from the associated illness, and side effects from treatment.[1,2] As chronic HIV infection becomes the norm, prolonged inflammation and immunodeficiency can combine to produce new disease associations, such as cardiovascular complications, and extended treatment may also induce novel side effects[3]; it is likely therefore that there is a still evolving pattern of endocrine abnormalities. This review focuses on thyroid abnormalities, which are usually asymptomatic or mild, but may cause diagnostic problems (**Table 1**). Approximately one third of patients with HIV infection may have biochemical disturbances of thyroid function, whereas only 1% to 3% develop overt thyroid disease.[4]

THYROID FUNCTION TESTS IN HIV-INFECTED INDIVIDUALS

In most patients with recent HIV infection, thyroid function tests are normal. However, as disease progresses and complications such as opportunistic infections ensue, a wide

Disclosure: The author has nothing to disclose.
Department of Human Metabolism, University of Sheffield, Beech Hill Road, Sheffield S10 2RX, UK
* Faculty of Medicine, Dentistry and Health, Barber House, 387 Glossop Road, Sheffield S10 2HQ, UK.
E-mail address: a.p.weetman@sheffield.ac.uk

Endocrinol Metab Clin N Am 43 (2014) 781–790
http://dx.doi.org/10.1016/j.ecl.2014.05.006
0889-8529/14/$ – see front matter © 2014 Elsevier Inc. All rights reserved.

Table 1	
Summary of the main types of thyroid disorders in HIV-infected individuals	
Disorder	Description
Infective thyroiditis	Caused by opportunistic infections that do not affect the thyroid in non–HIV-infected individuals
Thyroid neoplasm	Kaposi sarcoma; lymphoma
Nonthyroidal illness	Especially in the terminal phase in AIDS patients
Isolated low free T4	In treated individuals, especially children
Subclinical hypothyroidism	In treated individuals
Reconstitution disease	After treatment; especially Graves disease

Abbreviations: HIV, human immunodeficiency virus; T4, thyroxine.

variety of asymptomatic disturbances may occur, which are part of the spectrum of disorders termed nonthyroid illness or sick-euthyroid syndrome (SES). Any acute, severe illness may cause SES, including anorexia and psychiatric disorders. The alterations seen in thyroid hormones are primarily owing to the effects of cytokines on thyroid hormone deiodination and on the pituitary, and teleologically have been regarded as an adaptive mechanism to conserve energy and limit catabolism. It is increasingly clear this view is overly simplistic, with significant variations in the presentation and outcome of SES that depend on etiology, end-organ responses, and chronicity.[5]

Weight-stable patients with HIV have normal serum free tri-iodothyromine (FT3) levels, in contrast with those who lose weight, in whom serum FT3 and reverse T3 levels can decrease rapidly, in close relationship to nutritional status.[6,7] The lowering of reverse T3 is unusual, because altered thyroxine (T4) deiodination in SES is usually accompanied by an increase in reverse T3 production, which works together with reduced clearance to elevate serum levels of reverse T3. This increased production results from a decrease in 5'-deiodination of T4, leading to a decrease in T3 production and reverse T3 metabolism and an increase in 5-deiodination of T4, leading to an increase in reverse T3. The pattern of reduced levels of reverse T3 seen in HIV infection has been replicated in other studies, but the reasons for it are unknown.[8,9] Any decline in T3 levels in HIV-infected individuals probably occurs later than would be expected in typical SES, and is associated with an increased mortality.[9] It is conceivable that the failure of T3 to decrease in the SES associated with HIV infection contributes to weight loss.

Another distinctive feature of HIV infection is that serum levels of T4-binding globulin progressively increase; cortisol-binding globulin and sex hormone-binding globulin remain unaltered.[6,8,10] The reason for this increase in T4-binding globulin is unknown, but seems unrelated to estrogen levels or clearance of the protein. The only relevance of the change in T4-binding globulin is that alterations in the level of this protein have a significant effect on biochemical tests that measure total rather than free thyroid hormones; however, these tests are used rarely. Serum thyrotropin (TSH) levels in HIV-infected individuals are typically normal, but more detailed study has revealed that the response to thyrotropin-releasing hormone is exaggerated and there is an altered pattern to the normal circadian rhythm of TSH, with higher pulse amplitudes and a higher mean 24-hour TSH level.[11] These changes again differ from typical SES, in which serum TSH levels may decline or (less commonly) increase, and indicate a mild underlying subclinical hypothyroidism.

Most studies preceded effective treatment for HIV and more recent work has focused on thyroid abnormalities in treated patients. However, a recent study of

50 HIV-infected individuals from India found that 18% had low FT3 levels, 20% had low free T4 (FT4) levels and 24% had elevated TSH levels.[12] CD4+ T-cell counts correlated with FT3 and FT4 levels and indirectly correlated with TSH levels. In perinatally acquired HIV infection, thyroid abnormalities occur early and are pronounced in those with the highest viral load and the most severe immunosuppression.[13]

ISOLATED LOW FT4 LEVEL

One of the most distinctive thyroid abnormalities found in individuals with HIV infection is an isolated low serum FT4 level, without any elevation of the serum TSH level. The reported frequency of this finding is between 1.8% and 6.8% in adults.[14–16] Most of these patients had received highly active antiretroviral therapy (HAART) with multiple combinations of antiviral drugs. Typically, treatment is with at least 3 agents chosen from reverse transcriptase inhibitors, protease inhibitors, or drugs that prevent viral entry into T cells. A direct correlation between serum FT4 levels and CD4+ T-cell counts was found in 1 study,[15] suggesting that this abnormality may be cytokine mediated. However, in another study there was no obvious relationship.[16]

The prevalence of this FT4 abnormality is higher in children, with frequency figures as high as 31% being reported.[17] All of these children were receiving HAART, raising the possibility that the antiviral treatment itself is in some way responsible; an association has been demonstrated particularly with stavudine. The cumulative dose of other drugs was no different in patients with and without low FT4 levels.[14] However, in this particular pediatric study, a shorter duration of HAART was associated with low FT4 levels.[17] These children had a normal TSH response to thyrotropin-releasing hormone, which tends to rule against any secondary form of hypothyroidism as a cause for this abnormality. In a more recent study of adults from Kenya, lowering of FT4 occurred progressively with HAART; there was no change in TSH levels.[18] Perhaps some agents given in HAART regimens, alone or in combination or in particular settings, cause anomalies in certain assays for FT4, which are similar to those encountered with carbamazepine, phenytoin, and other drugs.

Although there remains uncertainty over the cause and effect of this anomaly, there is no reason at present to give any treatment. The serum TSH level seems to be a reliable guide to the presence of true hypothyroidism (see Hypothyroidism), and so it would be prudent to follow patients who are discovered to have a low FT4 level with repeat measurement of TSH and FT4 at 3- to 6-month intervals until the pattern of any further change becomes apparent.

HYPOTHYROIDISM

In untreated individuals with HIV, the prevalence of subclinical and clinical hypothyroidism is approximately twice that of the healthy population. The prevalence of subclinical hypothyroidism (elevated serum TSH level with normal serum FT3 and FT4 levels) is 4.3% among adults living in the United States; 0.3% have overt hypothyroidism (elevated serum TSH level with a low serum FT4 level).[19] Similar figures have been reported in other countries, such as Norway; women are more commonly affected than men.[20] Most cases are the result of autoimmunity, as shown by the association between TSH levels and thyroid autoantibodies in population studies.[21]

One study from Italy of HIV-infected individuals found a prevalence of 7.4% for subclinical hypothyroidism; all of these individuals were negative for thyroid autoantibodies and rates were similar for those who were untreated and those receiving HAART.[22] Men were almost as frequently affected as women. An earlier study in France found overt hypothyroidism in 2.6% of HIV-infected individuals and subclinical hypothyroidism in 6.6%, with more men than women affected.[14] Thyroid autoantibodies were not measured, but there was an association between hypothyroidism and the receipt of HAART, suggesting that at least some of these cases may have been owing to a reconstitution syndrome. This is borne out by findings of subclinical hypothyroidism only in HAART-treated patients, and in 1 case interruption of HAART was associated with normalization of thyroid function.[16]

Other studies have also found subclinical hypothyroidism to be confined to those receiving HAART, and to be present without detectable thyroid autoantibodies.[23,24] One other follow-up study, by contrast, found subclinical hypothyroidism to be present in 14.4% of HAART-treated patients and 9.6% of untreated patients; further cases developed both in those who were untreated for 2 years (7.1%) and in those receiving HAART (19.0%); thyroid autoantibodies were not measured.[25] Other cross-sectional studies have found variable hypothyroidism rates of 13.5% in Thailand[26] and 3.6% in older men in the United States.[27] In 1 study from the United Kingdom, 6.5% of HIV-infected individuals had hypothyroidism, but only 1% developed new hypothyroidism over 3 years and no independent variables were associated with the presence of hypothyroidism.[28]

Taken together, these results indicate that subclinical and overt hypothyroidism are more common in HIV-infected individuals and this does not seem to be the result of typical thyroid autoimmunity, although this has not been rigorously assessed, for instance by use of thyroid ultrasound. Moreover, the studies so far have not used contemporary local controls for comparison purposes. In addition, hypothyroidism is increased as a result of HAART. This may be a combined effect of the drugs used, as with the isolated low FT4 level abnormality noted, and immune reconstitution.

Treatment for hypothyroidism in HIV-infected individuals should follow the guidelines for those without infection,[28] although when hypothyroidism is associated with HAART that is subsequently changed, there could be a case for determining whether any levothyroxine treatment that has been given could be reduced or stopped, although there are no data to confirm this supposition. Establishing that hypothyroidism is permanent is most easily done by asking the patient to stop levothyroxine and measuring the TSH after 6 weeks.

IMMUNE RECONSTITUTION THYROID DISEASE

Immune reconstitution inflammatory syndrome refers to the phenomenon of an enhanced immune response seen when lymphopenia is reversed; this syndrome may manifest as worsening of an underlying opportunistic infection, a "paradoxic" symptomatic relapse of a previously treated infection or recurrence of Kaposi sarcoma.[29,30] In immune reconstitution inflammatory syndrome, it is thought that reversal of CD4+ T-cell depletion and dendritic cell dysfunction after commencing HAART results in a predominantly T helper cell 1 and T helper cell 17 response as the immune response is restored, and this in turn results in tissue inflammation with atypical presentations of any underlying infection. An imbalance in CD8+ T-cell responses may also contribute.[31]

Another feature of immune reconstitution is the appearance of autoimmune disorders and sarcoidosis. Immune reconstitution-related autoimmune disease occurs in 3 settings: (i) after HAART treatment of HIV-infected individuals, (ii) after treatment of multiple sclerosis with alemtuzumab, a monoclonal antibody that depletes lymphocytes, and (iii) after bone marrow transplantation when the donor has previously had Graves disease.[32] Although it is not yet established that these 3 entities have a common pathogenesis, the principle that some disorder of immunoregulation occurs during immune restoration seems a plausible thread, and this explanation mirrors the appearance of autoimmunity in rodents subjected to thymectomy and irradiation, which also produces lymphopenia.[33] In the latter setting, it is known that disease can be prevented by CD4[+] T regulatory cells. It is therefore possible that an imbalance in T regulatory cell function or in the cytokine milieu results in the appearance of reconstitution after reversal of lymphopenia in these patient groups (**Box 1**).

CD4[+] T cell levels rise rapidly in the first 3 months after commencing HAART; failure to achieve a CD4[+] T-cell count of 100 to 150/μL is regarded as evidence that the HAART regimen is not effective. This initial rise is in memory T cells; naïve T cells recover more slowly. Preexisting thyroid antibody levels are not affected by HAART.[16] However, the appearance of thyroid autoantibodies and thyroid disease is more common after HAART, the first reports being of 5 patients in whom Graves disease developed 14 to 22 months after HAART was commenced and 9 to 17 months after the rise in CD4[+] T cells.[34] In these patients, both thyroid peroxidase and TSH receptor antibodies became detectable; unusually, 4 of them were male and there was no family history of thyroid autoimmunity. Other case reports followed this initial description; in 1 patient, alopecia universalis and subclinical autoimmune hypothyroidism preceded the onset of Graves disease and in another the clinical presentation was with thyrotoxic periodic paralysis.[35,36]

A retrospective analysis of HIV-infected patients in the UK revealed more patients with Graves disease, with an estimated prevalence of 3% for women and 0.2% for men.[37] Most of these patients were black African, an ethnic group with a low incidence of Graves disease; the risk of Graves disease in these HIV-infected patients was therefore approximately 4-fold greater than expected. The average time onset of Graves disease was 17 months (range 8–33 months) after the start of HAART, at a time when there is an increasing ratio of naïve to memory T cells. Those individuals who developed Graves disease had lower CD4[+] T-cell counts before HAART than those who remained euthyroid.

The fact that other autoimmune disorders also occur after HAART supports the proposition that these cases of Graves disease are not merely coincidental.

Box 1
Pathogenic factors in the occurrence of reconstitution Graves disease after HAART treatment for HIV infection

- Immune restoration with increase in memory CD4[+] T cells released from sequestration in inflamed lymphoid tissue.

- Subsequent increase in naïve CD4[+] T cells newly produced in the thymus.

- Altered cytokine milieu with a bias toward a Th1 and Th17 profile, leading to a proinflammatory immune response; subsequent increase in the Th2 response may allow autoantibody formation.

- Dysregulation of CD4[+], CD25[+], and FoxP3[+] T regulatory cells.

- Variability in the clearance of abundant pathogenic antigens from persistent opportunistic infections may also be a determinant of the immune response.

- It is not yet known whether there is the same role for predisposing genetic and environmental factors that precipitate conventional Graves disease.

Abbreviations: HAART, highly active antiretroviral therapy; HIV, human immunodeficiency virus; Th, T helper cell.

Autoimmune hepatitis, rheumatoid arthritis, systemic lupus erythematosus, type 1 diabetes, and type B insulin resistance syndrome have all been found after immune reconstitution with HAART.[38–41] Further evidence for a causal relationship comes from a case report in which Graves disease occurred 21 months after starting HAART, resolved spontaneously when HAART was stopped, and then reappeared after a second course of HAART.[42] Graves disease has also been reported in a HIV-infected individual who received interleukin-2 therapy, which also results in T-cell expansion.[43] In 2 cases of Graves disease occurring after HAART, methimazole treatment was associated with a further increase in the CD4[+] T-cell count beyond that achieved by HAART and prompt resolution of the thyroid dysfunction.[44] There has also been a description of acute, painful thyroiditis owing to Hashimoto thyroiditis 10 months after commencing HAART.[45]

Graves disease occurs in around 2% of HIV-infected patients treated with HAART during the late phase of immune reconstitution.[24,37] The mechanism for this complication remains to be fully elucidated, but these are clear similarities to other types of reconstitution Graves disease.[32] It is associated with the recovery of naïve T cells derived from primary thymic emigration, which results in inappropriate autoantibody production.[46] Whether the clinical course of Graves disease in these patients differs from normal has not been systematically studied, although theoretically one might predict that continued recovery of the immune system could lead to spontaneous remission in some cases. Treatment should follow standard practice, with antithyroid drug treatment being a reasonable first-line choice.[47]

THYROID INFECTIONS

Opportunistic infection is an obvious consequence of HIV infection and the consequent immunodeficiency. Opportunistic infections may spread to include the thyroid in the late stage of HIV infection, but this is rarely significant clinically. In a prospective autopsy study of 100 patients who died of AIDS and were not in receipt of HAART, examination of the thyroid revealed *Mycobacterium tuberculosis* in 23%, cytomegalovirus in 17%, *Cryptococcus* in 5%, *Mycobacterium avium* in 5%, and *Pneumocystis* in 4%.[48] Other bacteria and fungi were found in 7%. Unfortunately no premortem thyroid function results were available.

Pneumocystis jiroveci infection of the thyroid presents with a painless or painful goiter, sometimes with fluctuating thyroid function as seen in subacute thyroiditis.[49] Most infections, however, occur as part of a disseminated infection without clinical manifestations, and are only evident at autopsy.[50] Patients most at risk are those with CD4[+] T-cell counts of less than 200/µL on prophylactic inhaled pentamidine. Diagnosis is usually made by fine needle aspiration and appropriate silver staining.

Suppurative thyroiditis is rare, but is likely to be increased in HIV-infected individuals, although there have been no systematic studies. Case reports of such thyroid infections include abscess formation owing to concomitant *M tuberculosis* and *C neoformans* infection,[51] *Rhodococcus equi*,[52] *Aspergillus*,[53] and *Coccidioides*.[54] In 1 case, a tuberculous abscess of the thyroid developed after starting HAART and may therefore have been a paradoxic worsening as a result of immune reconstitution inflammatory syndrome.[55]

Treatment for tuberculosis infection in HIV patients may also be associated with thyroid dysfunction. In a cohort of HIV-infected Indian patients with multidrug-resistant tuberculosis, the use of p-aminosalicylic acid and ethionamide doubled the risk of hypothyroidism, which occurred in 54% of 116 patients.[56] Screening for changes in serum TSH level at frequent intervals seems prudent in such patients.

THYROID NEOPLASMS

An autopsy study of 100 patients who died from AIDS found that 4% had papillary carcinoma of the thyroid and 2% had Kaposi sarcoma of the thyroid.[48] A case has been reported in which Kaposi sarcoma destroyed the majority of thyroid tissue, resulting in hypothyroidism.[57] The advent of HAART has led to a marked decline in Kaposi sarcoma,[58] so further cases afflicting the thyroid are likely to be rare.

It is not clear whether the high prevalence of papillary carcinoma found in the study cited[48] reflects a true effect of HIV infection. One case report has documented papillary carcinoma and micrometastases in an HIV-infected individual,[59] and 1 nondifferentiated thyroid carcinoma was found in 2560 Spanish patients with HIV infection.[60] Two patients with AIDS have been reported in whom the clinical presentation of thyroid lymphoma was with altered thyroid function.[61,62] Overall, it seems unlikely that there is a significant increased risk of thyroid malignancy in current HAART-treated patients with HIV.

SUMMARY

Thyroid abnormalities do occur in HIV-infected individuals, but are less common than other types of endocrine and metabolic dysfunction. Presentation has also changed over time with the advent of HAART, and some types of thyroid abnormality seen are the result of treatment rather than the HIV infection per se. There is no single pattern of thyroid dysfunction in HIV infection, but 2 distinctive features are the occurrence of low serum reverse T3 levels with normal T3 levels early in disease, and isolated low serum FT4 levels later. HAART therapy is associated with a greater risk of Graves disease during the later phase of immune reconstitution. Because of the lack of systematic data, it is difficult to make recommendations on routine screening for thyroid disease in HIV-infected individuals. At present, it seems preferable to maintain vigilance for the occurrence of thyroid dysfunction in this setting.

REFERENCES

1. Grinspoon SK, Donovan DS Jr, Bilezikian JP. Aetiology and pathogenesis of hormonal and metabolic disorders in HIV infection. Baillieres Clin Endocrinol Metab 1994;8:735–55.
2. Hofbauer LC, Heufelder AE. Endocrine implications of human immunodeficiency virus infection. Medicine (Baltimore) 1996;75:262–78.
3. Deeks SG, Lewin SR, Havlir DV. The end of AIDS: HIV infection as a chronic disease. Lancet 2013;382:1525–33.
4. Hoffmann CJ, Brown TT. Thyroid function abnormalities in HIV-infected patients. Clin Infect Dis 2007;45:488–94.
5. Boelen A, Kwakkel J, Fliers E. Beyond low plasma T3: local thyroid hormone metabolism during inflammation and infection. Endocr Rev 2011;32:670–93.
6. Grunfeld C, Pang M, Doerrler W, et al. Indices of thyroid function and weight loss in human immunodeficiency virus infection and the acquired immunodeficiency syndrome. Metabolism 1993;42:1270–6.
7. Ricart-Engel W, Fernández-Real JM, González-Huix F, et al. The relation between thyroid function and nutritional status in HIV-infected patients. Clin Endocrinol (Oxf) 1996;44:53–8.
8. LoPresti JS, Fried JC, Spencer CA, et al. Unique alterations of thyroid hormone indices in the acquired immunodeficiency syndrome (AIDS). Ann Intern Med 1989;110:970–5.

9. Sellmeyer DE, Grunfeld C. Endocrine and metabolic disturbances in human immunodeficiency virus infection and the acquired immune deficiency syndrome. Endocr Rev 1996;17:518–32.

10. Lambert M, Zech F, De Nayer P, et al. Elevation of serum thyroxine-binding globulin (but not of cortisol-binding globulin and sex hormone-binding globulin) associated with the progression of human immunodeficiency virus infection. Am J Med 1990;89:748–51.

11. Hommes MJ, Romijn JA, Endert E, et al. Hypothyroid-like regulation of the pituitary-thyroid axis in stable human immunodeficiency virus infection. Metabolism 1993;42:556–61.

12. Jain G, Devpura G, Gupta BS. Abnormalities in the thyroid function tests as surrogate marker of advancing HIV infection in infected adults. J Assoc Physicians India 2009;57:508–10.

13. Chiarelli F, Galli L, Verrotti A, et al. Thyroid function in children with perinatal human immunodeficiency virus type 1 infection. Thyroid 2000;10:499–505.

14. Beltran S, Lescure FX, El Esper I, et al. Subclinical hypothyroidism in HIV-infected patients is not an autoimmune disease. Horm Res 2006;66:21–6.

15. Collazos J, Ibarra S, Mayo J. Thyroid hormones in HIV-infected patients in the highly active antiretroviral therapy era: evidence of an interrelation between the thyroid axis and the immune system. AIDS 2003;17:763–5.

16. Madeddu G, Spanu A, Chessa F, et al. Thyroid function in human immunodeficiency virus patients treated with highly active antiretroviral therapy (HAART): a longitudinal study. Clin Endocrinol (Oxf) 2006;64(4):375–83.

17. Viganò A, Riboni S, Bianchi R, et al. Thyroid dysfunction in antiretroviral treated children. Pediatr Infect Dis J 2004;23:235–9.

18. Thaimuta ZL, Sekadde-Kigondu C, Makawiti DW, et al. Thyroid function among HIV/AIDS patients on highly active anti-retroviral therapy. East Afr Med J 2010; 87:474–80.

19. Hollowell JG, Staehling NW, Flanders WD, et al. Serum TSH, T(4), and thyroid antibodies in the United States population (1988 to 1994): National Health and Nutrition Examination Survey (NHANES III). J Clin Endocrinol Metab 2002;87: 489–99.

20. Bjoro T, Holmen J, Krüger O, et al. Prevalence of thyroid disease, thyroid dysfunction and thyroid peroxidase antibodies in a large, unselected population. The Health Study of Nord-Trondelag (HUNT). Eur J Endocrinol 2000;143:639–47.

21. Spencer CA, Hollowell JG, Kazarosyan M, et al. National Health and Nutrition Examination Survey III thyroid-stimulating hormone (TSH)-thyroperoxidase antibody relationships demonstrate that TSH upper reference limits may be skewed by occult thyroid dysfunction. J Clin Endocrinol Metab 2007;92:4236–40.

22. Quirino T, Bongiovanni M, Ricci E, et al. Hypothyroidism in HIV-infected patients who have or have not received HAART. Clin Infect Dis 2004;38:596–7.

23. Calza L, Manfredi R, Chiodo F. Subclinical hypothyroidism in HIV-infected patients receiving highly active antiretroviral therapy. J Acquir Immune Defic Syndr 2002;31:361–3.

24. de Carvalho LG, Teixeira Pde F, Panico AL, et al. Evaluation of thyroid function and autoimmunity in HIV-infected women. Arq Bras Endocrinol Metabol 2013; 57:450–6.

25. Bongiovanni M, Adorni F, Casana M, et al. Subclinical hypothyroidism in HIV-infected subjects. J Antimicrob Chemother 2006;58:1086–9.

26. Ketsamathi C, Jongjaroenprasert W, Chailurkit LO, et al. Prevalence of thyroid dysfunction in Thai HIV-infected patients. Curr HIV Res 2006;4:463–7.

27. Wiener M, Lo Y, Klein RS. Abnormal thyroid function in older men with or at risk for HIV infection. HIV Med 2008;9:544–9.
28. Garber JR, Cobin RH, Gharib H, et al. Clinical practice guidelines for hypothyroidism in adults: cosponsored by the American Association of Clinical Endocrinologists and the American Thyroid Association. Thyroid 2012;22:1200–35.
29. Müller M, Wandel S, Colebunders R, et al. Immune reconstitution inflammatory syndrome in patients starting antiretroviral therapy for HIV infection: a systematic review and meta-analysis. Lancet Infect Dis 2010;10:251–61.
30. Leidner RS, Aboulafia DM. Recrudescent Kaposi's sarcoma after initiation of HAART: a manifestation of immune reconstitution syndrome. AIDS Patient Care STDS 2005;19:635–44.
31. French MA. HIV/AIDS: immune reconstitution inflammatory syndrome: a reappraisal. Clin Infect Dis 2009;48:101–7.
32. Weetman A. Immune reconstitution syndrome and the thyroid. Best Pract Res Clin Endocrinol Metab 2009;23:693–702.
33. Gleeson PA, Toh BH, van Driel IR. Organ-specific autoimmunity induced by lymphopenia. Immunol Rev 1996;149:97–125.
34. Jubault V, Penfornis A, Schillo F, et al. Sequential occurrence of thyroid autoantibodies and Graves' disease after immune restoration in severely immunocompromised human immunodeficiency virus-1-infected patients. J Clin Endocrinol Metab 2000;85:4254–7.
35. Sereti I, Sarlis NJ, Arioglu E, et al. Alopecia universalis and Graves' disease in the setting of immune restoration after highly active antiretroviral therapy. AIDS 2001;15:138–40.
36. Brown JD, Kangwanprasert M, Tice A, et al. Thyrotoxic periodic paralysis in a Polynesian male following highly active antiretroviral therapy for HIV infection. Hawaii Med J 2007;66:60–3.
37. Chen F, Day SL, Metcalfe RA, et al. Characteristics of autoimmune thyroid disease occurring as a late complication of immune reconstitution in patients with advanced human immunodeficiency virus (HIV) disease. Medicine (Baltimore) 2005;84:98–106.
38. Calabrese LH, Kirchner E, Shrestha R. Rheumatic complications of human immunodeficiency virus infection in the era of highly active antiretroviral therapy: emergence of a new syndrome of immune reconstitution and changing patterns of disease. Semin Arthritis Rheum 2005;35:166–74.
39. O'Leary JG, Zachary K, Misdraji J, et al. De novo autoimmune hepatitis during immune reconstitution in an HIV-infected patient receiving highly active antiretroviral therapy. Clin Infect Dis 2008;46:e12–4.
40. Mohammedi K, Roussel R, El Dbouni O, et al. Type B insulin resistance syndrome associated with an immune reconstitution inflammatory syndrome in an HIV-infected woman. J Clin Endocrinol Metab 2011;96:E653–7.
41. Takarabe D, Rokukawa Y, Takahashi Y, et al. Autoimmune diabetes in HIV-infected patients on highly active antiretroviral therapy. J Clin Endocrinol Metab 2010;95:4056–60.
42. Visković K, Stemberger L, Brnić Z, et al. Repeated presentation of Graves' disease as a manifestation of immune reconstitution syndrome in an HIV-infected patient taking HAART: case report. Acta Clin Croat 2013;52:125–7.
43. Jimenez C, Moran SA, Sereti I, et al. Graves' disease after interleukin-2 therapy in a patient with human immunodeficiency virus infection. Thyroid 2004;14:1097–102.
44. Honda A, Kashiwazaki K, Tsunoda T, et al. Short communication: CD4 cell count increases during successful treatment of Graves' disease with methimazole in

HIV-infected patients on antiretroviral therapy. AIDS Res Hum Retroviruses 2012;28:1627–9.

45. Visser R, de Mast Q, Netea-Maier RT, et al. Hashimoto's thyroiditis presenting as acute painful thyroiditis and as a manifestation of an immune reconstitution inflammatory syndrome in a human immunodeficiency virus-seropositive patient. Thyroid 2012;22:853–5.
46. Sheikh V, Dersimonian R, Richterman AG, et al. Graves' disease as immune reconstitution disease in HIV-positive patients is associated with naive and primary thymic emigrant CD4(+) T-cell recovery. AIDS 2014;28:31–9.
47. Bahn RS, Burch HB, Cooper DS, et al. Hyperthyroidism and other causes of thyrotoxicosis: management guidelines of the American Thyroid Association and American Association of Clinical Endocrinologists. Endocr Pract 2011;17: 456–520.
48. Basílio-De-Oliveira CA. Infectious and neoplastic disorders of the thyroid in AIDS patients: an autopsy study. Braz J Infect Dis 2000;4:67–75.
49. Guttler R, Singer PA, Axline SG, et al. Pneumocystis carinii thyroiditis. Report of three cases and review of the literature. Arch Intern Med 1993;153:393–6.
50. Zavascki AP, Maia AL, Goldani LZ. Pneumocystis jiroveci thyroiditis: report of 15 cases in the literature. Mycoses 2007;50:443–6.
51. Kiertiburanakul S, Sungkanuparph S, Malathum K, et al. Concomitant tuberculous and cryptococcal thyroid abscess in a human immunodeficiency virus-infected patient. Scand J Infect Dis 2003;35:68–70.
52. Martín-Dávila P, Quereda C, Rodríguez H, et al. Thyroid abscess due to Rhodococcus equi in a patient infected with the human immunodeficiency virus. Eur J Clin Microbiol Infect Dis 1998;17:55–7.
53. Nguyen J, Manera R, Minutti C. Aspergillus thyroiditis: a review of the literature to highlight clinical challenges. Eur J Clin Microbiol Infect Dis 2012;31:3259–64.
54. Jinno S, Chang S, Jacobs MR. Coccidioides thyroiditis in an HIV-infected patient. J Clin Microbiol 2012;50:2535–7.
55. Katusiime C, Ocama P, Kambugu A. Initial description of immune reconstitution inflammatory syndrome involving the thyroid gland in an immunocompromised patient. BMJ Case Rep 2011; pii:bcr0420114053.
56. Andries A, Isaakidis P, Das M, et al. High rate of hypothyroidism in multidrug-resistant tuberculosis patients co-infected with HIV in Mumbai, India. PLoS One 2013;8:e78313.
57. Mollison LC, Mijch A, McBride G, et al. Hypothyroidism due to destruction of the thyroid by Kaposi's sarcoma. Rev Infect Dis 1991;13:826–7.
58. Engels EA, Biggar RJ, Hall HI, et al. Cancer risk in people infected with human immunodeficiency virus in the United States. Int J Cancer 2008;123:187–94.
59. Lloret Linares C, Troisvallets D, Sellier P, et al. Micrometastasis of papillary thyroid carcinoma in a human immunodeficiency virus-infected patient: a case report and discussion. Med Oncol 2010;27:756–9.
60. Santos J, Palacios R, Ruiz J, et al. Unusual malignant tumours in patients with HIV infection. Int J STD AIDS 2002;13:674–6.
61. Samuels MH, Launder T. Hyperthyroidism due to lymphoma involving the thyroid gland in a patient with acquired immunodeficiency syndrome: case report and review of the literature. Thyroid 1998;8:673–7.
62. Gochu J, Piper B, Montana J, et al. Lymphoma of the thyroid mimicking thyroiditis in a patient with the acquired immune deficiency syndrome. J Endocrinol Invest 1994;17:279–82.

Hypothalamic-Pituitary-Adrenal Axis in HIV Infection and Disease

George P. Chrousos, MD[a], Evangelia D. Zapanti, MD, PhD[b],*

KEYWORDS

• HIV • AIDS • Insulin resistance • HPA • Cortisol • Adrenals

KEY POINTS

- HIV infection is associated with hypothalamic-pituitary-adrenal axis stimulation and glucocorticoid hypersensitivity.
- Diagnosis of adrenal insufficiency, although challenging, is imperative because prompt treatment is life-saving.
- Unnecessary treatment with glucocorticoids in HIV infection is likely to accelerate the progression of disease.
- The pathogenesis of AIDS-related insulin resistance and lipodystrophy syndrome is multifactorial and might be related to the HIV infection itself, to the host, and/or to treatment with antiretroviral agents.

INTRODUCTION

The Hypothalamic-Pituitary-Adrenal Axis

Physical, psychological, and/or biological stimuli, such as bacterial or viral infection lead to the activation of the stress system and its resultant response. The stress system involves activation of the hypothalamic–pituitary–adrenal (HPA) axis, a major mediator of the stress response, which has a pivotal role in the maintenance of basal and stress-related homeostasis.[1,2]

Both central and peripheral nervous system tissues are components of the stress system and are involved in the mediation of the response to stress. The central components of the stress system are located in the hypothalamus and the brainstem. They include the hypophysiotropic neurons in the medial parvocellular nucleus, which synthesize and release corticotropin-releasing hormone (CRH), arginine vasopressin neurons of the paraventricular nuclei (PVN), medulla CRH neurons, the locus caeruleus (LC), and the

[a] First Department of Pediatrics, "Agia Sofia" Children's Hospital, University of Athens, Thivon and Papadiamantopoulou, Athens 11527, Greece; [b] First Endocrine Department and Diabetes Center, Alexandra Hospital, 80 Vassilisis Sofias Avenue, Athens 11528, Greece
* Corresponding author. 27 Plastira Street, Athens 17121.
E-mail address: liazapanti@yahoo.gr

Endocrinol Metab Clin N Am 43 (2014) 791–806
http://dx.doi.org/10.1016/j.ecl.2014.06.002
endo.theclinics.com

LC-norepinephrine (LC/NE) autonomic system nuclei. The peripheral components of the stress system include the HPA axis and the peripheral limbs, the systemic sympathetic and adrenomedullary systems and part of the parasympathetic system.[1–3]

The primary mediator of the stress response is hypothalamic CRH, a 41-amino acid peptide released into the pituitary portal vessels, which, by binding to its receptor, stimulates the secretion of adrenocorticotropic hormone (ACTH) from the anterior pituitary into the systemic circulation. Besides the stimulation of ACTH secretion, CRH has also been implicated in the regulation of the autonomic nervous system and in several other functions (memory, feeding, and reproductive behaviors).[4,5] The CRH family includes 3 other stress related peptides members of the urocortin (UCN) family (UCN1, UCN2, UCN3) expressed in the hypothalamus and the brain. The peptides of the CRH family exert their physiologic actions by binding to 2 distinct receptor subtypes belonging to the family of the G-protein coupled receptors[6]: CRH type 1 receptor (CRHR1) and CRH type 2 receptor (CRHR2). CRHR1 is expressed in the anterior pituitary and in the brain at high levels, and in peripheral tissues (adrenals, testis, ovaries) at lower levels, in contrast with CRHR2, which is expressed at higher levels in the periphery and at lower levels in the brain.[7] In humans, the CRHR1 gene encodes 1 functional variant (α), and the CRHR2 gene encodes 3 functional variants (α, β, and γ).[8] The neuroendocrine function of CRH is exerted through CRHR1 in the anterior pituitary. CRH, upon binding with CRHR1, activates cyclic adenosine monophosphate pathway events resulting in the release of ACTH from pituitary corticotropes.[9] Pituitary ACTH is a 39-amino acid peptide derived from pro-opiomelanocortin, which is processed into several biologically active peptides, including α-melanocyte-stimulating hormone, β-endorphin, and β-lipotropin hormone.[1] The main target of ACTH is the adrenal cortex, where it binds to its specific receptor melanocortin type 2 receptor and stimulates the secretion of glucocorticoids and adrenal androgens by the zonae fasciculata and reticularis, respectively.[10] ACTH also participates in the regulation of aldosterone secretion by the zona glomerulosa.[1]

Glucocorticoids are the final effectors of the HPA axis. In humans, they bind to the human glucocorticoid receptor-α, a cytosolic protein that belongs to the steroid/thyroid/retinoic acid nuclear receptor superfamily and is distributed throughout the brain and peripheral tissues. In the inactive state, the GRα is part of a hetero-oligomeric complex consisting of several molecules of heat shock proteins.[3] Ligand binding induces the dissociation of the receptor from the heat shock protein complex, dimerization, and translocation into the nucleus, where it binds to specific DNA sequences called glucocorticoid response elements in the regulatory regions of target genes. The GR, upon binding to the glucocorticoid response element, regulates expression through interaction with general transcription factors. Ligand activated hGRα can also regulate activation of target genes independent of glucocorticoid response element binding, by interacting with other transcription factors, including nuclear factor–κB and activating protein 1.[3,9] Glucocorticoids have metabolic, immune, cardiovascular, and behavioral effects, and play a prominent role in the regulation of HPA axis activity. Increased levels of glucocorticoids exert inhibitory effects on the HPA axis by acting at the level of extrahypothalamic centers, the hypothalamus and the pituitary.

REGULATION OF THE HPA AXIS
Neuronal Regulation of the HPA Axis

The neuronal regulation of the HPA axis is exerted by afferent projections from multiple brain regions to the PVN. The PVN receives information from the brain stem neurons, cell groups of the lamina terminalis, other hypothalamic nuclei, and the limbic system through intermediary neurons.[9] Catecholaminergic and nonaminergic neurons from the nucleus of the solitary tract and LC innervate the PVN and have stimulatory effects on the HPA axis. GLP1 and other neuropeptides (enkephalins, substance P, somatostatin) are also expressed in nucleus of the solitary tract neurons and they participate in the regulation of the HPA axis.[11,12] γ-Aminobutyric acid-ergic neurons of the dorsomedia hypothalamic nucleus and preoptic area and neurons of the arcuate nucleus (where feeding regulating neuropeptides are synthesized) also innervate the PVN, regulate CRH release, and play a central role in hypothalamic integration of stress and energy balance (**Fig. 1**).[9,13,14]

Immune Regulation of the HPA Axis

Complex interactions take place between the HPA axis and the immune system. Several inflammatory cytokines such as tumor necrosis factor (TNF)-α, interleukin

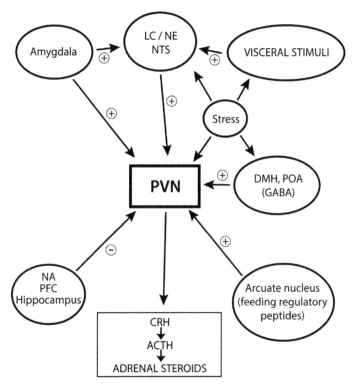

Fig. 1. Neural regulation of the hypothalamic-pituitary-adrenal (HPA) axis. Stress and visceral stimuli relay sensory information to the nucleus of the solitary tract (NTS) and locus caeruleus/norepinephrine (LC/NE) system and stimulate PVN CRH release. The paraventricular nucleus (PVN) receives information from the dorsomedial hypothalamic nucleus (DMH), preoptic area (POA) nuclei through γ-aminobutyric acid (GABA)-ergic neurons. The limbic system (amygdala, prefrontal cortex [PFC], hippocampus) regulate PVN function through intermediary neurons. The amygdala exerts stimulatory effects on the LC/NE and PVN. The PFC and hippocampus exert inhibitory effects on the PVN. Neurons of the arcuate nucleus, where "feeding" regulator peptides are synthesized, influence corticotropin-releasing hormone (CRH) and adrenocorticotropic hormone (ACTH) release and cortisol production.

(IL)-1, IL-6, and interferons (IFN-α/β), which mediate the innate immune response, have long been recognized as important modulators of HPA axis function.[1,15] They stimulate the classical pathway of CRH secretion and can act directly on the pituitary and adrenals. These cytokines are released early in the inflammatory process from a variety of cells, including macrophages, neurons, fibroblasts, and endothelial cells. Furthermore, T-cell cytokines such, as IFN-γ and IL-2, which mediate adaptive immunity and have antiviral effects, are released subsequently in the inflammatory cascade and activate the HPA axis.[15]

In addition to circulating cytokines, local production of cytokines has been demonstrated in the brain, the anterior pituitary, and the adrenals. Locally produced cytokines act in a paracrine manner to enhance and maintain HPA axis activity.[16] Other mediators released during the inflammatory process, like epidermal growth factor, transforming growth factor-β, arginine vasopressin, endothelin, and atrial natriuretic factor, may also participate in the regulation of the HPA axis directly or indirectly by stimulating the release of inflammatory cytokines.[1,2,17,18]

Cytokines acting synergistically promote the activation of the HPA axis and, hence, glucocorticoid secretion.[16] In turn, glucocorticoids further suppress cytokine synthesis and release, protecting the host from the effects of an overactive immune response.[16] Glucocorticoids under physiologic conditions exert permissive or proinflammatory effects. However, during acute illness, the increased concentrations of glucocorticoids are associated with well-known antiinflammatory effects[16,18,19]: Suppression of the immune activation of inflammatory cells, inhibition of cytokines (TNF-α, IL-1β, IL-6), and modulation of the immune response (shift of cellular T helper 1 cells [Th1] to humoral Th2 immune response). The immunomodulatory effect of glucocorticoids on target tissues is accomplished through modulation of the binding affinity to the GR, as well as through alteration of cytokine receptors in glucocorticoid-dependent cells.[17] Glucocorticoids can also alter the production by macrophages of other factors such as macrophage-migration inhibitory factor.[17] Macrophage-migration inhibitory factor is released in critical illness and has both inflammatory and antiinflammatory effects.[20]

HPA AXIS ACTIVITY IN HIV-INFECTED PATIENTS

HIV infection is characterized by an asymptomatic phase when peak viremia occurs but infection is controlled, followed by a symptomatic phase, associated with severe depletion of CD4+ T lymphocytes and a subsequent increase of viral load; these 2 phases constitute the 2 immunopathogenetic hallmarks of AIDS.[21] A principal factor preventing the progression of HIV infection to AIDS is a strong cell-mediated Th1 immune response to HIV.[22] In patients with HIV infection, an immune activation of all the components of the immune system occurs.[23] According to recent studies, HIV causes a profound disruption in the balance of the cytokine network between viral suppressors, such as type 1 IFNs and viral inducers, as for instance TNF-α, IL-1β, IL-6, and IL-15.[24] Progression of HIV infection was suggested as being associated with a reduction in Th1 and an increase in Th2 cytokine production.[22,25] Recently, it was shown that HIV infection can alter the TH17-Treg balance. HIV-infected patients demonstrate a rapid TH17 depletion and an expansion of Tregs associated with impaired gut mucosal immunity against pathogens.[26] Because glucocorticoids have immunomodulatory effects shifting Th1 to Th2 immunity, and also altering the balance of TH17/Treg,[27] the level of HPA axis activation in HIV patients could play a central role in the progression of the infection to manifestation of the disease.[16]

HPA axis activity has been examined extensively in AIDS and HIV-infected patients. Derangements of the HPA axis ranging from subclinical to frank adrenal insufficiency, depending on the stage of HIV infection, have been described.[28] On the other hand, in HIV-infected patients high levels of cortisol have been reportedly associated with either low or high levels of ACTH, suggesting a direct adrenal stimulation or stimulation of a local ACTH-like effect, respectively.[29]

Hypercortisolemia in HIV Infection

Many studies report increased basal ACTH/cortisol levels in a considerable number of symptomatic, as well as asymptomatic, HIV-infected patients, but a blunted ACTH and cortisol response to stress and CRH challenge, especially in advanced disease.[29,30] Several pathogenetic mechanisms have been proposed to explain the hypecortisolemia in HIV infection. This includes a shift of steroidogenesis from dehydroepiandrosterone (DHEA) and aldosterone to cortisol and the stimulation of hypothalamus, pituitary, and adrenal cortex by cytokines.[30,31] In patients with hypercortisolemia and increased ACTH levels, the stimulation of the HPA axis may result from the stimulatory effects of cytokines and viral proteins, like the HIV envelope protein gp-120 and the structural protein viral protein r (Vpr; **Fig. 2**). It has been shown that the protein gp-120 may increase serum levels of ACTH by stimulating CRH release.[32] Furthermore, Vpr can potentiate glucocorticoid receptor signaling, inducing glucocorticoid hypersensitivity by acting as a coactivator of the GR.[33,34] Glucocorticoid hypersensitivity mainly involves the immune system, manifested by reduction of Th1 immunity and IL-4 increase, but is also found in the brain, muscles, adipose tissue, and liver.[33]

Interestingly, the HPA axis is not influenced by glucocorticoid hypersensitivity, suggesting that appropriate negative feedback sensitivity is preserved.[35] However, whether cortisol effects are beneficial owing to their antiinflammatory properties or deleterious as a result of their immunosuppressive properties remains unclear. Recently, it was shown by Kino and colleagues[36] that glucocorticoids can suppress rather than stimulate the HIV-1 promoter, thus acting protectively to the host.

Another factor that could induce hypercortisolism in HIV-infected patients is the use of combined antiretroviral therapy (cART). Antiretroviral treatment usually includes therapeutic agents that have been shown to produce serious side effects involving immune function and metabolism. Therapeutic intervention with such agents could transform acute infection into a chronic inflammatory disease associated with increased levels of proinflammatory cytokines, such as TNF-α, IL-1, and IFN-γ. These cytokines stimulate the production of cortisol and, thereby, the shift of cytokine profile (Th1 to Th2) and the development of metabolic complications (insulin resistance [IR], dyslipidemia, lypodystrophy).[37] Furthermore, IL-1 and TNF-α can provoke an overexpression of the enzyme hydroxysteroid dehydrogenase type 1 (11-β HSD 1). This enzyme is found in many tissues, including liver and adipose tissue, and acts as a reductase, transforming inactive cortisone into active cortisol.[37]

HIV-infected patients demonstrate a characteristic pattern of high cortisol and low DHEA-S levels.[38] This pattern has been associated with a negative course of disease.[29,38] In fact, it has been shown that DHEA-S levels decline with the progression of the disease in parallel with the CD4 cell count.[38] The deterioration of the immune status in HIV-infected patients with high cortisol/DHEAS levels is apparently associated with a suppression of Th1 cytokines and an excessive production of cytokines by Th2 cells.[39] DHEAS supplementation seems to restore cytokine production and CD4 cell count in animal models.[40,41]

Glucocorticoid Resistance

A subset of AIDS patients develop adrenal insufficiency associated with hypercortisolemia and mildly elevated plasma ACTH. In these patients, the number of

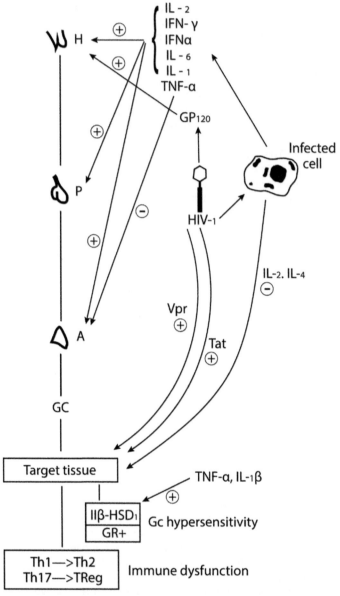

Fig. 2. Schematic representation of HIV-1 effects on the hypothalamic-pituitary-adrenal (HPA) axis. GP 120 induces cortisol secretion by direct stimulation of the HPA axis. HIV-1 accessory proteins Vpr and Tat stimulate glucocorticoid action (GR+) by increasing glucocorticoid sensitivity of target tissues. Inflammatory cytokines exert stimulatory effects on HPA activity at all 3 levels of the HPA axis, inducing cortisol secretion. Glucocorticoid hypersensitivity induces immune dysfunction. A subset of HIV-infected patients exhibits glucocorticoid resistance probably attributable to the suppressive effects of interleukin (IL)-2 and IL-4 on glucocorticoid action in target tissues. Interferon (IFN)-α and IL-1β cytokines have a stimulatory effect on hydroxysteroid dehydrogenase type 1 (11B HSD1) activity enhancing glucocorticoid hypersensitivity. Th, T helper cell; TNF, tumor necrosis factor; TReg, T regulatory cell.

glucocorticoid receptors is increased and the glucocorticoid affinity to its ligand is reduced, suggesting a partial glucocorticoid-resistant state.[42] This might be owing to HIV itself, to the HIV-1 Vpr gene, and/or to the simultaneous presence of Th1 (IL-2) and Th2 (IL-4) cytokines.[43] Another possible explanation for cortisol resistance is the altered proportion of the 2 isoforms of the GR, GRα, and GRβ, in favor of GRβ. The GRα isoform is the main mediator of glucocorticoid activity, whereas the GRβ isoform inhibits GRα action; thus, the increased intracellular proportion of GRβ leads to a decreased glucocorticoid effect.[44] It has been suggested that cortisol-resistant, HIV-infected patients have a prominent Th1 cytokine profile and, therefore, present a limited progression to AIDS.[16,43]

Adrenal Insufficiency in AIDS

Etiology

Adrenal insufficiency in HIV-infected patients is caused by infection, malignancy, hemorrhage, and necrosis at the level of pituitary or adrenals and by medication (**Table 1**). Before the introduction of cART, adrenal gland involvement was detected in 40% to 90% of cases and pituitary gland involvement in 30% of cases.[45] Glandular involvement has been, however, less common since the introduction of cART. The prevalence of adrenal insufficiency in the pre-cART era was reported to be 5% to 10%. In AIDS, the adrenal glands are the site of opportunistic infections caused by cytomegalovirus (CMV), *Mycobacterium avium*-intracellulare, *M tuberculosis*, *Cryptococcus neoformans*, *Toxoplasma gondii*, *Pneumocystis carinii*, and *Histoplasma capsulatum*.[46] In autopsy series, CMV adrenalitis was the most common infection, affecting up to 93% of untreated HIV-infected patients.[47]

CMV adrenalitis is characterized by the presence of intracytoplamic and intranuclear inclusion bodies in enlarged adrenal glands and leads to adrenal insufficiency when more than 80% of adrenal tissue has been destroyed.[29] Interestingly, in a small percentage of the autopsies performed in AIDS patients, CMV infection and necrosis was revealed in more than 80% of adrenal tissue.[48]

HIV infection of the adrenals, as well as adrenal neoplasms, such as Kaposi sarcoma and lymphoma, can impair adrenal function directly.[49] However, the use of cART has led to a reduction of the incidence of malignant infiltration of the adrenals.[50] On the other hand, protease inhibitors like ritonavir, used for advanced HIV infection, can interact with corticosteroids by inhibiting hepatic cytochrome P-450-CYP3A4 isoenzyme activity. The interaction of ritonavir with corticosteroids results in increased glucocorticoid levels, leading to a suppression of HPA activity. This is common in HIV patients on cART, who use inhaled corticosteroids for respiratory conditions.[51]

Medications commonly used in HIV patients, like ketoconazole, rifampin, and phenytoin, can interfere with adrenal function. Ketoconazole is used in the treatment of mycoses and directly inhibits steroidogenesis; rifampin and phenytoin increase

Table 1
Etiology of adrenal insufficiency

Primary Adrenal Insufficiency	Secondary/Tertiary Adrenal Insufficiency
Infection	Infection/infiltration
Malignancy: Kaposi sarcoma, non-Hodgkin lymphoma	Malignancy
Hemorrhage, fibrosis	Hemorrhage, fibrosis
Drugs: Ketoconazole, rifampin, phenytoin	Drugs: Corticosteroids, megestrol acetate

steroid clearance and may unmask adrenal insufficiency in patients with diminished adrenal reserve.[52] The progestational agent megestrol acetate used for the management of anorexia and muscle wasting in HIV-infected patients has an intrinsic glucocorticoid activity and can suppress the HPA axis. Abrupt discontinuation of the medication after prolonged administration can precipitate acute adrenal insufficiency.[53] Antiadrenal autoantibodies have been detected in HIV patients, probably linked to nonspecific B-cell activation or reflecting thymic dysfunction.[54]

Symptoms

Even though the classic picture of adrenal insufficiency is not always manifested, it should be suspected in HIV-infected patients when they present with unexplained fatigue, hypotension, anorexia, weight loss, and/or fever.[46] Laboratory abnormalities, such as hyponatremia, hyperkalemia, and hypoglycemia, should point to the correct diagnosis. However, hyperkalemia may not be manifested because of concurrent diarrhea or vomiting. Risk factors for the development of adrenal insufficiency in the pre-cART era were reported to be the CD4 count (<50 cells/mm^3), disease chronicity, and history of opportunistic infections.[46]

Diagnosis

Diagnosis of adrenal insufficiency in HIV-infected patients may be challenging, because HIV patients may have symptoms such as weight loss, nausea, and vomiting resembling those of adrenal insufficiency. Institution of appropriate therapy is imperative because treatment can be lifesaving. On the other hand, unnecessary treatment with cortisol can accelerate the progression of the disease and exacerbate underlying opportunistic infections. As in other forms of suspected adrenal insufficiency, tests evaluating adrenal function should be carried out. Baseline cortisol levels can be increased in HIV patients and, therefore, normal values are not reliable to exclude adrenal insufficiency. The most commonly used test for the diagnosis of adrenal insufficiency is the cosyntropin stimulation test. Serum cortisol is obtained before and 30 or 60 minutes after the administration of 250 μg of intravenous or intramuscular synthetic ACTH (cosyntropin). An abnormal response establishes the diagnosis of adrenal insufficiency, whereas a normal response (serum cortisol of >20 μg/mL) does not exclude the possibility of mild secondary adrenal insufficiency. Importantly, critically ill patients can achieve increased cortisol levels, which may complicate interpretation of the test results.[55]

Traditionally, the golden standard test for the diagnosis of adrenal insufficiency has been the insulin tolerance test. Insulin-induced hypoglycemia (serum glucose <40 mg/DL) stimulates the HPA axis and increases cortisol production. Serum glucose and cortisol are measured before and at 15, 30, 45, 60, 75, and 90 minutes after the IV administration of insulin. A normal response is considered a rise of serum cortisol of greater than 20 μg/mL. The insulin tolerance test is more sensitive than the cosyntropin stimulation test because it tests the integrity of the entire HPA axis. However, it might be dangerous and requires careful medical supervision. Another commonly used test for the assessment of the adrenal function is the overnight metyrapone test. Metyrapone inhibits the enzyme 11β hydroxylase, and consequently, the last step of cortisol production, and results in a compensatory rise in ACTH and 11-deoxycortisol. Normal response is an elevation of 11-deoxycortisol to more than 7 μg/dL with suppression of cortisol to less than 5 μg/dL. Although there are reports of precipitation of adrenal insufficiency, the test is considered safe with no serious side effects. The value of the CRH test in the diagnosis of adrenal insufficiency in HIV-infected patients is limited because acute or chronic inflammation can alter HPA axis activity.[46]

Imaging studies
In adrenal insufficiency imaging can reveal normal, large or small adrenal glands. Large adrenals are seen early in the course of tuberculosis, but they may become progressively small and fibrotic. Calcifications are suggestive of adrenal tuberculosis.[49] Large adrenals may also be associated with fungal disease.

Treatment
Patients with documented adrenal insufficiency should be treated with hydrocortisone. In patients with primary adrenal insufficiency, addition of mineralocorticoids (fludrocortisone acetate 0.05–0.2 mg/d) might be required. As in other forms of adrenal insufficiency, the dose of hydrocortisone ranges from 15 to 25 mg/d and should be increased up to 2 to 3 times in moderate stress states or during concomitant administration of other agents that increase cortisol clearance, such as rifampin or phenytoin.[56] In some cases, the agent that impairs adrenal function may be substituted or discontinued. Adrenal insufficiency induced by rifampin subsides after drug withdrawal.[28] During severe stress like major surgery, the dose of hydrocortisone should be increased up to 300 mg/d for 2 or 3 days.

Mineralocorticoids

Both hyperreninemic and hyporeninemic hypoaldosteronism have been described in HIV-infected patients.[57] Although frank hypoaldosteronism is rare, an impaired aldosterone response to ACTH has been described in these subjects.[58] Hyperkalemia and hyponatremia are commonly observed in AIDS patients. There are findings indicating that in HIV infection there is a significant abnormality in systemic K^+ equilibrium, in part related to an inhibited aldosterone response to hyperkalemia.[59] However, electrolyte abnormalities are most likely owing to drugs with amiloride-like properties.[60] Furthermore, it has been demonstrated in vitro that protease inhibitors can activate the renin-angiotensin system when incubated with murine adipocytes.[61] A few cases of primary hyperaldosteronism have also been reported in HIV patients.[62] However, the diagnosis of primary hyperaldosteronism in screened patients based on the aldosterone to renin ratio might be overestimated given the intrinsic renin-like properties of the HIV aspartic protease.[63]

IR AND LIPODYSTROPHY IN HIV INFECTION

The introduction of highly active antiretroviral therapy in the mid 1990s resulted in a dramatic reduction in HIV-associated mortality and transformed AIDS into a chronic disease. However, it also led to the emergence of a number of morbidities, central among them the AIDS-related insulin-resistance and lipodystrophy syndrome.

The most prominent feature of lipodystrophy in AIDS patients is a redistribution of adipose tissue with a loss of subcutaneous fat in the extremities and the face (lipoatrophy) and a gain in dorsocervical (buffalo hump) and visceral fat. Because the phenotype of lipodystrophy closely resembles the phenotype of chronic glucocorticoid excess, as seen in Cushing syndrome, the term pseudo-Cushing was initially used to describe this syndrome.[28,64]

The prevalence of IR in HIV-infected adults is estimated to be as high as 25% to 33%.[65] In a small percentage (5%–10%), IR progresses to overt diabetes. Reported prevalence of IR in HIV-infected children is 1.5% to 2% and is more closely linked with obesity.[66] Recently, it was demonstrated that HIV-infected children on antiretroviral therapy develop significant and persistent body composition changes and dyslipidemia but no overt abnormalities of glucose metabolism.[67]

Hypertriglyceridemia and increased free fatty acid concentrations were commonly observed in the pre-cART era in AIDS patients. This was related in part to increased visceral adipose tissue and to inflammation.[68] HIV infection per se can cause lipid abnormalities, including high triglyceride levels and low high-density lipoprotein cholesterol.[69] Similarities between AIDS-related IR and lipodystrophy syndrome and the metabolic syndrome in non–HIV-infected individuals have been reported.[70] The link between the 2 morbidities might be the chronic inflammation and the immune activation. However, the reports on the association between CD4+ T-cell count and the risk of metabolic syndrome are conflicting.[71,72] The results of a recent study have shown that the risk of the metabolic syndrome was decreased for each increasing level of CD4. According to the authors, the association of CD4+ count with the metabolic syndrome was explained by higher levels of inflammation among patients with more advanced HIV disease.[70]

Pathogenesis of IR and Lipodystrophy Syndrome

The pathogenesis of IR and lipodystrophy in HIV-infected patients is multifactorial. Pathogenetic factors might be related to the HIV infection itself, to the host, and to the treatment. Factors related to the infection and to the host include genetic predisposition, hormonal alterations, visceral obesity, aging, reduced physical activity, and chronic inflammation.[73–76]

The mechanisms underlying the AIDS-related IR and lipodystrophy syndrome are described in other articles in this issue. This section includes a review of the action of the viral proteins on glucocorticoid sensitivity and their potential contribution to the pathogenesis of IR and lipodystrophy (**Fig. 3**).

Viral proteins Vpr and Tat

The HIV1 accessory proteins like Vpr and Tat have central roles in mediating viral replication and host cell function. Vpr is a 96-amino acid virion associated accessory protein that acts as a modulator of the host cell activity. Vpr binds directly to the GR, via its conserved LXXLL motif sequence located at amino acids 64–68. This sequence is found in various coactivator molecules like P300/CREB-binding protein and is considered essential in nuclear receptor and coactivator molecule interaction.[77] Thus, Vpr potentiates the action of the GR and consequently increases tissue sensitivity to glucocorticoids by acting as a nuclear receptor coactivator.[34] Vpr may also reduce tissue sensitivity to insulin, not only via hypersensitivity to glucocorticoids, but also by modulating insulin transcriptional activity. It has been demonstrated that insulin exerts its function by regulating the activity of several FOXO proteins. These proteins, in the absence of insulin, activate the transcription rate of their target genes, thereby promoting gluconeogenesis and glycolysis. In the presence of insulin, FOXO proteins bind to the protein 14-3-3 and lose their transcriptional activity. Vpr inhibits the negative effect of insulin on FOXO proteins through interaction with the 14-3-3 protein and, thereby, induces IR.[34,78]

Another HIV-1 accessory protein, Tat, is considered the most potent transactivator protein of the HIV-1 LTR promoter. Tat may enhance tissue glucocorticoid sensitivity by interaction with coactivator molecules p300/CREB-binding protein and p160 and through accumulation of the positive transcription elongation factor-b on glucocorticoid responsive promoters.[34] Vpr and Tat could also contribute to viral proliferation indirectly by suppressing the host immune system activity, possibly via glucocorticoid hypersensitivity.[34]

HIV infection also contributes to adipocyte cell apoptosis and IR by inhibiting peroxisome proliferator activated (PPAR)-γ activity. In fact, it has been demonstrated that PPAR-γ expression is lower in HIV-infected patients with lipodystrophy and without treatment compared with PPAR-γ expression in healthy controls.[79] Interestingly,

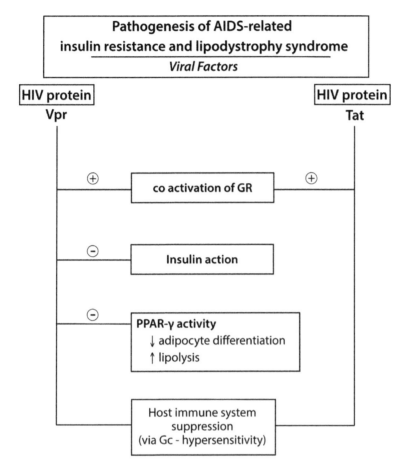

Fig. 3. Pathogenesis of AIDS-related insulin resistance (IR) and lipodystrophy syndrome: Viral factors. Vpr and Tat accessory HIV-1 proteins coactivate GR and potentially induce glucocorticoid (GC) hypersensitivity. In addition, Vpr may inhibit insulin action and peroxisome proliferator-activated receptor γ (PPAR-γ) activity, inducing IR and lipoatrophy. Vpr and Tat may induce host immune system suppression via GC hypersensitivity.

Vpr can be replicated during protease inhibitor therapy and is sequestered in tissue reservoirs (adipose tissue, liver) in treated patients.[80] Recently, in vivo studies in mouse models showed that Vpr arriving in adipocytes or hepatocytes can alter their transcriptional regulation and function by disrupting PPAR/GR coregulation: Vpr induces PPAR corepression, GR coactivation, and produces adipose dysfunction (blocked preadipocyte differentiation, increased lipolisis) and hepatosteatosis.[81]

Besides the effects of HIV infection itself, the immune activation and inflammation related to other viral infections, such as hepatitis C and CMV, is an additional risk factor for IR and diabetes in HIV-infected patients. HIV/hepatitis C coinfection in patients on cART has been associated with greater IR and higher endothelial dysfunction.[82]

FUTURE CONSIDERATIONS

The development of novel therapeutic approaches for the IR and lipodystrophy syndrome in HIV patients relies on the better comprehension and definition of the mechanisms (genetic, viral, drug interferences) responsible for the manifestation of the syndrome. The comprehension of mechanisms underlying the action of Vpr on PPARs and GR could lead to treatments with Vpr inhibitors, PPAR agonists, and compounds that antagonize the action of the GR.[81]

SUMMARY

HPA axis alterations in HIV infection comprise a spectrum of biochemical and clinical disturbances. Hypercortisolemia and cortisol hypersensitivity are prominent features of HIV infection and are owing to the stimulation of the HPA axis by proinflammatory cytokines (also stimulated by cART), and to the direct effects of HIV proteins. Adrenal insufficiency ranges from subclinical to frank, depending on the stage of HIV infection, and is caused by infection, malignancy, and necrosis at the level of pituitary and the adrenals. Several medications used to treat comorbidities in HIV-infected patients may suppress the HPA axis and unmask adrenal insufficiency in patients with a decreased adrenal reserve. In recent years, the introduction of novel therapies has transformed AIDS from a fatal disease into a chronic condition. The chronicity of the disease, cART, comorbidities, and lifestyle have led to the emergence of the AIDS-related IR and lipodystrophy syndrome. Ongoing research into the molecular mechanisms underlying this syndrome could lead to the development of targeted treatment options.

REFERENCES

1. Chrousos GP. The hypothalamic-pituitary-adrenal axis and immune-mediated inflammation. N Engl J Med 1995;332:1351–62.
2. Chrousos GP, Gold PW. The concepts of stress and stress system disorders. Overview of physical and behavioral homeostasis. JAMA 1992;267:1244–52.
3. Chrousos GP, Kino T, Charmandari E. Evaluation of the hypothalamic-pituitary-adrenal axis function in childhood and adolescence. Neuroimmunomodulation 2009;16:272–83.
4. Chatterton RT. The role of stress in female reproduction: animal and human considerations. Int J Fertil 1990;35:8–13.
5. Valentino RJ, Foote SL, Aston-Jones G. Corticotropin-releasing factor activates noradrenergic neurons of the locus coeruleus. Brain Res 1983;270:363–7.
6. Perrin MH, Vale WW. Corticotropin releasing factor receptors and their ligand family. Ann N Y Acad Sci 1999;885:312–28.
7. Van Pett K, Viau V, Bittencourt JC, et al. Distribution of mRNAs encoding CRF receptors in brain and pituitary of rat and mouse. J Comp Neurol 2000;428: 191–212.
8. Perrin M, Donaldson C, Chen R, et al. Identification of a second corticotropin-releasing factor receptor gene and characterization of a cDNA expressed in heart. Proc Natl Acad Sci U S A 1995;92:2969–73.
9. Smith SM, Vale WW. The role of the hypothalamic-pituitary-adrenal axis in neuro-endocrine responses to stress. Dialogues Clin Neurosci 2006;8:383–95.
10. Cone RD, Lu D, Koppula S, et al. The melanocortin receptors: agonists, antagonists, and the hormonal control of pigmentation. Recent Prog Horm Res 1996; 51:287–317 [discussion: 318].
11. Rinaman L. Interoceptive stress activates glucagon-like peptide-1 neurons that project to the hypothalamus. Am J Physiol 1999;277:R582–90.
12. Sawchenko PE, Arias C, Bittencourt JC. Inhibin beta, somatostatin, and enkephalin immunoreactivities coexist in caudal medullary neurons that project to the paraventricular nucleus of the hypothalamus. J Comp Neurol 1990;291:269–80.

13. Roland BL, Sawchenko PE. Local origins of some GABAergic projections to the paraventricular and supraoptic nuclei of the hypothalamus in the rat. J Comp Neurol 1993;332:123–43.

14. Mastorakos G, Zapanti E. The hypothalamic-pituitary-adrenal axis in the neuro-endocrine regulation of food intake and obesity: the role of corticotropin releasing hormone. Nutr Neurosci 2004;7:271–80.

15. Mastorakos G, Magiakou MA, Chrousos GP. Effects of the immune/inflammatory reaction on the hypothalamic-pituitary-adrenal axis. Ann N Y Acad Sci 1995;771: 438–48.

16. Silverman MN, Pearce BD, Biron CA, et al. Immune modulation of the hypothalamic-pituitary-adrenal (HPA) axis during viral infection. Viral Immunol 2005;18:41–78.

17. Arafah BM. Hypothalamic pituitary adrenal function during critical illness: limitations of current assessment methods. J Clin Endocrinol Metab 2006;91: 3725–45.

18. Vermes I, Beishuizen A, Hampsink RM, et al. Dissociation of plasma adrenocorticotropin and cortisol levels in critically ill patients: possible role of endothelin and atrial natriuretic hormone. J Clin Endocrinol Metab 1995;80:1238–42.

19. Charmandari E, Kino T, Chrousos GP. Glucocorticoids and their actions: an introduction. Ann N Y Acad Sci 2004;1024:1–8.

20. Fingerle-Rowson G, Koch P, Bikoff R, et al. Regulation of macrophage migration inhibitory factor expression by glucocorticoids in vivo. Am J Pathol 2003;162: 47–56.

21. Tasca KI, Calvi SA, Souza Ldo R. Immunovirological parameters and cytokines in HIV infection. Rev Soc Bras Med Trop 2012;45:663–9.

22. Clerici M, Fusi ML, Ruzzante S, et al. Type 1 and type 2 cytokines in HIV infection – a possible role in apoptosis and disease progression. Ann Med 1997;29:185–8.

23. Catalfamo M, Le Saout C, Lane HC. The role of cytokines in the pathogenesis and treatment of HIV infection. Cytokine Growth Factor Rev 2012;23:207–14.

24. Keating SM, Jacobs ES, Norris PJ. Soluble mediators of inflammation in HIV and their implications for therapeutics and vaccine development. Cytokine Growth Factor Rev 2012;23:193–206.

25. Reuter MA, Pombo C, Betts MR. Cytokine production and dysregulation in HIV pathogenesis: lessons for development of therapeutics and vaccines. Cytokine Growth Factor Rev 2012;23:181–91.

26. Ancuta P, Monteiro P, Sekaly RP. Th17 lineage commitment and HIV-1 pathogenesis. Curr Opin HIV AIDS 2010;5:158–65.

27. Liu LL, Qin Y, Cai JF, et al. Th17/Treg imbalance in adult patients with minimal change nephrotic syndrome. Clin Immunol 2011;139:314–20.

28. Zapanti E, Terzidis K, Chrousos G. Dysfunction of the hypothalamic-pituitary-adrenal axis in HIV infection and disease. Hormones (Athens) 2008;7:205–16.

29. Mayo J, Collazos J, Martinez E, et al. Adrenal function in the human immunodeficiency virus-infected patient. Arch Intern Med 2002;162:1095–8.

30. Azar ST, Melby JC. Hypothalamic-pituitary-adrenal function in non-AIDS patients with advanced HIV infection. Am J Med Sci 1993;305:321–5.

31. Christeff N, Gherbi N, Mammes O, et al. Serum cortisol and DHEA concentrations during HIV infection. Psychoneuroendocrinology 1997;22(Suppl 1):S11–8.

32. Costa A, Nappi RE, Polatti F, et al. Stimulating effect of HIV-1 coat protein gp120 on corticotropin-releasing hormone and arginine vasopressin in the rat hypothalamus: involvement of nitric oxide. Exp Neurol 2000;166:376–84.

33. Kino T, Chrousos GP. Glucocorticoid and mineralocorticoid resistance/hypersensitivity syndromes. J Endocrinol 2001;169:437–45.

34. Kino T, Chrousos GP. Human immunodeficiency virus type-1 accessory protein Vpr: a causative agent of the AIDS-related insulin resistance/lipodystrophy syndrome? Ann N Y Acad Sci 2004;1024:153–67.

35. Yanovski JA, Miller KD, Kino T, et al. Endocrine and metabolic evaluation of human immunodeficiency virus-infected patients with evidence of protease inhibitor-associated lipodystrophy. J Clin Endocrinol Metab 1999;84:1925–31.

36. Kino T, Gragerov A, Slobodskaya O, et al. Human immunodeficiency virus type 1 (HIV-1) accessory protein Vpr induces transcription of the HIV-1 and glucocorticoid-responsive promoters by binding directly to p300/CBP coactivators. J Virol 2002;76:9724–34.

37. Norbiato G. Endocrine, metabolic, and immunologic components of HIV infection. Ann N Y Acad Sci 2012;1262:51–5.

38. Wisniewski TL, Hilton CW, Morse EV, et al. The relationship of serum DHEA-S and cortisol levels to measures of immune function in human immunodeficiency virus-related illness. Am J Med Sci 1993;305:79–83.

39. Clerici M, Trabattoni D, Piconi S, et al. A possible role for the cortisol/anticortisols imbalance in the progression of human immunodeficiency virus. Psychoneuroendocrinology 1997;22(Suppl 1):S27–31.

40. Maingat FG, Polyak MJ, Paul AM. Neurosteroid-mediated regulation of brain innate immunity in HIV/AIDS: DHEA-S suppresses neurovirulence. FASEB J 2013;27:725–37.

41. Araneo BA, Woods ML 2nd, Daynes RA. Reversal of the immunosenescent phenotype by dehydroepiandrosterone: hormone treatment provides an adjuvant effect on the immunization of aged mice with recombinant hepatitis B surface antigen. J Infect Dis 1993;167:830–40.

42. Norbiato G, Bevilacqua M, Vago T, et al. Cortisol resistance in acquired immunodeficiency syndrome. J Clin Endocrinol Metab 1992;74:608–13.

43. Norbiato G, Bevilacqua M, Vago T, et al. Glucocorticoid resistance and the immune function in the immunodeficiency syndrome. Ann N Y Acad Sci 1998;840:835–47.

44. Charmandari E, Chrousos GP, Ichijo T, et al. The human glucocorticoid receptor (hGR) beta isoform suppresses the transcriptional activity of hGRalpha by interfering with formation of active coactivator complexes. Mol Endocrinol 2005;19:52–64.

45. Tapper ML, Rotterdam HZ, Lerner CW, et al. Adrenal necrosis in the acquired immunodeficiency syndrome. Ann Intern Med 1984;100:239–41.

46. Eledrisi MS, Verghese AC. Adrenal insufficiency in HIV infection: a review and recommendations. Am J Med Sci 2001;321:137–44.

47. Hoshino Y, Nagata Y, Gatanaga H, et al. Cytomegalovirus (CMV) retinitis and CMV antigenemia as a clue to impaired adrenocortical function in patients with AIDS. AIDS 1997;11:1719–24.

48. McKenzie R, Travis WD, Dolan SA, et al. The causes of death in patients with human immunodeficiency virus infection: a clinical and pathologic study with emphasis on the role of pulmonary diseases. Medicine (Baltimore) 1991;70:326–43.

49. Freda PU, Bilezikian JP. The hypothalamus-pituitary-adrenal axis in HIV disease. AIDS Read 1999;9:43–50.

50. George MM, Bhangoo A. Human immune deficiency virus (HIV) infection and the hypothalamic pituitary adrenal axis. Rev Endocr Metab Disord 2013;14:105–12.

51. Foisy MM, Yakiwchuk EM, Chiu I, et al. Adrenal suppression and Cushing's syndrome secondary to an interaction between ritonavir and fluticasone: a review of the literature. HIV Med 2008;9:389–96.
52. Putignano P, Kaltsas GA, Satta MA, et al. The effects of anti-convulsant drugs on adrenal function. Horm Metab Res 1998;30:389–97.
53. Leinung MC, Liporace R, Miller CH. Induction of adrenal suppression by megestrol acetate in patients with AIDS. Ann Intern Med 1995;122:843–5.
54. Salim YS, Faber V, Wiik A, et al. Anti-corticosteroid antibodies in AIDS patients. APMIS 1988;96:889–94.
55. Prasanthai V, Sunthornyothin S, Phowthongkum P, et al. Prevalence of adrenal insufficiency in critically ill patients with AIDS. J Med Assoc Thai 2007;90: 1768–74.
56. Kyriazopoulou V, Parparousi O, Vagenakis AG. Rifampicin-induced adrenal crisis in addisonian patients receiving corticosteroid replacement therapy. J Clin Endocrinol Metab 1984;59:1204–6.
57. Seney FD Jr, Burns DK, Silva FG. Acquired immunodeficiency syndrome and the kidney. Am J Kidney Dis 1990;16:1–13.
58. Findling JW, Buggy BP, Gilson IH, et al. Longitudinal evaluation of adrenocortical function in patients infected with the human immunodeficiency virus. J Clin Endocrinol Metab 1994;79:1091–6.
59. Caramelo C, Bello E, Ruiz E, et al. Hyperkalemia in patients infected with the human immunodeficiency virus: involvement of a systemic mechanism. Kidney Int 1999;56:198–205.
60. Greenberg S, Reiser IW, Chou SY, et al. Trimethoprim-sulfamethoxazole induces reversible hyperkalemia. Ann Intern Med 1993;119:291–5.
61. Boccara F, Auclair M, Cohen A, et al. HIV protease inhibitors activate the adipocyte renin angiotensin system. Antivir Ther 2010;15:363–75.
62. Stricker RB, Goldberg DA, Hu C, et al. A syndrome resembling primary aldosteronism (Conn syndrome) in untreated HIV disease. AIDS 1999;13:1791–2.
63. Fradley M, Liu J, Atta MG. Primary aldosteronism with HIV infection: important considerations when using the aldosterone:renin ratio to screen this unique population. Am J Ther 2005;12:368–74.
64. Singhania R, Kotler DP. Lipodystrophy in HIV patients: its challenges and management approaches. HIV AIDS (Auckl) 2011;3:135–43.
65. Domingos H, Cunha RV, Paniago AM, et al. Metabolic effects associated to the highly active antiretroviral therapy (HAART) in AIDS patients. Braz J Infect Dis 2009;13:130–6.
66. Geffner ME, Patel K, Miller TL, et al. Factors associated with insulin resistance among children and adolescents perinatally infected with HIV-1 in the pediatric HIV/AIDS cohort study. Horm Res Paediatr 2011;76:386–91.
67. Spoulou V, Kanaka-Gantenbein C, Bathrellou I, et al. Monitoring of lipodystrophic and metabolic abnormalities in HIV-1 infected children on antiretroviral therapy. Hormones (Athens) 2011;10:149–55.
68. Florescu D, Kotler DP. Insulin resistance, glucose intolerance and diabetes mellitus in HIV-infected patients. Antivir Ther 2007;12:149–62.
69. Grunfeld C, Pang M, Doerrler W, et al. Lipids, lipoproteins, triglyceride clearance, and cytokines in human immunodeficiency virus infection and the acquired immunodeficiency syndrome. J Clin Endocrinol Metab 1992;74:1045–52.
70. Krishnan S, Schouten JT, Atkinson B, et al. Metabolic syndrome before and after initiation of antiretroviral therapy in treatment-naive HIV-infected individuals. J Acquir Immune Defic Syndr 2012;61:381–9.

71. Mondy K, Overton ET, Grubb J, et al. Metabolic syndrome in HIV-infected patients from an urban, midwestern US outpatient population. Clin Infect Dis 2007;44:726–34.
72. Bonfanti P, De Socio GL, Marconi P, et al. Is metabolic syndrome associated to HIV infection per se? Results from the HERMES study. Curr HIV Res 2010;8: 165–71.
73. Mulligan K, Grunfeld C, Tai VW, et al. Hyperlipidemia and insulin resistance are induced by protease inhibitors independent of changes in body composition in patients with HIV infection. J Acquir Immune Defic Syndr 2000;23:35–43.
74. Murata H, Hruz PW, Mueckler M. The mechanism of insulin resistance caused by HIV protease inhibitor therapy. J Biol Chem 2000;275:20251–4.
75. Noor MA, Lo JC, Mulligan K, et al. Metabolic effects of indinavir in healthy HIV-seronegative men. AIDS 2001;15:F11–8.
76. Grunfeld C, Rimland D, Gibert CL, et al. Association of upper trunk and visceral adipose tissue volume with insulin resistance in control and HIV-infected subjects in the FRAM study. J Acquir Immune Defic Syndr 2007;46:283–90.
77. Heery DM, Kalkhoven E, Hoare S, et al. A signature motif in transcriptional co-activators mediates binding to nuclear receptors. Nature 1997;387:733–6.
78. Kino T, De Martino MU, Charmandari E, et al. HIV-1 accessory protein Vpr inhibits the effect of insulin on the Foxo subfamily of forkhead transcription factors by interfering with their binding to 14-3-3 proteins: potential clinical implications regarding the insulin resistance of HIV-1-infected patients. Diabetes 2005;54: 23–31.
79. Giralt M, Domingo P, Villarroya F. HIV-1 infection and the PPARgamma-dependent control of adipose tissue physiology. PPAR Res 2009;2009:607902.
80. Poon B, Grovit-Ferbas K, Stewart SA, et al. Cell cycle arrest by Vpr in HIV-1 virions and insensitivity to antiretroviral agents. Science 1998;281:266–9.
81. Agarwal N, Iyer D, Patel SG, et al. HIV-1 Vpr induces adipose dysfunction in vivo through reciprocal effects on PPAR/GR co-regulation. Sci Transl Med 2013;5: 213ra164.
82. de Larranaga GF, Wingeyer SD, Puga LM, et al. Relationship between hepatitis C virus (HCV) and insulin resistance, endothelial perturbation, and platelet activation in HIV-HCV-coinfected patients under highly active antiretroviral treatment. Eur J Clin Microbiol Infect Dis 2006;25:98–103.

Endocrinopathies in Children Infected with Human Immunodeficiency Virus

Lindsey A. Loomba-Albrecht, MD[a,*], Thea Bregman, MD[b], Caroline J. Chantry, MD[c]

KEYWORDS

- HIV • Endocrinopathy • Children • Lipodystrophy • Dyslipidemia • Insulin resistance
- Thyroid • Adrenal

KEY POINTS

- Direct viral effects, chronic inflammation, and antiretroviral therapy may all lead to endocrine dysfunction in children infected with human immunodeficiency virus (HIV).
- Adrenal insufficiency is extremely rare in children with HIV but a high index of suspicion is indicated given the potential morbidity and mortality.
- Growth failure is often multifactorial and may be associated with hormonal abnormalities; it is best addressed with a multidisciplinary team.
- Children infected with HIV have an increased likelihood of lipodystrophy, dyslipidemia, and insulin resistance.
- Bone mineral density is often reduced in pediatric patients with HIV.

INTRODUCTION

There were 3.3 million children living with HIV globally and 260,000 new pediatric infections in 2012,[1] more than 90% of whom acquired the infection perinatally. Combined antiretroviral therapy (cART), introduced in 1996, has resulted in dramatic reductions in HIV-related mortality in both children and adults. Prenatally infected infants are now surviving into adulthood and the care of the patient with HIV has transitioned from treatment of life-threatening illness to management of chronic disease. Although mortality has decreased, access to antiretroviral therapy (ART) among

Conflicts of interest or financial interests: None.
[a] Section of Endocrinology, Department of Pediatrics, University of California Davis Medical Center, 2516 Stockton Boulevard, Suite 384, Sacramento, CA 95817-2208, USA; [b] Department of Pediatrics, University of California Davis Medical Center, 2516 Stockton Boulevard, Suite 216, Sacramento, CA 95817, USA; [c] Department of Pediatrics, University of California Davis Medical Center, 2516 Stockton Boulevard, Suite 334, Sacramento, CA 95817-2208, USA
* Corresponding author.
E-mail address: lindsey.albrecht@ucdmc.ucdavis.edu

Endocrinol Metab Clin N Am 43 (2014) 807–828
http://dx.doi.org/10.1016/j.ecl.2014.06.001
0889-8529/14/$ – see front matter Published by Elsevier Inc.

children is problematic in some regions, and complications from acquired immunodeficiency syndrome (AIDS) are still a reality for many. Among children receiving ART, complications from HIV infection and/or its treatment(s) can still affect many aspects of health, including endocrine function. Pediatric patients may be at particular risk for these complications given what is often lifelong exposure to HIV and cART. Children additionally undergo unique developmental changes (such as puberty) that give them a unique set of potential complications compared with adults. The proper diagnosis of endocrine dysfunction requires a high index of suspicion, because signs and symptoms of hormone abnormalities can be difficult to recognize.

ADRENAL DYSFUNCTION

The most common endocrine effect of HIV infection is dysregulation of the hypothalamic-pituitary-adrenal (HPA) axis.[2–4] This dysregulation, resulting occasionally in overt adrenal insufficiency, occurs by direct glandular invasion of infectious organisms or infiltrate, inflammation associated with chronic viral infection, or drug effects. As with all cases of adrenal insufficiency, a high degree of suspicion is required to avoid morbidity and mortality related to unrecognized adrenal insufficiency or crisis. A challenge arises for treating physicians given that signs and symptoms of adrenal insufficiency (eg, fatigue, weakness, weight loss, and nausea) may be indistinguishable from the signs of HIV infection.[5,6] Hyponatremia, resulting from mineralocorticoid deficiency associated with primary adrenal disease, should raise suspicion for underlying adrenal insufficiency.

Direct Invasion

Direct invasion of the adrenal gland by cytomegalovirus (CMV) in untreated adults is common and is associated with a wide range of histologic findings, from asymptomatic adrenalitis to adrenal necrosis. Other organisms that infect the adrenal gland include *Cryptococcus*, *Nocardia*, *Mycobacterium avium-intracellulare*, *Mycobacterium tuberculosis*, and *Histoplasma capsulatum*.[4] CMV infection causing clinically recognized adrenal insufficiency seems to be extremely rare in children infected with HIV.[7] Malignant infiltrate by Kaposi sarcoma and lymphoma are reported in adults infected with HIV but not to our knowledge in children. Secondary adrenal insufficiency caused by hypothalamic or pituitary destruction arising from opportunistic central nervous system (CNS) infection is a theoretic possibility but also seems to be very rare.

Medication Effects

The antiretroviral agents used for initial therapy are not commonly associated with HPA axis dysregulation in children.[8] However, the protease inhibitor (PI) ritonavir is a potent inhibitor of the hepatic cytochrome P450-CYP3A4 isozyme and may thus increase the levels of certain concomitantly administered drugs, including glucocorticoids. Ritonavir is used as a pharmacokinetic enhancer of other PIs in more advanced disease. This interaction decreases pill burden and increases dosing intervals, improving adherence to ART. Ritonavir's use in children infected with HIV taking inhaled glucocorticoids for pulmonary disease may cause severe cortisol excess (iatrogenic Cushing syndrome) and adrenal insufficiency with the discontinuation of the inhaled glucocorticoid (**Table 1**).[9–11] Prescribers should be aware of this interaction, particularly given the widespread use of inhaled glucocorticoids in the pediatric population.

Ketoconazole was widely used in the past to treat candidal infection in children with HIV and AIDS. Its use is now limited because of the recognition of potential life-threatening hepatotoxicity. Ketoconazole inhibits adrenal steroidogenesis by

Table 1
Endocrinopathies associated with ART

Drug Category	Endocrine Effects	Mechanism	Comments
NRTIs			
Stavudine	Lipodystrophy	Mitochondrial toxicity	Also direct action by HIV
	Lipoatrophy	—	—
Tenofovir	Possible growth impairment with prenatal exposure	—	—
	Reduced bone mineral density	Phosphate wasting caused by proximal tubule toxicity	—
NNRTIs			
Efavirenz	Low vitamin D levels	—	—
PIs			
	Dyslipidemia	Inhibition of LDLRP	Other drug classes also implicated; atazanavir has more favorable profile
	Lipodystrophy	Homology between HIV-1 protease and cytoplasmic retinoic acid binding protein 1	—
	Insulin resistance	Inhibition of GLUT4	Data conflicting; other drug classes implicated
	Reduced bone mineral density, especially boosted regimens	—	Data conflicting
Ritonavir	Cortisol excess and adrenal insufficiency with concomitantly administered glucocorticoids	Inhibitor of P450-CPY3A4	—

Abbreviations: LDLRP, lipoprotein receptor-related protein; NNRTI, non-nucleoside reverse transcriptase inhibitor.

inhibiting 11-hydroxylase activity, resulting in such a significant reduction in circulating cortisol levels that ketoconazole is used therapeutically for patients with Cushing syndrome. Fluconazole, now more widely used, inhibits steroidogenesis in vitro and may also put patients at increased risk for HPA axis dysfunction.[12]

Rifampin, used to treat children with HIV and tuberculosis, increases cortisol metabolism and can thereby induce adrenal insufficiency.[13] Megesterol acetate, used for anorexia and wasting associated with HIV infection, has glucocorticoidlike properties and may cause Cushing syndrome. Abrupt withdrawal can precipitate adrenal insufficiency.

Prophylactic treatment of exposed, uninfected infants with a ritonavir-boosted PI regimen was associated with biochemical evidence of adrenal dysfunction in 14% (increased 17-hydroxyprogesterone concentrations); dehydroepiandrosterone-sulfate concentrations were also increased in some subjects who were additionally exposed in utero. Term infants were asymptomatic, but 3 premature infants experienced life-threatening symptoms of adrenal insufficiency.[14]

Inflammatory Effects

Increased cortisol levels occur as part of the stress response to illness. Cytokines, released in response to viral infection, as well as direct effect of viral proteins, may cause alterations in the HPA axis. Proinflammatory cytokines, including interleukin (IL)-1, IL-6, tumor necrosis factor (TNF) alpha, and type 1 interferons (IFNα and IFNβ) activate the HPA axis at each level, increasing glucocorticoid production. Increased cortisol levels in turn dampen the immune response, helping to protect the host from toxicity related to an overly robust immune response. Adults infected with HIV, including those with AIDS, have higher mean morning cortisol levels than normal controls.[15,16] However, patients with advanced disease may also develop cortisol resistance, leading to clinical signs of adrenal insufficiency in the face of normal or increased basal cortisol levels. Symptomatic and advanced disease in adults can frequently result in diminished response to corticotropin-releasing hormone, adrenocorticotropic hormone (ACTH) deficiency, or primary adrenal insufficiency[4,15,17]; data in children are scarce.

Evaluation and Management

Studies have shown normal cortisol response to ACTH or glucagon in nearly all children with HIV, even in those with low morning cortisol levels.[18–20] These and other data are reassuring for the rarity of overt adrenal insufficiency in children infected with HIV, particularly in the modern era of cART. However, extreme caution is required because unrecognized adrenal insufficiency may result in increased morbidity and mortality. The possibility of primary adrenal insufficiency should be considered in patients with advanced disease or symptoms including refractory hypotension or critical illness and is typically evaluated by a morning cortisol level and, if abnormal, stimulation testing of the HPA axis. Mineralocorticoid function can be assessed by obtaining electrolytes, aldosterone, and plasma renin activity levels.

Treatment of adrenal insufficiency in children consists of physiologic replacement doses of hydrocortisone (10–15 mg/m^2/d) divided 3 times daily. Higher stress doses may be temporarily required in some instances, such as acute illness or surgery. Mineralocorticoid replacement, when indicated, is given as oral fludrocortisone.

GROWTH

In childhood, disruption of linear growth may provide the first clue of underlying disease. Monitoring of growth is critical in HIV infection: growth velocity predicts survival, regardless of viral load and CD4 count in symptomatic children with HIV.[21] Despite advances in therapy, poor growth remains a common finding among children with HIV. Early initiation of therapy is associated with more rapid, but not more complete, growth recovery.[22]

Prenatal and Infant Growth

Birth weight is usually normal in perinatally acquired HIV infection, consistent with the typical timing of transmission late in gestation or at delivery. Infants infected with HIV with birth weights less than 2400 g have an earlier onset of severe conditions than children with higher birth weights.[23] Infants infected with HIV have a reduced linear growth rate, decreased weight gain, and decreased head circumference compared with uninfected infants; this is usually apparent by 3 months of age and is progressive over time.[24,25] Infants with severe disease often show growth failure before the development of severe immune dysfunction. Uninfected infants born to mothers with HIV also have higher rates of poor postnatal growth than the normal population; multiple caregivers is one reported association[26]; prenatal antiretroviral drug exposure to tenofovir, a nucleoside reverse transcriptase inhibitor (NRTI), has more recently been implicated.[27]

Childhood

Failure to thrive may progress to complete growth failure and wasting syndrome in children with AIDS. Growth failure was a feature of the earliest reported pediatric AIDS cases and wasting syndrome is recognized as an AIDS-defining illness in childhood. The cause of growth failure in AIDS is likely multifactorial, including effects of chronic illness, malnutrition, enteropathy, increased tissue catabolism, and pubertal delay.[28]

Before the use of highly active ART (HAART), children with hemophilia and HIV were noted to have reduced adult heights compared with controls.[28] With the availability of HAART, most (but not all) studies show continued reduction in final adult height.[29–33] Kessler and colleagues[34] recently showed that the final adult height of patients infected with HIV was significantly shorter than that of controls (with a standard deviation [SD] score of -0.78 ± 1.1) despite normal timing and magnitude of the pubertal growth spurt. This finding may indicate that the greatest negative effect of HIV on height occurs before puberty. Final height was additionally seen to be positively correlated with CD4 count ($P = .019$), confirming prior reports and underscoring the importance of good immunologic control in maximizing final adult height.

Endocrine Abnormalities

Hormonal abnormalities, including deficiencies of growth hormone (GH), thyroid hormones, and pubertal hormones, may partially contribute to the growth impairment observed in pediatric HIV disease. Thyroid abnormalities are discussed further later. GH is a pulsatile hormone that exerts its effect on linear growth primarily through insulinlike growth factor (IGF) 1. Measurement of IGF-1 and its binding protein IGFBP-3 are typically used as proxy measurements of GH activity. However, these levels may be difficult to interpret given the reduction of IGF-1 that occurs with malnutrition and the enhanced proteolysis of IGFBP-3 (leading to low levels of IGFBP-3) in pediatric patients with HIV.[35,36]

Studies of the GH–IGF-1 axis in children infected with HIV have shown lower IGF-1 and IGFBP-3 levels in children infected with HIV with impaired growth.[36,37] However, basal and stimulated GH levels are normal in most children with HIV,[20,38,39] and frank GH deficiency as a cause of growth failure is only rarely reported.[40,41] IGF-1 levels increase on initiation or change in ART, but these changes are associated with improved muscle mass and not increased linear growth.[42]

GH resistance may underlie some of the growth impairment seen in children with HIV. Geffner and colleagues[43] reported resistance to IGF-1 and GH in vitro in erythroid progenitor cells. In a cohort of children infected with HIV, Rondanelli and colleagues[38] reported normal GH secretion but impaired IGF-1 and IGFBP-3 response to exogenous GH, indicating a degree of GH insensitivity. In a study of 27 children with HIV, Van Rossum and colleagues[44] reported increases in IGF-1 and IGFBP-3 in children initiating a PI-containing ART regimen; greater increases in IGF-1 were found in those with greater improvement in linear growth, consistent with the possibility of a treatment-associated decrease in GH resistance. GH resistance in both prepubertal and pubertal children infected with HIV may be related to increased IGFBP-1, which increases in catabolic states and renders IGF-1 unavailable to binding sites.[34,42] Treatment with a PI-containing regimen resulted in changes suggesting the return of normal GH sensitivity.

GH changes are additionally associated with metabolic effects in patients with HIV. Lipodystrophy associated with HAART therapy and increased visceral adiposity seems to be associated with decreased GH secretion in adolescents and adults.[45,46]

The degree of contribution of these GH axis perturbations to height outcomes is unclear. Kessler and colleagues[34] reported no correlation of IGF-1, IGFBP-3, and the cytokines IL-1α, IL-6, and TNF-α to final adult height. However, given the frequency of growth disturbances in children infected with HIV, further longitudinal studies are indicated.

Management

The goal is to maintain normal growth. Linear and ponderal growth should be routinely measured and plotted on age-specific and gender-specific growth charts. Poor weight gain or reduced height velocity should prompt thorough evaluation of nutritional status (both macronutrients and micronutrients, in addition to body composition) and potentially of hormone levels (including thyroid hormone, pubertal hormones, and IGF-1 and IGFBP3). Given that growth failure is often multifactorial, it is best addressed with a multidisciplinary team, including the primary care provider in conjunction with a dietitian, social worker, and specialists in pediatric endocrinology, infectious disease, and gastroenterology, depending on the presenting signs and symptoms and results of initial evaluation. GH therapy is indicated in the rare cases of GH deficiency but is not effective in GH resistance. Anabolic steroids (eg, oxandrolone) have increased lean body mass in HIV-associated wasting.[47] Children with HIV may also warrant evaluation for unrelated disorders leading to growth arrest (eg, a coincidental CNS tumor).

PUBERTY

Puberty is a complex process of developmental change regulated by multiple genetic, environmental, and endocrine controls. Central puberty describes the portion of pubertal development marked by increasing levels of luteinizing hormone (LH) and follicle-stimulating hormone and then by increasing levels of the gonadal steroids (estradiol in women and testosterone in men). The increase of gonadal steroids can be recognized clinically by the initial physical changes of puberty: breast development in women and testicular enlargement in men. Adrenarche refers to the increasing levels of adrenal androgens that cause pubic hair and axillary hair and odor in both sexes. Pubertal delay is associated with impaired quality of life and may worsen the psychological distress that an adolescent infected with HIV may already face.

Pubertal Delay

Multiple studies have shown delayed pubertal onset in youth infected with HIV, both with perinatally acquired and transfusion-acquired infection.[28,48–50] The largest and most recent study to date[48] found delays in pubertal onset of 6 to 11 months in children infected with HIV compared with HIV-exposed but noninfected controls. The delays were significant for all aspects of puberty, including both central puberty and adrenarche in both sexes. Increasing pubertal delay occurs with more advanced disease, as measured by CD4 count and viral load.[48,51] Pubertal delay and concomitant delay in skeletal maturity may exacerbate the effects of poor growth in this population. Combination ART seems to be associated with more normal pubertal timing; future studies may reveal a near normalization of pubertal onset in most children infected with HIV with viral suppression.

The mechanism of pubertal delay in children infected with HIV is unknown. In adult men with AIDS, hypogonadism is common and is mainly caused by testicular dysfunction associated with wasting and opportunistic infection.[52] In the modern era of cART, premature decline in serum testosterone may be one element in the process of premature aging associated with HIV infection. Testosterone deficiency is often associated with low or inappropriately normal LH levels, implying a major role of the hypothalamic-pituitary axis.[53] However, no studies to date have evaluated pubertal hormones over time in children infected with HIV.

Management

There are no specific recommendations for children infected with HIV with delayed puberty. Optimization of nutritional and virologic status is critical, and hormonal evaluation may be indicated for delayed pubertal onset beyond the upper limits of normal (age 13 years in girls and age 14 years in boys).

THYROID

Thyroid hormone plays a critical role in the growth and neurodevelopment of young children, and may manifest as linear growth failure with relative preservation of somatic growth. In older children, hypothyroidism is often associated with fatigue, cold intolerance, dry skin, constipation, and weight gain. Abnormal thyroid function tests are common in adults and children with HIV,[54,55] although overt hypothyroidism is extremely rare. A variety of thyroid abnormalities have been described in children with HIV (summarized in **Table 2**) but understanding of the frequency and nature of thyroid disturbance in children infected with HIV is limited. The cause of thyroid dysfunction is also unclear but hypotheses include autoimmune disease, concurrent infections, destruction by opportunistic infections, and drug reactions.[54] Thyroid abnormalities are associated with disease progression, including severe immunosuppression and high viral load.[56,57]

Table 2
Thyroid dysregulation in children with HIV infection

	TSH	FT4	T3	Comments
Euthyroid sick syndrome (nonthyroid illness)	Normal	Normal	Decreased	Caused by decreased peripheral conversion of T4 to T3
Hypothyroidism	Increased	Decreased	Decreased	Rarely seen in children with HIV infection; unclear contribution of autoantibodies and may be associated with immune reconstitution inflammatory syndrome
Subclinical hypothyroidism	Increased	Normal	Normal	Unclear clinical significance
Isolated low FT4	Normal	Low	Normal	May have similar mechanism of energy conservation to euthyroid sick syndrome
Hyperthyroidism	Decreased	Increased	Increased	Rarely seen in children with HIV but may be associated with immune reconstitution inflammatory syndrome

Abbreviations: FT4, free thyroxine; T3, triiodothyronine; TSH, thyroid-stimulating hormone.

Euthyroid Sick Syndrome

Euthyroid sick syndrome (or nonthyroid illness) is an adaptive mechanism to conserve energy during times of stress caused by illness. Decreased peripheral conversion of thyroxine (T4) to triiodothyronine (T3) by 5′ deiodination results in low T3 levels and a relative buildup of T4 that decreases as T4 converts into reverse T3, an inactive form of thyroid hormone. In a study by Panamonta and colleagues,[58] 14% of Thai children with HIV had low serum T3 and normal thyroid-stimulating hormone (TSH; also called thyrotropin), and free thyroxine (FT4) levels consistent with euthyroid sick syndrome. All were clinically euthyroid. 72% of these patients were classified as severely immunosuppressed by low CD4+ counts, presumably accounting for the high percentage of patients with euthyroid sick syndrome.

Hypothyroidism

Clinically evident hypothyroidism is rarely seen in children with HIV infection. Subclinical hypothyroidism, defined as increased TSH with normal T4, T3, and FT4, occurs more frequently. Reported frequencies vary from 2%[54] to 14%[58]; the clinical significance remains unclear. High TSH values are more frequently observed in patients with moderate to severe immunosuppression[59] and an inverse correlation exists between CD4+ cell count and TSH. Many children with HIV have normal to high levels of T3 and T4, normal to increased TSH, and increased thyroid-binding globulin (TBG) with normal to low levels of FT4.[56] These changes may be explained by a progressive increase in TBG levels, a finding that has been confirmed by other investigators.[57,59] These abnormalities in thyroid function become more significant as CD4 count decreases. TBG remains increased even after treatment with thyroid hormone and normalization of other thyroid indices.

Isolated low FT4 has been described in both adults and children with HIV infection. Vigano and colleagues[54] found that 31% of 52 children infected with HIV had isolated low FT4 values with normal TSH and normal response to thyrotropin releasing hormone. Isolated low FT4 is positively correlated with CD4+ cell percentage[56] and a shorter duration of HAART compared with children with normal FT4.[54] The investigators postulated that low FT4 in the setting of incomplete disease recovery is a mechanism to conserve energy, similar to the euthyroid sick syndrome.

The literature is mixed with respect to the effect of autoantibodies on thyroid function in HIV disease. Thyroid autoantibodies have been described in up to 34% of children with HIV infection.[59] However, other studies fail to confirm this association.[56–58] Hashimoto thyroiditis has also been reported in an adult after initiation of HAART, and is considered a potential complication of immune reconstitution inflammatory syndrome (IRIS).[60]

Hyperthyroidism

Graves disease is an autoimmune hyperthyroid state caused by the production of anti-TSH receptor antibodies; it is the leading cause of hyperthyroidism in the general pediatric population. Clinical signs include heat intolerance, warm/moist skin, palpitations/tachycardia, anxiety, hyperreflexia, and diarrhea. Thyroid function studies reveal increased FT4 and T3 with suppressed TSH.

Graves disease may also occur as a complication of IRIS.[55] IRIS is characterized by worsening symptoms of inflammation associated with the initiation of HAART through stimulation of CD4+ cells in a biphasic manner. Children with very low CD4+ T-cell values before initiation of combination ARV therapy seem to be at greatest risk. In the first 3 to 6 months after HAART initiation, there is an increase in CD4+ memory cells that is associated with reactivation of latent viral and mycobacterial infection. The second phase of IRIS typically occurs 12 to 36 months after initiation of HAART and is hypothesized to be dominated by expansion of naive CD4+ cells. This second phase correlates with the onset of Graves disease, because the pathogenic antibodies causing Graves disease may be created during this repopulation of CD+-naive cells.[61] The prevalence of Graves disease following HAART initiation in the pediatric HIV population is unknown, although it seems rare based on the single identified reported case in the pediatric literature.[62]

Management

Given the increased prevalence of thyroid hormone abnormalities in children with HIV, providers should have a low threshold for thyroid function screening with FT4 and TSH testing, particularly in patients with poor growth. It is unclear whether or not treatment with thyroid hormone for subclinical thyroid disease would benefit overall growth. In one study, Rana and colleagues[63] provided thyroid hormone replacement to a small sample of children 0.7 to 3.7 years old infected with HIV with increased TSH and normal or increased T4. Increased height velocity was noted in 3 of the 4 patients. The fourth patient died of candida sepsis 2 weeks after initiation of thyroid replacement and thus the effects of thyroid hormone therapy on growth could not be evaluated. This study suggests that there may be some benefit to treatment of subclinical thyroid disease, but newer post–HAART era studies with larger sample sizes are indicated.

METABOLIC COMPLICATIONS

Unfavorable changes in lipid and glucose metabolism (including lipodystrophy, dyslipidemia, and glucose intolerance) occur in adults and children with HIV. These changes are associated with an increased incidence of cardiovascular disease; children with HIV show early atherosclerotic changes on carotid artery imaging, measured both by intima media thickness[64] and stiffness assessed by pulse wave velocity.[65] Effects of ART are largely responsible for these metabolic changes, although HIV infection also plays a role. The use of NRTIs is primarily associated with lipodystrophy, whereas PIs have greater association with dyslipidemias (see **Table 1**).[30,66] Lipoatrophy and lipohypertrophy can be disfiguring and stigmatizing and therefore may cause psychosocial morbidity in addition to medical complications, particularly in adolescents.[67] Again, given that the pediatric HIV population may have lifelong exposure to ART, these associations are of particular importance in children.

Lipodystrophy

Lipodystrophy, or abnormal body fat distribution, occurs alone or in combination with insulin resistance or dyslipidemia. Fat loss, or lipoatrophy, often localizes to the face, limbs, and/or buttocks and should be differentiated from AIDS-related wasting. Fat accumulation, or lipohypertrophy, tends to localize to the base of the neck/back (dorsocervical fat pad), abdomen, and/or breasts. A mixed pattern of both lipoatrophy and lipohypertrophy may occur. Lipodystrophy syndrome is variably defined, but typically refers to abnormal body fat distribution in combination with one or more metabolic abnormalities.[68] Alam and colleagues[69] studied a large cohort of European children (median age 12.2 years and duration of ART use 5.2 years) and reported a 42% prevalence of body fat abnormality and 57% prevalence of lipodystrophy syndrome (defined therein as body fat abnormalities and/or metabolic abnormalities). The proportions of children with lipohypertrophy, lipoatrophy, and the mixed lipohypertrophy-lipoatrophy phenotype were roughly equivalent at 13% to 14% each. Dapena and colleagues[70] followed a Spanish cohort of pediatric patients infected with HIV (median age 13 years) and reported abnormal fat distribution in 40.5% of their subjects; half of these were isolated lipoatrophy. Other studies vary widely in their prevalence estimates. In 2 recent studies of younger children in Tanzania (mean age 9.7 years) and Uganda (median age 8 years), prevalence of lipodystrophy was 30% and 27% respectively.[71,72] An earlier prospective study of an even younger cohort of children and adolescents in Thailand (mean age 7.6 years at entry) revealed a prevalence of lipodystrophy of 65% after 144 weeks of non-nucleoside reverse transcriptase inhibitor (NNRTI)–based cART.[73] These differences in reported lipodystrophy prevalence likely reflect differences in type of therapeutic regimen(s), duration of treatment, population differences (eg, age, race-ethnicity), and inconsistencies in methodologies and case definitions.

Lipodystrophy is associated with ART duration and specific agents and drug classes; it has been most closely associated with NRTIs as well as with PIs.[74] Alam and colleagues[69] showed that stavudine was highly associated with lipoatrophy, a finding consistent with numerous earlier studies. The investigators additionally reported an increased risk of lipodystrophy syndrome with white ethnicity, higher body mass index, exposure to lopinavir/ritonavir and NNRTIs, and an increased risk of lipoatrophy with white ethnicity and history of US Centers for Disease Control and Prevention (CDC) stage B/C disease. In an earlier study, independent predictors of fat redistribution included CDC class C disease, female gender, and ever versus never use of PIs and of stavudine use.[75] Other studies have shown higher prevalence of lipodystrophy in men; thus, there is no consensus at this time regarding the role of gender. Fat redistribution and hyperlipidemia is also associated with sexual maturity with the likelihood of lipodystrophy increasing during puberty.[72,76]

The cause of lipodystrophy is multifactorial and poorly understood. NRTIs such as stavudine have mitochondrial toxicity via effects on mitochondrial DNA. Decreased ATP resulting from mitochondrial dysfunction may decrease lipogenesis and increase proapoptotic mediators, culminating in fat loss.[77,78] PIs may inhibit proteins involved in lipid metabolism, possibly via homology between HIV-1 protease and a protein involved in lipid metabolism, cytoplasmic retinoic acid binding protein type 1, which leads to decreased fat storage and adipocyte apoptosis,[79] but their underlying mechanism in lipodystrophy is poorly understood. Children naive to ART have also been reported with lipodystrophy, consistent with a possible direct action of HIV.[80]

As noted earlier, both diagnosis and prevalence estimates of lipodystrophy in children are hampered by a lack of clear case definition. In adults, a validated model of severity is in widespread use.[81] In pediatric studies, physical examination scores have been commonly used to define and quantify lipodystrophy, although concern exists for high inter-rater variability. Other techniques have included anthropometric measurements, bioelectrical impedence, dual energy X-ray absorptiometry (DEXA), computed tomography (CT), and magnetic resonance imaging (MRI). Anthropometric measurements are noninvasive and inexpensive, but cannot measure visceral fat and require an experienced evaluator. Bioelectrical impedance measures lean body mass and total body fat, but cannot assess regional fat distribution. DEXA measures regional fat distribution and is considered ideal for longitudinal studies. Abdominal CT scan and MRI both discriminate well between subcutaneous fat and visceral fat but are expensive and raise concern for radiation effects and the need for sedation respectively.[76]

Management

The principle treatment of lipodystrophy is to discontinue the causative agent, but few studies have assessed the effect of treatment-switching strategies in children. Vigano and colleagues[82] followed a small cohort of children with HIV after switching from stavudine to tenofovir and from a PI to the NNRTI efavirenz. The children showed normalization of physiologic fat accrual with no further progression of lipoatrophy 1.8 years after the switch. This same cohort was reevaluated again 8 years after the treatment switch and showed no frankly pathologic abnormalities of body composition.[83]

Recommended treatment strategies include lifestyle changes such as a calorically appropriate low-fat diet; exercise (especially strength training); and smoking cessation, if applicable, to decrease future cardiovascular risk. Proposed treatments include metformin and thiazolidinediones, but data regarding their efficacy are lacking in children.[84] GH may be effective for treating visceral adiposity in adolescents[85] but may increase the risk of glucose intolerance. Surgical interventions such as fillers, fat transplantation, and resection of localized adipose tissue have been considered as treatment of the disfiguring effects of lipodystrophy. Adolescents with facial lipoatrophy reported satisfaction and increased self-confidence after facial autologous fat transplantation.[67] However, surgical intervention is reserved for severe cases because of its inherent risks.

Dyslipidemia

Children with HIV are at increased risk for dyslipidemia (including hypertriglyceridemia, increased low-density lipoprotein [LDL] and total cholesterol levels, and reduced high-density lipoprotein [HDL] levels). The Pediatric AIDS Clinical Trials Group reported a 13% prevalence of hypercholesterolemia (defined as cholesterol levels greater than the 95th percentile for age and gender) in a large cohort of 1812 children with HIV.[86] More recently, Brewinski and colleagues[66] reported a 20.5% prevalence of hypercholesterolemia and 29.4% prevalence of hypertriglyceridemia. Current overall estimates are that from 20% to 50% of treated children have abnormal lipid profiles.[8] However, prospective studies comparing the effects of various treatment regimens on lipid profiles in children have been limited.

The pathogenesis of dyslipidemia in children with HIV is complex and includes direct effects of the virus as well as medication toxicity. Chantry and colleagues[87] reported that antiretroviral-naive patients are more likely than uninfected controls to have low HDL (30% vs 4%, respectively). Strehlau and colleagues[88] later reported higher risk of dyslipidemia in treatment-naive subjects (93% with low HDL and 63% with increased triglyceride) likely caused by the preponderance of those subjects with advanced disease. In both studies, HDL levels improved with antiretroviral initiation. On cART initiation, HDL changes correlate with immune reconstitution,[87] and total cholesterol/HDL improvements relate to decreased TNF-α[89]; thus, both HIV-associated immunodeficiency and inflammation seem to have detrimental effects on lipid levels.

However, initiation or change in ART in infected children is associated with significant increases in multiple other lipid measures in addition to HDL that can be detrimental. PIs are strongly implicated (both boosted and nonboosted), and all available PIs are associated with dyslipidemia (including hypertriglyceridemia and increased LDL and total cholesterol levels).[90,91] This effect may be caused by PI inhibition of low-density lipoprotein receptor–related protein, resulting in hyperlipidemia caused by ineffective removal of triglycerides from the circulation. However, other antiretroviral drug classes are also implicated,[92] including NRTIs (stavudine), and the combination of certain drugs may be particularly deleterious: ART regimens that contain both a PI and NNRTI seem to be associated with worse lipid profiles than regimens that contain 1 but not both of these drug classes.[87]

Management

Management strategies for dyslipidemia include lifestyle modifications such as low-fat diet, aerobic exercise, and avoidance of smoking. A switch to an alternate therapy (a different agent within the same class, or a different class) may improve the lipid profile but care must be taken to avoid compromising antiviral efficacy. Among PIs, dyslipidemia seems worst with lopinavir/ritonavir combinations. Atazanavir has a more favorable lipid profile and a switch to atazanavir has been shown to reduce lipid levels in children.[93] Strehalau and colleagues[88] reported that with initiation of a lopinavir/ritonavir-based regimen, children infected with HIV had increases in HDL, LDL, and total cholesterol, and decreases in total cholesterol/HDL ratio and triglyceride (TG) levels, a pattern that corresponds with prior descriptions. After switching to nevirapine, HDL was significantly higher and total cholesterol/HDL ratio and TG significantly lower compared with the group remaining on the PI-based regimen. Arpadi and colleagues[94] similarly reported unfavorable changes in lipid profiles in young South African children infected with HIV and receiving PI therapy (lopinavir/ritonavir-based regimens) versus those switched to nevirapine-based regimens. The lopinavir/ritonavir group had lower mean HDL and higher mean total cholesterol, LDL, and triglycerides than the nevirapine group. Gonzalez-Tome and colleagues[95] also noted a trend toward decreased total cholesterol with significantly improved HDL in children who substituted PI-based regimens with nevirapine. Switches from a PI-based regimen to the NNRTI efavirenz have also resulted in improvements in lipid profiles in children.[96,97]

The National Institutes of Health Panel of Antiretroviral Therapy and Medical Management of HIV-Infected Children recommend a fasting lipid panel every 6 to 12 months in adolescents and a nonfasting screening panel every 6 to 12 months in children more than 2 years old (with follow-up fasting testing if TG or LDL is increased). Before initiating or changing lipid-lowering therapy in adolescents, a fasting lipid panel should be obtained twice (2 weeks–3 months apart) and results averaged (**Table 3**).[8]

There is no consensus for treatment of dyslipidemia in children on ART and complete discussion is beyond the scope of this article. For young children and children or adolescents with severe dyslipidemia (TG>500 mg/dL or LDL>250 mg/dL), consultation with a lipid specialist is indicated. For less severe dyslipidemia, a 6-month to 12-month trial of lifestyle modification may be warranted. Lipid-lowering drug therapy with statins may be considered for children more than 10 years old with LDL greater than or equal to 190 mg/dL who have failed lifestyle management, or greater than or equal to 160 mg/dL with a strong family history of cardiovascular disease or who have additional other risk factors in addition to HIV infection. Children 8 to 10 years of age may also warrant treatment of LDL greater than or equal to 190 mg/dL in certain circumstances.[98] Therapy may also be considered in children with triglycerides that remain increased at greater than or equal to 200 mg/dL despite lifestyle management. Care must be taken when prescribing statins to children on ART, because PIs may increase statin levels and thus increase the risk of side effects such as muscle damage (caused by the drugs' similar hepatic metabolism via the P450-CYP3A4 pathway). Consultation with a lipid specialist is recommended.

Table 3		
Monitoring for dyslipidemia		
	Regular Monitoring	**Before Initiating or Changing Therapy**
Children ≥2 y old without known lipid abnormalities	Nonfasting screening lipid panel every 6–12 mo. If any abnormalities, then obtain 12-h fasting sample	Nonfasting screening lipid panel. If any abnormalities, then obtain 12-h fasting sample
Children with known lipid abnormalities and/or other risk factors	12-h fasting screening lipid panel every 6 mo	12-h fasting screening lipid panel
Adolescents	12-h fasting screening lipid panel every 6–12 mo	12-h fasting screening lipid panel obtained twice (>2 wk and ≤3 mo apart) and averaged together

Adapted from Panel on Antiretroviral Therapy and Medical Management of HIV-Infected Children. Guidelines for the use of antiretroviral agents in pediatric HIV infections. Available at: http://aidsinfo.nih.gov/contentfiles/lvguidelines/pediatricguidelines.pdf. Accessed April 2, 2014.

Insulin Resistance

Insulin resistance is characterized by increase in pancreatic insulin level caused by a decreased ability of insulin to stimulate glucose use and suppress hepatic glucose production. With insulin resistance, progressive limitations in pancreatic insulin secretion may result in impairments in glucose tolerance and fasting glucose and frank type 2 diabetes mellitus. In patients without HIV, insulin resistance is associated with multiple factors, including genetic factors, obesity, and physical inactivity. HIV infection and ART are associated with disturbed glucose metabolism, most often presenting as impaired fasting glucose and less often impaired glucose tolerance or type 2 diabetes mellitus. Insulin resistance occurs less frequently in children with HIV than in adults, perhaps because of less visceral fat in prepubertal children compared with pubertal children and adults.[99] Glucose disorders may occur independently or in conjunction with fat maldistribution or dyslipidemia.

Insulin resistance is diagnosed in multiple ways, including via measurements of fasting glucose, fasting insulin, C peptide, oral glucose tolerance tests, and/or by combining them to calculate the homeostatic model assessment of insulin resistance (HOMA-IR) or quantitative insulin sensitivity check index.[79] Hyperinsulinemic euglycemic clamp remains the gold standard but is rarely performed in clinical practice.

Overall, prevalence estimates of impaired glucose homeostasis in children range from 8% to 35%.[79] Geffner and colleagues[100] reported that insulin resistance occurred in 15.2% of children infected with HIV and was associated with Tanner stage 5 pubertal status. Dapena and colleagues[70] recently reported insulin resistance in nearly 20% of subjects in a cross-sectional Spanish cohort and noted associations with hepatitis C coinfection, current use of stavudine, and hypertriglyceridemia. Rosso and colleagues[101] noted insulin resistance with normal fasting glucose but increased fasting insulin in 60% of subjects, but most were postpubertal. Longitudinal data regarding the development of insulin resistance in children infected with HIV are sparse. Chantry and colleagues[87] reported a significant increase in insulin resistance and abnormal glucose tolerance (as measured by HOMA-IR) in prepubertal children over 48 weeks after beginning or changing cART, although no statistically significant difference in frankly abnormal values were detected. Similarly, Vigano and colleagues[102] reported higher rates of insulin resistance in a small group of Italian children with HIV versus healthy controls, but the subjects had normal fasting glucose concentration and glucose tolerance tests. Thus, the progression of these early metabolic changes to clinically significant disease is poorly understood and further longitudinal studies are needed.

The underlying mechanism of disordered glucose metabolism is complex and includes ART effects, HIV-related viral and immunologic factors, genetic influences, physical inactivity, and diet.[101] PIs affect insulin sensitivity by direct inhibition of the glucose transporter type 4 (GLUT4) in myocytes and adipocytes, as well as inhibiting the response of the beta cells of the pancreas.[103] However, studies conflict regarding the association of insulin resistance with PIs.

Management

Clinicians should monitor for clinical signs of hyperglycemia and hyperinsulinism (polydipsia, polyuria, polyphagia, unintentional weight loss, and acanthosis nigricans). Monitoring of random blood glucose concentration at initiation of ART and 3 to 6 months after initiation, and then yearly afterward, has been recommended (Table 4).[8] Treatment of insulin resistance includes lifestyle changes as a first intervention. Simultaneous switching of the ART regimen to a PI-sparing regimen including efavirenz and from stavudine to tenofovir has been reported to improve insulin sensitivity,[104] but again not all studies confirm the association between PI use and insulin resistance. Metformin is approved for use in children more than 10 years old (although it is used in younger children) but must be monitored closely given the risk of lactic acidosis when used in combination with NRTIs.[79]

CALCIUM METABOLISM AND BONE DISEASE
Normal Bone Accretion

The most important phases of bone accretion occur during infancy and during puberty.[105] Girls reach peak calcium accretion around 12.5 years of age, whereas boys reach this stage at about 14 years; one study estimated that 26% of total skeletal calcium is laid down during the 2 peak pubertal years of bone growth.[106] Sex steroids are critical for bone maturation and for attainment and maintenance of normal bone mineral density (BMD). In both sexes, hypogonadism leads to osteoporosis. Estrogen plays the critical role in stimulating new bone formation and augmenting mineralization; androgens play a more minor role. In addition to the gonadal steroids, GH and IGF-1 contribute to attainment of peak bone mass.[107]

Table 4 Monitoring for insulin resistance	
Signs and symptoms	Polydipsia, polyuria, polyphagia, change in body habitus, acanthosis nigricans
Obtain random plasma glucose (values ≥140 mg/dL, obtain 8-h fasting plasma glucose)	Before initiation of ART 3–6 mo after initiation of ART Every 12 mo while on ART

Adapted from Panel on Antiretroviral Therapy and Medical Management of HIV-Infected Children. Guidelines for the use of antiretroviral agents in pediatric HIV infections. Available at: http://aidsinfo.nih.gov/contentfiles/lvguidelines/pediatricguidelines.pdf. Accessed April 2, 2014.

Effects of HIV on BMD

Low BMD is common in adults infected with HIV.[108] Osteopenia occurs in more than 50% of adults with HIV and osteoporosis in 15%.[109] The cause of low BMD in patients with HIV is likely multifactorial. The HIV envelope glycoprotein gp120 seems to promote osteoblast apoptosis and osteoclast proliferation[110]; animal studies provide further evidence that the HIV infection leads to an increase in osteoclastogenic cytokine-related bone resorption.[111] Other contributors include ART and presumably traditional risk factors such as low weight and poor nutritional status. Furthermore, HIV infection is associated with low vitamin D levels in many patients in a variety of settings.[112] Although less studied than adults, children with HIV may be more susceptible to developing osteopenia or osteoporosis than adults, given that perinatally infected individuals may have lifelong exposure to HIV infection and medication effects. Furthermore, the effects of HIV and ART on growth and puberty may secondarily lead to deleterious effects on bone health caused by interruption of the normal processes for bone accrual described earlier.

Multiple studies have shown lower than expected bone mass in children infected with HIV.[113–115] Much of the difference can be attributed to lower weight and height in these children, but not universally. Adolescents who were infected perinatally have lower BMD at the end of puberty than their uninfected peers.[114] One recent, representative study by DiMeglio and colleagues[115] showed that reduced total body and lumbar spine BMD z scores in children aged 7 to 15 years who were perinatally infected with HIV were largely attributable to differences in weight-for-age and height-for-age z scores compared with their exposed, uninfected counterparts. These children nonetheless had a significantly increased prevalence of low age–adjusted and bone age–adjusted total body BMD (z score <-2) compared with controls. However, fracture data in these subjects were unknown. A recent large, case-control study of Danish adults with HIV showed a 3-fold increase in fracture risk compared with uninfected controls.[116]

Children treated with HAART also have lower BMD and increased bone turnover (assessed by serologic markers) compared with controls (see **Table 1**). The study by DiMeglio and colleagues[115] also found that, consistent with adult studies, boosted PI regimens, lamivudine, and indinavir (known to increase osteoclast activity) were associated with lower BMD, as were CD4% (percentage of total lymphocytes that are CD4 cells), peak viral load, and more years on HAART. Adults treated with HAART have a 2.5-fold increased risk of osteoporosis compared with HAART-naive patients.[108] Tenofovir is associated with reduced BMD in both adults and children, which may be the result of phosphate wasting and increased bone turnover associated with proximal tubule toxicity.[117] Efavirenz, an NNRTI, is highly associated with low vitamin D levels[118] and may affect BMD indirectly via vitamin D metabolism. PIs have also been implicated, but data are conflicting.

Management

Universal DEXA screening in pediatric patients with HIV is not currently recommended, although it may be warranted in special cases (such as prior fragility fracture or before and during therapy with an antiretroviral known to have greater risk, eg tenofovir).[8] DEXA standards exist for evaluating bone mineralization in children, but it is imperative that the correct standards for age are used. Adequate vitamin D and calcium intake, weight-bearing exercise, and smoking cessation are recommended, along with reducing other modifiable risk factors such as corticosteroids and medroxyprogesterone. Vigorous physical activity is shown to be protective for spine BMD in children infected with HIV.[115] Vitamin D levels of greater than 30 mmol/L are recommended for the HIV-positive population; data are lacking on the effect of vitamin D replacement therapy on bone mass accrual. Safety and efficacy data of bisphosphonates therapy in children infected with HIV are inadequate.

SUMMARY

Endocrine changes (with and without clinically significant effect) accompany HIV infection in pediatric patients. The cause of these changes is multifactorial and includes effects of HIV, chronic inflammation, and ART (ART effects are summarized in **Table 1**). These effects may be of particular importance in childhood given the critical developmental processes that occur during this time period and the likelihood of prolonged exposure to the virus and to medication therapy. The proper diagnosis of endocrine dysfunction requires a high index of suspicion and often specialized laboratory testing. Future longitudinal work is indicated to help clarify the risks and natural course of endocrine dysfunction in HIV-positive children.

REFERENCES

1. Joint United Nations Programme on HIV/AIDS (UNAIDS). Global report. UNAIDS report on the global AIDS epidemic. 2013. Available at: http://www.unaids.org/en/media/unaids/contentassets/documents/epidemiology/2013/gr2013/UNAIDS_Global_Report_2013_en.pdf. Accessed March 20, 2014.
2. Eledrisi MS, Verghese AC. Adrenal insufficiency in HIV infection: a review and recommendations. Am J Med Sci 2001;321(2):137–44.
3. Grinspoon SK, Bilezikian JP. HIV disease and the endocrine system. N Engl J Med 1992;327(19):1360–5.
4. George MM, Bhangoo A. Human immune deficiency virus (HIV) infection and the hypothalamic pituitary adrenal axis. Rev Endocr Metab Disord 2013;14(2):105–12.
5. Danoff A. Endocrinologic complications of HIV infection. Med Clin North Am 1996;80(6):1453–69.
6. Sellmeyer DE, Grunfeld C. Endocrine and metabolic disturbances in human immunodeficiency virus infection and the acquired immune deficiency syndrome. Endocr Rev 1996;17(5):518–32.
7. Seel K, Guschmann M, van Landeghem F, et al. Addison-disease - an unusual clinical manifestation of CMV-end organ disease in pediatric AIDS. Eur J Med Res 2000;5(6):247–50.
8. Panel on Antiretroviral Therapy and Medical Management of HIV-Infected Children. Guidelines for the use of antiretroviral agents in pediatric HIV infections. Available at: http://aidsinfo.nih.gov/contentfiles/lvguidelines/pediatricguidelines.pdf. Accessed April 2, 2014.
9. Johnson S, Marion AA, Vrchoticky T, et al. Cushing syndrome with secondary adrenal insufficiency from concomitant therapy with ritonavir and fluticasone. J Pediatr 2006;148:386–8.
10. St Germain RM, Yigit S, Wells L, et al. Cushing syndrome and severe adrenal suppression caused by fluticasone and protease inhibitor combination in an HIV-infected adolescent. AIDS Patient Care STDS 2007;21:373–7.
11. Bhumbra NA, Sahloff EG, Oehrtman SJ, et al. Exogenous cushing syndrome with inhaled fluticasone in a child receiving lopinavir/ritonavir. The Annals of Pharmacotherapy 2007;41(7):1306–9.
12. van der Pas R, Hofland LJ, Hofland J, et al. Fluconazole inhibits human adrenocortical steroidogenesis in vitro. J Endocrinol 2012;215(3):403–12.

13. Meya DB, Katabira E, Otim M, et al. Functional adrenal insufficiency among critically ill patients with human immunodeficiency virus in a resource-limited setting. Afr Health Sci 2007;7(2):101–7.

14. Simon A, Warszawski J, Kariyawasam D, et al. Association of prenatal and postnatal exposure to lopinavir-ritonavir and adrenal dysfunction among uninfected infants of HIV-infected mothers. JAMA 2011;306(1):70–8.

15. Verges B, Chavanet P, Desgres J, et al. Adrenal function in HIV infected patients. Acta Endocrinol (Copenh) 1989;121(5):633–7.

16. Membreno L, Irony I, Dere W, et al. Adrenocortical function in acquired immunodeficiency syndrome. J Clin Endocrinol Metab 1987;65(3):482–7.

17. Wolff FH, Nhuch C, Cadore LP, et al. Low-dose adrenocorticotropin test in patients with the acquired immunodeficiency syndrome. Braz J Infect Dis 2001; 5(2):53–9.

18. Oberfield SE, Kairam R, Bakshi S, et al. Steroid response to adrenocorticotropin stimulation in children with human immunodeficiency virus infection. J Clin Endocrinol Metab 1990;70(3):578–81.

19. Laue L, Pizzo PA, Butler K. Growth and neuroendocrine dysfunction in children with acquired immunodeficiency syndrome. J Pediatr 1990;117(4):541–5.

20. Schwartz LJ, St Louis Y, Wu R, et al. Endocrine function in children with human immunodeficiency virus infection. Am J Dis Child 1991;145(3):330–3.

21. Chantry CJ, Byrd RS, Englund JA, et al, Pediatric AIDS Clinical Trials Group Protocol 152 Study Team. Growth, survival and viral load in symptomatic childhood human immunodeficiency virus infection. Pediatr Infect Dis J 2003;22(12):1033–9.

22. Shiau S, Arpadi S, Strehlau R, et al. Initiation of antiretroviral therapy before 6 months of age is associated with faster growth recovery in South African children perinatally infected with human immunodeficiency virus. J Pediatr 2013; 162(6):1138–45, 1145.e1–2.

23. Galli L, de Martino M, Tovo PA. Onset of clinical signs in children with HIV-1 perinatal infection. Italian Register for HIV Infection in Children. AIDS 1995;9(5): 455–61.

24. Isanaka S, Duggan C, Fawzi WW. Patterns of postnatal growth in HIV-infected and HIV-exposed children. Nutr Rev 2009;67(6):343–59.

25. Moye J Jr, Rich KC, Kalish LA, et al. Natural history of somatic growth in infants born to women infected by human immunodeficiency virus. Women and Infants Transmission Study Group. J Pediatr 1996;128(1):58–69.

26. Paul ME, Chantry CJ, Read JS, et al. Morbidity and mortality during the first two years of life among uninfected children born to human immunodeficiency virus type 1-infected women: the women and infants transmission study. Pediatr Infect Dis J 2005;24(1):46–56.

27. Ransom CE, Huo Y, Patel K, et al. Infant growth outcomes after maternal tenofovir disoproxil fumarate use during pregnancy. J Acquir Immune Defic Syndr 2013;64(4):374–81.

28. Gertner JM, Kaufman FR, Donfield SM, et al. Delayed somatic growth and pubertal development in human immunodeficiency virus-infected hemophiliac boys: Hemophilia Growth and Development Study. J Pediatr 1994;124(6):896–902.

29. Nachman SA, Lindsey JC, Moye J, et al. Growth of human immunodeficiency virus-infected children receiving highly active antiretroviral therapy. Pediatr Infect Dis J 2005;24(4):352–7.

30. Aldrovandi GM, Lindsey JC, Jacobson DL, et al. Morphologic and metabolic abnormalities in vertically HIV-infected children and youth. AIDS 2009;23(6): 661–72.

31. Miller TL, Mawn BE, Orav EJ, et al. The effect of protease inhibitor therapy on growth and body composition in human immunodeficiency virus type 1-infected children. Pediatrics 2001;107(5):E77.

32. Buchacz K, Cervia JS, Lindsey JC, et al. Impact of protease inhibitor-containing combination antiretroviral therapies on height and weight growth in HIV-infected children. Pediatrics 2001;108(4):E72.

33. Verweel G, van Rossum AM, Hartwig NG, et al. Treatment with highly active antiretroviral therapy in human immunodeficiency virus type 1-infected children is associated with a sustained effect on growth. Pediatrics 2002;109(2):E25.

34. Kessler M, Kaul A, Santos-Malava C. Growth patterns in pubertal HIV-infected adolescents and their correlation with cytokines, IGF-1 IGFBP-1, and IGFBP-3. J Pediatr Endocrinol Metab 2013;26:639–44.

35. Frost RA, Nachman SA, Lang CH, et al. Proteolysis of insulin-like growth factor-binding protein-3 in human immunodeficiency virus-positive children who fail to thrive. J Clin Endocrinol Metab 1996;81(8):2957–62.

36. Chantry CJ, Frederick MM, Meyer WA, et al. Endocrine abnormalities and impaired growth in human immunodeficiency virus-infected children. Pediatr Infect Dis J 2007;26(1):53–60.

37. Arpadi SM. Growth failure in children with HIV infection. J Acquir Immune Defic Syndr 2000;25(Suppl 1):S37–42.

38. Rondanelli M, Caselli D, Arico M, et al. Insulin-like growth factor I (IGF-I) and IGF-binding protein 3 response to growth hormone is impaired in HIV-infected children. AIDS Res Hum Retroviruses 2002;18(5):331–9.

39. Laue L, Pizzo PA, Butler K, et al. Growth and neuroendocrine dysfunction in children with acquired immunodeficiency syndrome. J Pediatr 1990;117(4):541–5.

40. Jospe N, Powell KR. Growth hormone deficiency in an 8-year-old girl with human immunodeficiency virus infection. Pediatrics 1990;86(2):309–12.

41. Watson DC, Counts DR. Growth hormone deficiency in HIV-infected children following successful treatment with highly active antiretroviral therapy. J Pediatr 2004;145(4):549–51.

42. Chantry CJ, Hughes MD, Alvero C, et al. Insulin-like growth factor-1 and lean body mass in HIV-infected children. J Acquir Immune Defic Syndr 2008;48(4):437–43.

43. Geffner ME, Yeh DY, Landaw EM, et al. In vitro insulin-like growth factor-I, growth hormone, and insulin resistance occurs in symptomatic human immunodeficiency virus-1-infected children. Pediatr Res 1993;34(1):66–72.

44. Van Rossum AM, Gaakeer MI, Verweel S, et al. Endocrinologic and immunologic factors associated with recovery of growth in children with human immunodeficiency virus type 1 infection treated with protease inhibitors. Pediatr Infect Dis J 2003;22(1):70–6.

45. Rietschel P, Hadigan C, Corcoran C, et al. Assessment of growth hormone dynamics in human immunodeficiency virus-related lipodystrophy. J Clin Endocrinol Metab 2001;86(2):504–10.

46. Vigano A, Mora S, Brambilla P, et al. Impaired growth hormone secretion correlates with visceral adiposity in highly active antiretroviral treated HIV-infected adolescents. AIDS 2003;17(10):1435–41.

47. Fox-Wheeler S, Heller L, Salata CM, et al. Evaluation of the effects of oxandrolone on malnourished HIV-positive pediatric patients. Pediatrics 1999;104(6):e73.

48. Williams PL, Abzug MJ, Jacobson DL, et al. Pubertal onset in children with perinatal HIV infection in the era of combination antiretroviral treatment. AIDS 2013;27(12):1959–70.

49. Buchacz K, Rogol AD, Lindsey JC, et al. Delayed onset of pubertal development in children and adolescents with perinatally acquired HIV infection. J Acquir Immune Defic Syndr 2003;33(1):56–65.
50. de Martino M, Tovo PA, Galli L, et al. Puberty in perinatal HIV-1 infection: a multicentre longitudinal study of 212 children. AIDS 2001;15(12):1527–34.
51. Mahoney EM, Donfield SM, Howard C, et al. HIV-associated immune dysfunction and delayed pubertal development in a cohort of young hemophiliacs. Hemophilia Growth and Development Study. J Acquir Immune Defic Syndr 1999; 21(4):333–7.
52. Crum NF, Furtek KJ, Olson PE, et al. A review of hypogonadism and erectile dysfunction among HIV-infected men during the pre- and post-HAART eras: diagnosis, pathogenesis, and management. AIDS Patient Care STDS 2005; 19(10):655–71.
53. Rochira V, Zirilli L, Orlando G, et al. Premature decline of serum total testosterone in HIV-infected men in the HAART-era. PLoS One 2011;6(12):e28512.
54. Vigano A, Riboni S, Bianchi R. Thyroid dysfunction in antiretroviral treated children. Pediatr Infect Dis J 2004;23(3):235–9.
55. Hoffmann CJ, Brown TT. Thyroid function abnormalities in HIV-infected patients. Clin Infect Dis 2007;45(4):488–94.
56. Hirschfeld S, Laue L, Cutler GB, et al. Thyroid abnormalities in children infected with human immunodeficiency virus. J Pediatr 1996;128(1):70–4.
57. Chiarelli F, Galli L, Verrotti A, et al. Thyroid function in children with perinatal human immunodeficiency virus type 1 infection. Thyroid 2000;10(6):499–505.
58. Panamonta O, Kosalaraksa P, Thinkhamrop B, et al. Endocrine function in Thai children infected with human immunodeficiency virus. J Pediatr Endocrinol Metab 2004;17(1):33–40.
59. Fundaro C, Olivieri A, Rendeli C. Occurrence of anti-thyroid autoantibodies in children vertically infected with HIV-1. J Pediatr Endocrinol Metab 1998;11(6): 745–50.
60. Visser R, de Mast Q, Netea-Maier RT, et al. Hashimoto's thyroiditis presenting as acute painful thyroiditis and as a manifestation of an immune reconstitution inflammatory syndrome in a human immunodeficiency virus-seropositive patient. Thyroid 2012;22(8):853–5.
61. Parsa AA, Bhangoo A. HIV and thyroid dysfunction. Rev Endocr Metab Disord 2013;14(2):127–31.
62. Perez N, Del R, Bianco G, et al. Graves' disease following successful HAART of a perinatally HIV-infected 11-year-old. AIDS 2009;23(5):645–6.
63. Rana S, Nunlee-Bland G, Valyasevi R, et al. Thyroid dysfunction in HIV-infected children: is L-thyroxine therapy beneficial? Pediatr AIDS HIV Infect 1996;7(6):424–8.
64. McComsey GA, O'Riordan M, Hazen SL, et al. Increased carotid intima media thickness and cardiac biomarkers in HIV infected children. AIDS 2007;21(8): 921–7.
65. Charakida M, Loukogeorgakis SP, Okorie MI, et al. Increased arterial stiffness in HIV-infected children: risk factors and antiretroviral therapy. Antivir Ther 2009; 14(8):1075–9.
66. Brewinski M, Megazzini K, Hance LF, et al. Dyslipidemia in a cohort of HIV-infected Latin American children receiving highly active antiretroviral therapy. J Trop Pediatr 2011;57(5):324–32.
67. Dollfus C, Blanche S, Trocme N, et al. Correction of facial lipoatrophy using autologous fat transplants in HIV-infected adolescents. HIV Med 2009;10(5): 263–8.

68. Loonam CR, Mullen A. Nutrition and the HIV-associated lipodystrophy syndrome. Nutr Res Rev 2012;25(2):267–87.
69. Alam N, Cortina-Borja M, Goetghebuer T, et al. Body fat abnormality in HIV-infected children and adolescents living in Europe: prevalence and risk factors. J Acquir Immune Defic Syndr 2012;59(3):314–24.
70. Dapena M, Jimenez B, Noguera-Julian A, et al. Metabolic disorders in vertically HIV-infected children: future adults at risk for cardiovascular disease. J Pediatr Endocrinol Metab 2012;25(5–6):529–35.
71. Kinabo GD, Sprengers M, Msuya LJ, et al. Prevalence of lipodystrophy in HIV-infected children in Tanzania on highly active antiretroviral therapy. Pediatr Infect Dis J 2013;32(1):39–44.
72. Piloya T, Bakeera-Kitaka S, Kekitiinwa A, et al. Lipodystrophy among HIV-infected children and adolescents on highly active antiretroviral therapy in Uganda: a cross sectional study. J Int AIDS Soc 2012;15(2):17427.
73. Aurpibul L, Puthanakit T, Lee B, et al. Lipodystrophy and metabolic changes in HIV-infected children on non-nucleoside reverse transcriptase inhibitor-based antiretroviral therapy. Antivir Ther 2007;12(8):1247–54.
74. Mallewa JE, Wilkins E, Vilar J, et al. HIV-associated lipodystrophy: a review of underlying mechanisms and therapeutic options. J Antimicrob Chemother 2008;62(4):648–60.
75. European Paediatric Lipodystrophy Group. Antiretroviral therapy, fat redistribution and hyperlipidaemia in HIV-infected children in Europe. AIDS 2004;18(10):1443–51.
76. McComsey GA, Leonard E. Metabolic complications of HIV therapy in children. AIDS 2004;18(13):1753–68.
77. Kakuda TN, Brundage RC, Anderson PL, et al. Nucleoside reverse transcriptase inhibitor-induced mitochondrial toxicity as an etiology for lipodystrophy. AIDS 1999;13(16):2311–2.
78. Oh J, Hegele RA. HIV-associated dyslipidaemia: pathogenesis and treatment. Lancet Infect Dis 2007;7(12):787–96.
79. Barlow-Mosha L, Eckard AR, McComsey GA, et al. Metabolic complications and treatment of perinatally HIV-infected children and adolescents. J Int AIDS Soc 2013;16:18600.
80. Safrin S, Grunfeld C. Fat distribution and metabolic changes in patients with HIV infection. AIDS 1999;13(18):2493–505.
81. Carr A, Law M, HIV Lipodystrophy Case Definition Study Group. An objective lipodystrophy severity grading scale derived from the lipodystrophy case definition score. J Acquir Immune Defic Syndr 2003;33(5):571–6.
82. Vigano A, Brambilla P, Cafarelli L, et al. Normalization of fat accrual in lipoatrophic, HIV-infected children switched from stavudine to tenofovir and from protease inhibitor to efavirenz. Antivir Ther 2007;12(3):297–302.
83. Fabiano V, Giacomet V, Vigano A, et al. Long-term body composition and metabolic changes in HIV-infected children switched from stavudine to tenofovir and from protease inhibitors to efavirenz. Eur J Pediatr 2013;172(8):1089–96.
84. Vigano A, Cerini C, Pattarino G, et al. Metabolic complications associated with antiretroviral therapy in HIV-infected and HIV-exposed uninfected paediatric patients. Expert Opin Drug Saf 2010;9(3):431–45.
85. Vigano A, Mora S, Manzoni P, et al. Effects of recombinant growth hormone on visceral fat accumulation: pilot study in human immunodeficiency virus-infected adolescents. J Clin Endocrinol Metab 2005;90(7):4075–80.

86. Farley J, Gona P, Crain M, et al. Prevalence of elevated cholesterol and associated risk factors among perinatally HIV-infected children (4-19 years old) in Pediatric AIDS Clinical Trials Group 219C. J Acquir Immune Defic Syndr 2005;38(4):480–7.
87. Chantry CJ, Hughes MD, Alvero C, et al. Lipid and glucose alterations in HIV-infected children beginning or changing antiretroviral therapy. Pediatrics 2008;122(1):e129–38.
88. Strehlau R, Coovadia A, Abrams EJ, et al. Lipid profiles in young HIV-infected children initiating and changing antiretroviral therapy. J Acquir Immune Defic Syndr 2012;60(4):369–76.
89. Cervia JS, Chantry CJ, Hughes MD, et al. Associations of proinflammatory cytokine levels with lipid profiles, growth, and body composition in HIV-infected children initiating or changing antiretroviral therapy. Pediatr Infect Dis J 2010; 29(12):1118–22.
90. Tassiopoulos K, Williams PL, Seage GR 3rd, et al. Association of hypercholesterolemia incidence with antiretroviral treatment, including protease inhibitors, among perinatally HIV-infected children. J Acquir Immune Defic Syndr 2008; 47(5):607–14.
91. Sax PE, Kumar P. Tolerability and safety of HIV protease inhibitors in adults. J Acquir Immune Defic Syndr 2004;37(1):1111–24.
92. Fontas E, van Leth F, Sabin CA, et al. Lipid profiles in HIV-infected patients receiving combination antiretroviral therapy: are different antiretroviral drugs associated with different lipid profiles? J Infect Dis 2004;189(6):1056–74.
93. Mobius U, Lubach-Ruitman M, Castro-Frenzel B, et al. Switching to atazanavir improves metabolic disorders in antiretroviral-experienced patients with severe hyperlipidemia. J Acquir Immune Defic Syndr 2005;39(2):174–80.
94. Arpadi S, Shiau S, Strehlau R, et al. Metabolic abnormalities and body composition of HIV-infected children on Lopinavir or Nevirapine-based antiretroviral therapy. Arch Dis Child 2013;98(4):258–64.
95. Gonzalez-Tome MI, Amador JT, Pena MJ, et al. Outcome of protease inhibitor substitution with nevirapine in HIV-1 infected children. BMC Infect Dis 2008;8:144.
96. McComsey G, Bhumbra N, Ma JF, et al, First Pediatric Switch Study. Impact of protease inhibitor substitution with efavirenz in HIV-infected children: results of the First Pediatric Switch Study. Pediatrics 2003;111(3):e275–81.
97. Vigano A, Aldrovandi GM, Giacomet V, et al. Improvement in dyslipidaemia after switching stavudine to tenofovir and replacing protease inhibitors with efavirenz in HIV-infected children. Antivir Ther 2005;10(8):917–24.
98. Expert Panel on Integrated Guidelines for Cardiovascular Health and Risk Reduction in Children and Adolescents, National Heart, Lung, and Blood Institute. Expert panel on integrated guidelines for cardiovascular health and risk reduction in children and adolescents: summary report. Pediatrics 2011; 128(Suppl 5):S213–56.
99. Eley B. Metabolic complications of antiretroviral therapy in HIV-infected children. Expert Opin Drug Metab Toxicol 2008;4(1):37–49.
100. Geffner ME, Patel K, Miller TL, et al. Factors associated with insulin resistance among children and adolescents perinatally infected with HIV-1 in the pediatric HIV/AIDS cohort study. Horm Res Paediatr 2011;76(6):386–91.
101. Rosso R, Parodi A, d'Annunzio G, et al. Evaluation of insulin resistance in a cohort of HIV-infected youth. Eur J Endocrinol 2007;157(5):655–9.
102. Vigano A, Zuccotti GV, Cerini C, et al. Lipodystrophy, insulin resistance, and adiponectin concentration in HIV-infected children and adolescents. Curr HIV Res 2011;9(5):321–6.

103. Bitnun A, Sochett E, Dick PT, et al. Insulin sensitivity and beta-cell function in protease inhibitor-treated and -naive human immunodeficiency virus-infected children. J Clin Endocrinol Metab 2005;90(1):168–74.

104. Vigano A, Brambilla P, Pattarino G, et al. Long-term evaluation of glucose homeostasis in a cohort of HAART-treated HIV-infected children: a longitudinal, observational cohort study. Clin Drug Investig 2009;29(2):101–9.

105. Leonard MB, Zemel BS. Current concepts in pediatric bone disease. Pediatr Clin North Am 2002;49(1):143–73.

106. Bailey DA, Martin AD, McKay HA, et al. Calcium accretion in girls and boys during puberty: a longitudinal analysis. J Bone Miner Res 2000;15(11):2245–50.

107. Soyka LA, Fairfield WP, Klibanski A. Clinical review 117: hormonal determinants and disorders of peak bone mass in children. J Clin Endocrinol Metab 2000; 85(11):3951–63.

108. Brown TT, Qaqish RB. Antiretroviral therapy and the prevalence of osteopenia and osteoporosis: a meta-analytic review. AIDS 2006;20(17):2165–74.

109. Paccou J, Viget N, Legrout-Gérot I, et al. Bone loss in patients with HIV infection. Joint Bone Spine 2009;76(6):637–41.

110. Gibellini D, De Crignis E, Ponti C, et al. HIV-1 triggers apoptosis in primary osteoblasts and HOBIT cells through TNFalpha activation. J Med Virol 2008;80(9): 1507–14.

111. Vikulina T, Fan X, Yamaguchi M, et al. Alterations in the immuno-skeletal interface drive bone destruction in HIV-1 transgenic rats. Proc Natl Acad Sci U S A 2010;107(31):13848–53.

112. Eckard AR, Tangpricha V, Seydafkan S, et al. The relationship between vitamin D status and HIV-related complications in HIV-infected children and young adults. Pediatr Infect Dis J 2013;32(11):1224–9.

113. Arpadi S, Horlick M, Shane E. Metabolic bone disease in human immunodeficiency virus-infected children. J Clin Endocrinol Metab 2004;89(1):21–3.

114. Jacobson DL, Lindsey JC, Gordon CM, et al. Total body and spinal bone mineral density across Tanner stage in perinatally HIV-infected and uninfected children and youth in PACTG 1045. AIDS 2010;24(5):687–96.

115. DiMeglio L, Wang J, Siberry GK, et al. Bone mineral density in children and adolescents with perinatal HIV infection. AIDS 2013;27(2):211–20.

116. Prieto-Alhambra D, Guerri-Fernandez R, De Vries F, et al. HIV infection and its association with an excess risk of clinical fractures: a nationwide case-control study. J Acquir Immune Defic Syndr 2014;66(1):90–5.

117. Fux CA, Rauch A, Simcock M, et al. Tenofovir use is associated with an increase in serum alkaline phosphatase in the Swiss HIV Cohort Study. Antivir Ther 2008; 13(8):1077–82.

118. Dao C, Patel P, Overton E, et al. Low vitamin D among HIV-infected adults: prevalence of and risk factors for low vitamin in a cohort of HIV-infected adults and comparison to prevalence among adults in the US general population. Clin Infect Dis 2011;52(3):396–405.

Index

Note: Page numbers of article titles are in **boldface** type.

Endocrinol Metab Clin N Am 43 (2014) 829–867
http://dx.doi.org/10.1016/S0889-8529(14)00065-6
0889-8529/14/$ – see front matter © 2014 Elsevier Inc. All rights reserved.

Z

Printed and bound by CPI Group (UK) Ltd, Croydon, CR0 4YY

03/10/2024

01040485-0002